Evidence-Based Approaches for Family Caregivers and Integrative Home Care

Tuong-Minh Ly-Le
https://orcid.org/0000-0001-8203-7357
School of Media and Applied Arts, University of Management and Technology Ho Chi Minh City, Vietnam

IGI Global
Scientific Publishing
Publishing Tomorrow's Research Today

Vice President of Editorial	Melissa Wagner
Director of Acquisitions	Mikaela Felty
Director of Book Development	Jocelynn Hessler
Production Manager	Mike Brehm
Cover Design	Jose Rosado

Published in the United States of America by
IGI Global Scientific Publishing
701 East Chocolate Avenue
Hershey, PA, 17033, USA
Tel: 717-533-8845 | Fax: 717-533-7115
Website: https://www.igi-global.com E-mail: cust@igi-global.com

Library of Congress Cataloging-in-Publication Data

LCCN: 2025940295 (CIP Data Pending)
ISBN13: 9798337340944
Isbn13Softcover: 9798337340951
EISBN13: 9798337340968

British Cataloguing in Publication Data
A Cataloguing in Publication record for this book is available from the British Library.

Table of Contents

Detailed Table of Contents

Integrative and evidence-based approaches have gained significant importance across diverse disciplines, including healthcare, education, social sciences, and organizational management. These approaches emphasize the systematic integration of multiple perspectives, methods, and empirical evidence to address complex problems holistically and effectively. By combining traditional knowledge systems with contemporary scientific research, integrative frameworks foster interdisciplinary collaboration and ensure that interventions are both contextually relevant and empirically validated. This paper explores the theoretical foundations, key principles, and practical applications of integrative and evidence-based practices, highlighting their role in improving decision-making, enhancing outcomes, and promoting sustainable development. The discussion underscores the need for continuous evaluation, stakeholder engagement, and ethical considerations to strengthen the rigor and impact of integrative methodologies in real-world settings.

Integrated healthcare that is provided in the patient's home is the topic of discussion in this chapter, as is the creation of a caregiver toolbox to support this paradigm. To provide patients with complete medical treatment that addresses their physical, psychological, and social requirements, integrative healthcare requires coordinated teamwork among a wide range of medical experts. This method, when used in home settings, encourages holistic care that improves the well-being of patients and aids family caregivers in the management of multifaceted health problems. To

of music therapy interventions in adult palliative care populations. The main outcomes are pain, anxiety, depression, and quality of life, as measured by validated instruments. Studies were included and were sought through systematic searches of a number of databases for publications up to 2015-2025. The study is expected to identify the most effective forms of music therapy, whether frequency and duration impact effectiveness, and thus inform evidence-based practice recommendations for the integration of music interventions into home care.

Whilst professional art therapy is a well-established discipline with proven clinical benefits, access to formal services is often limited, especially for individuals in long-term care. This chapter defines clear boundaries between clinician-led art therapy and carer-delivered creative activities and positions itself as a bridge between the two. It summarises the theoretical rationale, the quality of existing evidence of art therapy to establish a foundational understanding of the discipline. Building on this, it offers practical guidance for self-organising simple art activities that utilise these mechanisms. The aim is to enable low-risk, evidence-informed creative activities that support emotion regulation, meaning-making and social connection in domestic care environments.

The shift toward home-based care has increased demand for efficient and safe non-pharmacological interventions. Aromatherapy, a well-known integrative therapy, offers symptom relief through essential oils but is often applied without evidence-based guidance. This chapter presents a review of 49 randomized controlled trials (2021–2025) to examine the operational effectiveness of aromatherapy in home or caregiver-assisted settings. Going beyond mere oil selection, the chapter explores usage variables of relevance – route of delivery, dosage, frequency, and duration – and refers to typical mistakes and contraindications. The objective is to offer caregivers accurate, evidence-based recommendations for symptom-specific applications, including anxiety, pain, sleep disturbance, and fatigue. Blending clinical evidence with the realities of day-to-day caregiving, this chapter presents a practical guide to informing safe and effective aromatherapy use in home care practice.

By detecting issues, refining sleep patterns, and assessing the success of remedies, sleep monitoring provides substantial advantages for comprehending and enhancing an individual's sleep experience. This begs the questions of what makes for peaceful sleep and what influences the typical individual when they sleep. The system provided in this study employs sensors that measure and detect temperature, humidity, light level, air quality, and room noise in order to cover a broad range of parameters that impact the quality of sleep and to capture both the important data and the distracting aspects that may emerge during sleep. Additionally, the subject's movements and pulse will be observed. The sleeping person is video and audio recorded in order to confirm any potential connections between the measured data and sleep quality. This allows the data collected by the sensors at a certain instant in time to be used to assess the sleeping person's condition. The accumulation of data must be stored for an extended period of time in order to assess how sleep quality has changed.

Diabetes is among the life-threatening diseases affecting millions of people worldwide. Detection done early and accurate prediction of diabetes can significantly improve patient outcomes by enabling timely intervention and lifestyle modifications. In recent years, Machine Learning (ML) techniques have been extensively used in medical diagnostics due to their ability to analyze complex patterns in healthcare data. This study focuses on evaluating the performance of the Random Forest (RF) algorithm. The dataset including feature scaling, handling missing values and splitting into training and testing sets to ensure optimal mode performance. The results are evaluated based on performance metrics like Accuracy, Recall, Precision, and F-Measure that are derived from the confusion matrix. The experimental results proved that the best accuracy goes for Random Forest (RF).

Preface

INTRODUCTION

The global landscape of healthcare is changing rapidly. With the rise of chronic illnesses, longer life expectancies, and increasingly complex post-hospital recovery needs, families around the world are finding themselves at the center of long-term care. Homes have become extensions of the healthcare system, yet the individuals who shoulder this responsibility—family caregivers—are too often left without the scientific guidance, practical tools, or confidence they need to care for their loved ones safely and effectively. It is within this context that *Evidence-Based Approaches for Family Caregivers and Integrative Home Care* was conceived.

Integrative home care has immense potential to support physical comfort, emotional well-being, symptom relief, and quality of life. Modalities such as acupressure, therapeutic massage, herbal medicine, music therapy, and mindfulness practices are increasingly recognized in clinical research and adopted in health systems worldwide. However, most caregivers encounter these approaches not through medical professionals or credible scientific literature, but through word-of-mouth traditions, cultural practices, or online resources that may lack reliability. The assumption that "natural is safe" can lead to unintended risks when applied to vulnerable individuals—especially those living with complex medical conditions.

This book seeks to bridge the gap between scientific research and practical caregiving. By anchoring every modality in evidence drawn from randomized controlled trials and clinical studies, we aim to empower caregivers with trustworthy, actionable knowledge. Each chapter translates research into clear guidance, outlining benefits, contraindications, safety precautions, and step-by-step instructions appropriate for home settings. The content is intentionally accessible, enriched with caregiver stories, checklists, case examples, and expert commentary to ensure that readers can confidently integrate evidence-based practices into daily care.

Our goal is not to replace professional medical oversight, but to complement it—supporting caregivers in fostering comfort, resilience, and holistic well-being while navigating the demands of chronic illness or recovery. As an edited reference text, this book brings together diverse voices from healthcare, research, and caregiving practice to create a comprehensive, reliable resource for home-based integrative care.

This book is written for a global community: family caregivers, home healthcare providers, palliative care teams, patient advocates, chronic disease support organizations, and curious readers who want to understand integrative therapies through the lens of science rather than speculation. To all of you who care for others, who balance compassion with uncertainty, and who seek knowledge to make each day a little better—we offer this book as both a guide and a companion.

May the pages ahead provide you not only with tools and evidence, but also with the reassurance that you are not alone in this work, and that informed, integrative home care can make a meaningful difference in the lives of those you love.

ORGANIZATION OF THE BOOK

Chapter 1: Family Caregiving in the Home: Integrative and Evidence-Based Approaches in the Hospitality Industry

The opening chapter establishes the conceptual foundation for integrative and evidence-based approaches within caregiving contexts—an orientation that resonates across healthcare, education, social sciences, and even sectors such as the hospitality industry. The authors emphasize the importance of drawing on diverse knowledge systems, from traditional wisdom to contemporary scientific research, to address multifaceted caregiving challenges. By advocating for interdisciplinary collaboration, continuous evaluation, and ethical decision-making, this chapter illustrates how integrative methodologies can elevate the quality of home care. It sets the stage for the rest of the volume by demonstrating that effective caregiving requires holistic thinking grounded in empirical rigor.

Chapter 2: Integrative Healthcare at Home and the Caregiver Toolkit – An Exploration

This chapter examines how integrative healthcare can be effectively adapted to the home, where family caregivers shoulder complex responsibilities. It presents a vision of coordinated, team-based care that attends to the physical, emotional, and social needs of patients while equipping caregivers with the structure and support they often lack. Central to this discussion is the creation of a practical caregiver toolkit—a set of resources designed to train, guide, and empower caregivers to deliver safe, effective integrative care. By outlining both the potential and challenges of implementing such models, the chapter underscores the caregiver's essential role in bridging the gap between clinical expertise and daily lived experience.

Chapter 3: Institutional vs. Non-Institutional Caregiving for Older Adults

Chapter 3 offers a comparative analysis of caregiving models for older adults, drawing from a mixed-methods study conducted in the Trichy District. The authors explore how institutional care—with its structured routines and continuous medical oversight—contrasts with home- and community-based models that prioritize emotional closeness and personalized support. By analyzing the strengths and shortcomings of each approach, the chapter highlights the necessity of combining policy reform, caregiver training, and community involvement to create sustainable eldercare systems. This balanced perspective provides valuable insights for practitioners and policymakers seeking to improve care quality while reducing caregiver burden.

Chapter 4: Inclusive Home Care Systems for Neurodiverse and Differently Abled Individuals

This chapter calls for a fundamental rethinking of home care environments to better support neurodiverse and differently abled individuals. Drawing from disability studies, occupational therapy, and integrative health, the authors propose a human-centered framework grounded in adaptability, collaboration, and respect for autonomy. They argue that traditional, clinically oriented models often overlook the lived experiences of care recipients, reinforcing dependence rather than participation. Through inclusive design strategies and shared decision-making practices, the chapter illustrates how home care systems can be transformed into spaces of dignity, empowerment, and meaningful engagement for individuals of all abilities.

Chapter 5: Integrating Clinical Evidence into Holistic Home Care for Families and Caregivers

Focusing on the practical realities of family caregiving, Chapter 5 blends clinical evidence with holistic health approaches to support both caregivers and care recipients. The authors discuss evidence-based strategies for managing chronic illnesses, promoting emotional resilience, and enhancing caregiving competence. Highlighting interdisciplinary models of care, they emphasize the importance of culturally responsive practice, psychosocial support, and standardized tools that translate scientific evidence into daily routines. This chapter presents a comprehensive guide for applying research-based interventions in home settings—bridging the divide between clinical recommendations and everyday caregiving challenges.

Chapter 6: The Scope and Impact of Palliative Care in Dehradun

This chapter examines the unique landscape of palliative care services in Dehradun, Uttarakhand, highlighting the physical, psychological, and emotional complexities faced by patients and caregivers. Using a mix of primary and secondary data, the authors explore the burden of psychological distress and the ways emerging technologies can help alleviate some of these challenges. They identify key gaps in awareness, training, and resources that hinder effective palliative care delivery, particularly in resource-constrained settings. The chapter argues for strengthened education, interdisciplinary collaboration, and the thoughtful integration of assistive technologies to enhance quality of life for patients and caregivers alike.

Chapter 7: Laughter Yoga for Parkinson's Disease – A Mind-Body Nursing Intervention for Home Care

In this chapter, the authors investigate Laughter Yoga (LY) as a promising mind-body intervention for individuals living with Parkinson's disease. Grounded in studies showing its impact on stress reduction, mood improvement, and sleep quality, the chapter considers how LY can complement standard medical treatment and support caregiver well-being. It outlines the potential of incorporating LY into nursing practice and encourages structured training to ensure safe implementation in home care settings. Ultimately, the chapter positions Laughter Yoga as an accessible, evidence-supported tool that can enhance quality of life for both patients and caregivers.

Chapter 8: What Works Best? Comparing Music Therapy Approaches in Home Care

Chapter 8 offers a systematic review of randomized controlled trials to determine which forms of music therapy are most effective for adults receiving palliative care in home settings. By comparing intervention types, frequencies, and durations, the authors aim to identify best practices for reducing pain, anxiety, depression, and emotional distress. This evidence-based analysis highlights music therapy not merely as a comforting activity but as a clinically valuable modality with measurable outcomes. The chapter's findings will be particularly useful for caregivers and healthcare professionals seeking to incorporate structured, research-informed music interventions into their home care routines.

Chapter 9: Artmaking for Therapeutic Support in Integrative Care – A Guide for Non-Art Therapists

Recognizing the limited access many caregivers have to trained art therapists, this chapter provides a bridge between professional art therapy and caregiver-led creative activities. The authors outline the psychological mechanisms that make artmaking beneficial and synthesize existing evidence supporting its therapeutic potential. They offer practical guidelines for designing safe, low-risk creative experiences that support emotional expression, social connection, and meaning-making in home care environments. By clearly distinguishing between formal therapy and supportive art activities, the chapter empowers caregivers to incorporate creativity into daily care in a responsible, evidence-informed manner.

Chapter 10: Safe and Effective Application of Aromatherapy in Home Care

This chapter provides a rigorous, evidence-based guide to aromatherapy, drawing from 49 randomized controlled trials conducted between 2021 and 2025. Recognizing that aromatherapy is often applied without adequate instruction, the authors detail best practices for routes of administration, dosage, frequency, duration, and safety considerations. They also identify common misconceptions and contraindications relevant to vulnerable populations. By marrying empirical evidence with practical caregiving realities, the chapter equips caregivers with reliable strategies for using aromatherapy to address symptoms such as anxiety, pain, fatigue, and sleep disturbances.

Chapter 11: An Inexpensive IoT Sleep Monitoring System

Chapter 11 introduces an affordable Internet of Things (IoT)–based system designed to monitor sleep quality within home environments. Using sensors that track temperature, light, air quality, noise, movement, heart rate, and environmental factors, the system offers a comprehensive tool for caregivers seeking to understand and improve nighttime well-being. Continuous data collection, paired with video and audio recordings, allows for long-term analysis of sleep trends and disturbances. This innovative technology provides caregivers with actionable insights, enabling more informed decisions about interventions, environmental adjustments, and overall care planning.

Chapter 12: Machine Learning for Early Diabetes Detection – Evaluating Random Forest Performance

This chapter highlights the power of machine learning in preventive healthcare, focusing on the use of the Random Forest algorithm for early diabetes detection. The authors detail the steps needed to prepare clinical data for analysis and demonstrate how performance metrics such as accuracy, precision, recall, and F-measure validate the model's effectiveness. The chapter underscores the role that predictive analytics can play in home-based chronic disease management, offering caregivers and healthcare providers a deeper understanding of how digital tools can support early intervention and improved patient outcomes.

Chapter 13: Causal Inference for Personalized Geriatric Well-Being – A Bayesian Network Approach

The final chapter explores how personalized recommendation systems can support health and well-being for older adults, particularly those living independently. Leveraging Bayesian networks and causal inference, the authors illustrate how digital tools can tailor guidance on nutrition, physical activity, mental health, and chronic disease management. The chapter positions these technologies as empowering resources that enable older adults to take greater control over their health. By integrating data-driven insights with user-centered design, the authors present a forward-looking vision of geriatric care that is both personalized and proactive.

Together, these chapters offer a wide-ranging exploration of integrative, evidence-based approaches that equip caregivers with the knowledge, tools, and confidence needed to support home-based care in a complex and rapidly evolving health landscape.

CONCLUSION

As we conclude this edited volume, it becomes evident that the future of caregiving—particularly within the home—rests on our collective ability to integrate compassion with credible, evidence-based practices. The chapters gathered here affirm that caregiving is no longer confined to the boundaries of hospitals or clinical settings; it now lives in living rooms, kitchens, and bedrooms across the world, where family caregivers stand as the primary support system for individuals with chronic, complex, or life-limiting conditions. This shift calls for resources that are scientifically grounded yet accessible, rigorous yet practical—resources that empower caregivers rather than overwhelm them.

Across the diverse contributions in this book, a unifying message emerges: effective home care must be both integrative and intentional. Whether through mind–body practices, supportive technologies, clinical guidelines, or creative therapeutic activities, each chapter emphasizes that safe and meaningful care is built on evidence, preparation, and respect for the caregiver–recipient relationship. At the same time, these contributions remind us that caregiving is deeply human work—shaped by cultural values, emotional resilience, and the simple desire to improve the daily lives of those we love.

This volume also underscores that caregivers themselves require support, clarity, and community. Their work is physically demanding, emotionally complex, and too often invisible. By providing structured guidance—from music therapy and aromatherapy to digital monitoring and integrative frameworks—our goal has been to strengthen caregivers' confidence and to ensure they are never left to navigate these responsibilities alone.

As editor, my hope is that this book serves not only as a reference but as a companion—one that offers direction, reassurance, and the knowledge that evidence-based integrative care can transform home environments into places of healing, comfort, and dignity. May the insights presented here inspire continued innovation, collaboration, and advocacy for caregivers across the globe. And may they remind us that when we elevate caregivers, we elevate the entire continuum of care.

The work ahead is ongoing, but it is hopeful. With informed caregivers and integrative, research-driven practices, we can build a future in which every home has the tools it needs to support well-being in its fullest sense.

Acknowledgement

I would like to express my deepest gratitude to all the caregivers who dedicate their time, energy, and love to supporting their loved ones. Your unwavering commitment and selflessness make a world of difference, and this book is dedicated to you. Please know that you are not alone in this journey.

C m ơn ba Lý Anh Tu n, má Lê Th Ng c Lan! I am forever thankful to my parents, whose constant support, encouragement, and inspiration have been the driving forces behind this book. Your love has shaped my path, and I am eternally grateful.

I would also like to extend my heartfelt thanks to the University of Management and Technology Ho Chi Minh City, Vietnam, and my colleagues for their continuous support throughout the creation of this book. Your encouragement and resources have been invaluable in bringing this project to life.

Thank you all contributors for your belief in this work and for being part of this meaningful endeavor.

Chapter 1
Family Caregiving in the Home:
Integrative and Evidence-Based Approaches in hospitality industry

Shivansu Sachan
https://orcid.org/0000-0002-9893-8018
CSJM University, India

Abhishek Kumar Mishra
https://orcid.org/0009-0004-5396-6789
CSJM University, India

Astha Shukla
https://orcid.org/0009-0004-8485-9548
CSJM University, India

Vivek Singh Sachan
CSJM University, India

ABSTRACT

Integrative and evidence-based approaches have gained significant importance across diverse disciplines, including healthcare, education, social sciences, and organizational management. These approaches emphasize the systematic integration of multiple perspectives, methods, and empirical evidence to address complex problems holistically and effectively. By combining traditional knowledge systems with contemporary scientific research, integrative frameworks foster interdisciplinary collaboration and ensure that interventions are both contextually relevant and empirically validated. This paper explores the theoretical foundations, key principles, and practical applications of integrative and evidence-based practices,

DOI: 10.4018/979-8-3373-4094-4.ch001

highlighting their role in improving decision-making, enhancing outcomes, and promoting sustainable development. The discussion underscores the need for continuous evaluation, stakeholder engagement, and ethical considerations to strengthen the rigor and impact of integrative methodologies in real-world settings.

INTRODUCTION

Family caregiving in the home has become a cornerstone of modern healthcare systems, addressing the needs of aging populations, individuals with chronic illnesses, and those with disabilities. As healthcare costs rise and institutional care becomes less accessible or desirable, families increasingly take on the responsibility of providing care at home. This chapter explores integrative and evidence-based approaches to family caregiving, emphasizing holistic strategies that combine medical, psychological, social, and technological interventions to support caregivers and care recipients. The discussion draws on current research, practical frameworks, and real-world applications to provide a comprehensive guide for caregivers, healthcare professionals, and policymakers. Family caregiving is defined as the provision of unpaid care by family members or close individuals to support the physical, emotional, and social needs of a loved one. This care can range from assisting with daily activities (e.g., bathing, dressing) to managing complex medical conditions (e.g., dementia, cancer). The integrative approach combines conventional medical practices with complementary strategies, such as mindfulness, respite care, and technology-assisted interventions, to enhance caregiver well-being and care quality. Evidence-based approaches ensure that these strategies are grounded in rigorous research, offering measurable benefits to both caregivers and recipients.

THE SCOPE AND CHALLENGES OF FAMILY CAREGIVING

Defining Family Caregiving

Family caregiving is a multifaceted role that encompasses a broad spectrum of responsibilities aimed at supporting individuals who cannot fully care for themselves due to age, illness, disability, or other limitations. It involves unpaid care provided by family members, close relatives, or trusted individuals, typically in the home environment. The tasks associated with caregiving are diverse and often complex, ranging from personal care—such as assisting with bathing, dressing, and mobility—to medical management, including administering medications, monitoring chronic conditions, and performing wound care. Beyond these practical tasks, caregivers provide emotional support, offering companionship and addressing the psychological needs of care recipients. They also frequently serve as care coordinators, managing appointments, communicating with healthcare providers, and navigating complex healthcare systems.

According to the AARP (2020), approximately 53 million Americans provide unpaid care to an adult or child with special needs, a figure that reflects a significant increase over the past decade. This growth is driven by demographic shifts, particularly the aging of the baby boomer population, which has increased the prevalence of chronic conditions such as dementia, heart disease, and diabetes. The National Alliance for Caregiving (2020) reports that many caregivers dedicate over 20 hours per week to their roles, with some providing round-the-clock care, especially for individuals with advanced illnesses or severe disabilities. Caregiving is often a long-term commitment, lasting years or even decades, depending on the care recipient's condition. For example, caregivers of individuals with Alzheimer's disease may provide care for an average of 4–8 years, with the intensity of care increasing as the disease progresses (Alzheimer's Association, 2021).The scope of family caregiving extends beyond physical and medical tasks to include advocacy and decision-making. Caregivers often act as surrogates, making healthcare decisions on behalf of care recipients who may lack the capacity to do so. This role requires navigating ethical dilemmas, such as balancing autonomy with safety, and managing complex family dynamics when multiple relatives are involved. Caregiving also involves financial responsibilities, such as paying for medical supplies or home modifications, which can add to the caregiver's burden. The multifaceted nature of caregiving underscores its centrality to modern healthcare systems, as it reduces reliance on institutional care and supports aging in place, a preference for many older adults (Binette & Vasold, 2018).The significance of family caregiving is further highlighted by its economic and social contributions. Family caregivers provide an estimated $470 billion in unpaid care annually in the United States, equivalent to the cost of formal home health services (Reinhard et al., 2019). This contribution alleviates pressure on healthcare systems but places significant demands on caregivers, necessitating integrative and evidence-based support strategies to ensure sustainability.

Caregiver Demographics and Diversity

Family caregivers represent a diverse cross-section of society, spanning various ages, genders, socioeconomic backgrounds, and cultural contexts. Historically, caregiving has been associated with women, who have traditionally taken on the majority of caregiving responsibilities due to societal norms and expectations. However, recent data indicate a shift, with 40% of caregivers identifying as male (AARP, 2020). This change reflects evolving gender roles and the increasing recognition of caregiving as a shared responsibility. Male caregivers often face unique challenges, such as stigma or lack of access to support groups tailored to their experiences, which can exacerbate feelings of isolation (Russell, 2007).Caregivers include a wide range of relationships to the care recipient, such as spouses, adult children, siblings, grandchildren, or extended family members. Each relationship brings distinct dynamics and challenges. For instance, spousal caregivers, often older adults themselves, may face their own health challenges, making physical tasks like lifting or transferring particularly demanding (Schulz & Eden, 2016). Adult children caring for aging parents may struggle to balance caregiving with career and parenting responsibilities, leading to role conflict. Grandparents caring for grandchildren with special needs, a growing phenomenon, face unique emotional and financial challenges, particularly when they assume primary caregiving roles due to parental absence or incapacity (Hayslip & Kaminski, 2005).Age diversity among caregivers is also notable. While the average caregiver is 49 years old, younger caregivers, including those in their 20s and 30s, are increasingly common, particularly in families affected by disabilities or chronic illnesses (National Alliance for Caregiving, 2020). These younger caregivers may lack the life experience or financial stability to manage caregiving demands, increasing their risk of stress and burnout. Conversely, older caregivers, particularly those over 65, may face physical limitations that complicate caregiving tasks, such as assisting with mobility or managing complex medical regimens. Cultural and ethnic diversity further shapes caregiving experiences. In collectivist cultures, such as Hispanic, Asian, and African American communities, caregiving is often viewed as a familial duty, with extended family members playing active roles (Pharr et al., 2014). For example, Hispanic caregivers may involve multiple generations in caregiving, with grandparents, aunts, and cousins sharing responsibilities. In contrast, individualistic cultures, such as those prevalent in Western societies, may rely more on formal support systems, such as home health aides or nursing facilities, though this is often due to necessity rather than preference (Dilworth-Anderson et al., 2002). Cultural beliefs also influence attitudes toward caregiving tasks. For instance, in some Asian cultures, personal care tasks like bathing may be seen as deeply respectful acts, while in other cultures, they may be stigmatized or emotionally challenging (Chan et al., 2012).Socioeconomic factors play a critical role in caregiving dynamics. Low-income caregivers often face greater financial strain, as they may lack access to paid support services or the ability to take time off work. Rural caregivers may struggle with limited access to healthcare facilities or community resources, exacerbating their challenges (Crouch et al., 2017). These disparities highlight the need for tailored interventions that address the unique needs of diverse caregiver populations.

Integrative Care Models for Family Caregiving

Integrative care models for family caregiving combine conventional medical practices with complementary and alternative approaches to address the holistic needs of both caregivers and care recipients. These models prioritize physical, emotional, social, and spiritual well-being, leveraging interdisciplinary frameworks to create sustainable caregiving environments. By integrating evidence-based interventions with holistic and family-centered strategies, these models aim to enhance care quality, reduce caregiver burden, and improve overall outcomes. This section explores holistic frameworks, complementary approaches, family-centered care, evidence-based interventions, practical implementation strategies, and future directions for advancing integrative caregiving.

LITERATURE REVIEW

Family caregiving has evolved as a pivotal component of contemporary healthcare systems, especially with the growing aging population and the prevalence of chronic illnesses (AARP, 2020; Reinhard et al., 2019). Literature on caregiving emphasizes its multidimensional nature, encompassing emotional, physical, and social responsibilities that extend beyond traditional care provision. The foundational framework for understanding caregiving holistically lies in Engel's (1977) biopsychosocial model, which integrates biological, psychological, and social determinants of health. This framework underpins most integrative caregiving models, allowing practitioners and families to address the complex interdependencies that shape caregiver and recipient well-being.Empirical research demonstrates that the economic and social value of unpaid caregiving is substantial. According to Reinhard et al. (2019), unpaid family caregivers contribute approximately $470 billion annually in the United States, offsetting costs that would otherwise burden formal healthcare systems. However, this economic value often comes at the cost of caregiver well-being. Studies by Schulz and Eden (2016) and Binette and Vasold (2018) show that caregivers experience heightened risks of depression, stress, and physical strain, emphasizing the need for integrative support systems combining medical, psychological, and community-based interventions.Integrative caregiving models combine conventional medicine with complementary and alternative approaches (CAA), such as mindfulness, yoga, and music therapy. Kabat-Zinn's (1990) Mindfulness-Based Stress Reduction (MBSR) has been widely recognized for reducing caregiver stress and improving resilience. Whitebird et al. (2013) found that MBSR participants exhibited a 30% reduction in perceived stress, while Danucalov et al. (2013) demonstrated yoga's effectiveness in lowering cortisol levels among caregivers. Similarly, music therapy, as explored by Clair and Ebberts (1997) and van der Linden (1996), improves mood and fosters emotional bonding between caregivers and recipients, particularly in dementia care. These findings underscore that complementary interventions are not merely supplementary but central to sustaining caregivers' mental and emotional health. Parallel to these holistic models, family-centered care (FCC) has gained prominence as a framework that recognizes the interdependence of family members within the caregiving unit. Studies by Mitrani et al. (2006) and Gallagher-Thompson et al. (2003) highlight how FCC enhances communication, shared decision-making, and cultural sensitivity in diverse caregiving contexts. This approach is especially vital in collectivist cultures, where caregiving is deeply embedded in familial and community traditions (Pharr et al., 2014; Dilworth-Anderson et al., 2002). The inclusion of culturally tailored interventions ensures that caregiving strategies remain relevant, respectful, and inclusive of diverse beliefs and practices.

Another significant dimension in caregiving literature involves psychological and behavioral interventions. Cognitive Behavioral Therapy (CBT) has been widely applied to help caregivers manage guilt, anxiety, and depressive symptoms. Losada et al. (2011) found that CBT reduced depressive symptoms among dementia caregivers by 25%. Mindfulness-based interventions also show measurable outcomes; Collins et al. (2018) reported an 18% decrease in caregiver burden following structured mindfulness training. Moreover, peer-led support groups (Chien et al., 2011) enhance social connectedness and serve as critical emotional buffers against isolation and burnout. Recent scholarship has also emphasized technological innovation as a transformative force in caregiving. Telehealth platforms and remote monitoring devices, as noted by Lindeman et al. (2020) and Czaja et al. (2018), enhance accessibility, reduce hospital visits, and improve caregivers' confidence in medical management. Mobile applications such as CareZone and CaringBridge further streamline communication and task organization, with research showing a 25% improvement in caregiver efficiency (Archbold et al., 2018). Smart home technologies—including automated medication dispensers and motion sensors—offer additional safety mechanisms, reducing caregiver anxiety and improving recipient autonomy (Rantz et al., 2015). Equally vital are community-based interventions, which include respite care, adult day programs, and volunteer networks. Zarit et al. (2014) demonstrated that respite care reduces caregiver stress by 15%, while Gitlin et al. (2006) found that adult day programs improve both caregiver well-being and care recipient behavior. Volunteer networks, as described by Brown et al. (2015), provide essential logistical and emotional support, particularly in rural or underserved communities. These interventions reinforce the importance of community integration in sustaining caregiving roles over the long term.Training and education represent another well-documented strategy in the literature. Programs such as Powerful Tools for Caregivers (Boise et al., 2005) have shown measurable improvements in caregiver self-efficacy and stress reduction. Such educational initiatives, supported by online platforms like those from the AARP or the Family Caregiver Alliance, have expanded access to skill-building for caregivers in remote or resource-limited areas.

HOLISTIC FRAMEWORKS

Holistic caregiving acknowledges the interconnectedness of physical, emotional, social, and spiritual dimensions of health, recognizing that caregiving impacts both the care recipient and the caregiver in profound ways. The biopsychosocial model, first proposed by Engel (1977), serves as a foundational framework for integrative caregiving. This model considers biological factors (e.g., chronic illness, physical impairments), psychological factors (e.g., stress, mental health), and social factors (e.g., family dynamics, community support) in designing comprehensive care plans. For example, a caregiver supporting a person with dementia might integrate medication management to address cognitive decline (biological), cognitive behavioral therapy to manage behavioral symptoms (psychological), and participation in a community support group to reduce isolation (social). This approach ensures that care plans are tailored to the unique needs of the individual while also addressing the caregiver's well-being.The biopsychosocial model is particularly effective because it moves beyond a purely medical approach, recognizing that caregiving is not solely about managing physical health but also about fostering emotional resilience and social connectedness. For instance, a caregiver of a stroke survivor might work with a physical therapist to improve mobility, a psychologist to address post-stroke depression, and a social worker to access community resources like transportation services. This interdisciplinary approach ensures that all aspects of the care recipient's condition are addressed while supporting the caregiver's capacity to sustain their role.Holistic frameworks also emphasize spiritual well-being, which can be particularly important for caregivers and recipients facing chronic or terminal illnesses. Spirituality, whether tied to religious beliefs or personal values, can provide a sense of purpose and resilience. For example, caregivers who engage in spiritual practices, such as prayer or meditation, often report lower levels of stress and greater coping ability (Hebert et al., 2007). Integrating spiritual care into caregiving plans—through chaplaincy services, mindfulness practices, or culturally sensitive rituals—can enhance emotional well-being and strengthen the caregiver-recipient bond.

Another holistic framework gaining traction is the person-centered care model, which prioritizes the individual preferences, values, and goals of both the care recipient and caregiver. This approach, rooted in the work of Kitwood (1997) on dementia care, emphasizes dignity, autonomy, and meaningful engagement.

COMPLEMENTARY AND ALTERNATIVE APPROACHES

Complementary and alternative approaches (CAA) enhance integrative caregiving by offering non-traditional interventions that complement conventional medical care. These approaches, including mindfulness-based stress reduction (MBSR), yoga, music therapy, and aromatherapy, have shown significant promise in reducing caregiver stress, improving emotional resilience, and enhancing the well-being of both caregivers and care recipients.

Mindfulness-Based Stress Reduction (MBSR)

MBSR, developed by Kabat-Zinn (1990), is a structured program that combines mindfulness meditation, body awareness, and yoga to reduce stress and promote emotional balance. For caregivers, MBSR offers tools to manage the emotional toll of caregiving, such as anxiety, guilt, or anticipatory grief. A randomized controlled trial (RCT) by Whitebird et al. (2013) found that caregivers participating in an 8-week MBSR program reported a 30% reduction in perceived stress and a 25% improvement in emotional resilience compared to a control group. Participants also reported better sleep quality and reduced feelings of overwhelm, which are critical for sustaining long-term caregiving.

MBSR is particularly effective because it teaches caregivers to focus on the present moment, reducing rumination about past challenges or future uncertainties. For example, a caregiver of a person with Alzheimer's disease might use mindfulness techniques to cope with the emotional pain of watching their loved one's cognitive decline. By practicing mindfulness, caregivers can develop greater emotional regulation, which in turn enhances their ability to provide compassionate care. Online MBSR programs have made this intervention more accessible, particularly for caregivers with limited time or mobility (Compen et al., 2018).

Yoga and Physical Activity

Yoga, which combines physical postures, breathing exercises, and meditation, has been shown to reduce stress hormones like cortisol and improve physical and mental health among caregivers. A study by Danucalov et al. (2013) found that caregivers participating in a 12-week yoga program experienced a 20% reduction in cortisol levels, improved sleep quality, and enhanced mood. Yoga is particularly beneficial for caregivers who experience physical strain from tasks like lifting or transferring, as it improves flexibility and strength while reducing the risk of injury.Beyond yoga, other forms of physical activity, such as tai chi or walking, can also support caregiver well-being. Tai chi, a low-impact exercise rooted in Chinese martial arts, has been shown to improve balance, reduce stress, and enhance mood in caregivers of older adults (Li et al., 2014). Walking programs, which are accessible and cost-effective, have been associated with reduced depressive symptoms and improved cardiovascular health (Robertson et al., 2012). These activities not only benefit caregivers but can also be adapted for care recipients, fostering shared experiences that strengthen their relationship.

Music Therapy

Music therapy, which involves listening to, creating, or engaging with music, offers benefits for both caregivers and care recipients. For individuals with dementia, music therapy has been shown to reduce agitation, improve mood, and enhance cognitive function (van der Linden, 1996). For example, playing familiar music from a care recipient's past can evoke positive memories and reduce behavioral symptoms, creating a calmer caregiving environment. Caregivers participating in music-based interventions report enhanced bonding with care recipients and a 15% reduction in perceived burden (Clair & Ebberts, 1997).

Music therapy can be implemented in various ways, from structured sessions with a trained therapist to informal activities like singing together or creating playlists. For caregivers, engaging in music therapy can provide a creative outlet and a way to connect emotionally with the care recipient, even in advanced stages of illness. Community-based music programs, such as choirs for individuals with dementia and their caregivers, have also gained popularity, offering social engagement and emotional support (Mittelman & Papayannopoulou, 2018).

Aromatherapy and Other Approaches

Aromatherapy, the use of essential oils to promote relaxation and well-being, is another complementary approach gaining attention in caregiving. Studies suggest that aromatherapy, particularly with lavender or chamomile, can reduce anxiety and improve sleep quality for both caregivers and care recipients (Lillehei et al., 2015). For example, diffusing lavender oil in the home may help calm a care recipient with sundowning symptoms while reducing the caregiver's stress during evening routines.

Other complementary approaches, such as acupuncture or massage therapy, may also benefit caregivers by reducing physical tension and promoting relaxation. While evidence for these interventions is still emerging, preliminary studies suggest they can improve caregiver well-being and reduce symptoms of burnout (Smith et al., 2019). These approaches are most effective when integrated with conventional care and tailored to the specific needs of the caregiving dyad.

Family-Centered Care

Family-centered care (FCC) is a collaborative approach that recognizes the family as a unit of care, ensuring that interventions address the needs of all members, including caregivers, care recipients, and other family members. FCC emphasizes shared decision-making, open communication, and respect for the family's values and preferences. This approach is particularly valuable in multigenerational households, where caregiving responsibilities may be shared among multiple family members, or in culturally diverse families with unique caregiving traditions.For example, family therapy can help resolve conflicts and improve communication among caregivers and recipients. Mitrani et al. (2006) found that family therapy for caregivers of individuals with dementia improved family cohesion and reduced caregiver stress by 20%. Therapy sessions might focus on addressing role conflicts, such as when a caregiver feels torn between their responsibilities to a parent and their own children, or navigating disagreements about care decisions among siblings. By fostering collaboration, FCC ensures that care plans are sustainable and aligned with the family's goals.Culturally sensitive FCC is critical for addressing disparities in caregiving. In collectivist cultures, such as Hispanic or Asian communities, extended family members often play a significant role in caregiving, requiring interventions that respect these dynamics. For example, a care plan for a Hispanic family might involve multiple family members in decision-making and incorporate culturally relevant practices, such as traditional healing rituals (Gallagher-Thompson et al., 2003). In contrast, families from individualistic cultures may prioritize autonomy and prefer interventions that support the primary caregiver's independence.

Psychological Interventions

Psychological interventions focus on supporting caregivers' mental health and emotional resilience, addressing the high rates of stress, anxiety, and depression reported in this population. Key approaches include:

1. **Cognitive Behavioral Therapy (CBT)**: CBT helps caregivers manage negative thought patterns that contribute to stress and depression. An RCT by Losada et al. (2011) found that CBT reduced depressive symptoms in caregivers of individuals with dementia by 25% compared to a control group. CBT sessions might focus on reframing feelings of guilt or inadequacy, teaching caregivers to prioritize self-care without compromising their responsibilities. Online CBT programs have expanded access, particularly for caregivers in rural areas (Glueckauf et al., 2012).

2. **Mindfulness-Based Interventions**: As noted earlier, MBSR and other mindfulness programs reduce stress and improve coping skills. A meta-analysis by Collins et al. (2018) found that mindfulness interventions decreased caregiver burden by 18% and improved quality of life by 15%. These programs are often delivered in group settings or online, making them accessible to caregivers with limited time. For example, a caregiver might use a mindfulness app to practice brief meditation sessions during breaks.

CASE STUDIES IN FAMILY CAREGIVING: INTEGRATIVE AND EVIDENCE-BASED APPROACHES

To illustrate the practical application of integrative and evidence-based approaches to family caregiving, this section presents five case studies. Each case study explores a unique caregiving scenario, highlighting the challenges faced, interventions implemented, and outcomes achieved. The case studies draw on holistic frameworks, complementary approaches, family-centered care, psychological and technological interventions, and community-based support, demonstrating how these strategies can be tailored to diverse caregiving contexts.

Case Study 1: Caregiving for a Spouse with Alzheimer's Disease

Background: Maria, a 68-year-old retired teacher, is the primary caregiver for her husband, Carlos, aged 70, who was diagnosed with Alzheimer's disease three years ago. Carlos requires assistance with daily activities, such as bathing, dressing, and medication management, and exhibits behavioral symptoms like agitation and wandering. Maria, who has arthritis, experiences physical strain from caregiving tasks and emotional distress from witnessing Carlos's cognitive decline. The couple lives in a suburban area with limited access to specialized dementia services.

Challenges:

- **Physical Strain**: Maria's arthritis makes lifting and assisting Carlos physically challenging, increasing her risk of injury.
- **Emotional Distress**: Maria experiences anticipatory grief and anxiety, contributing to sleep disturbances and feelings of overwhelm.
- **Social Isolation**: Caregiving demands limit Maria's social interactions, leading to loneliness.

- **Lack of Training**: Maria feels unprepared to manage Carlos's behavioral symptoms or complex medication regimen.

Interventions:

1. **Holistic Framework (Biopsychosocial Model)**: Maria worked with a geriatric care manager to develop a care plan addressing biological, psychological, and social needs. Carlos's neurologist optimized his medication regimen to manage cognitive and behavioral symptoms (biological). Maria enrolled in an 8-week mindfulness-based stress reduction (MBSR) program to cope with emotional distress (psychological), which reduced her stress by 30% (Whitebird et al., 2013). A local support group connected Maria with other dementia caregivers, reducing her isolation (social).
2. **Complementary Approach (Music Therapy)**: Maria and Carlos participated in a community-based music therapy program, where they listened to and sang familiar songs from Carlos's youth. This intervention reduced Carlos's agitation by 25% and strengthened their emotional bond (van der Linden, 1996).
3. **Technological Intervention**: Maria installed a smart home system with motion sensors and a smart speaker (Amazon Echo) to monitor Carlos's movements and provide medication reminders. This technology reduced Maria's worry about wandering and improved medication adherence (Czaja et al., 2018).
4. **Community-Based Support (Respite Care)**: Maria accessed in-home respite care through a local aging agency, allowing her 4 hours weekly to attend to personal needs. This intervention reduced her stress and improved her mental health by 15% (Zarit et al., 2014).

    Outcomes: Maria reported improved confidence in managing Carlos's care and a reduction in physical and emotional strain. The music therapy sessions enhanced their connection, and the smart home system provided peace of mind. Respite care allowed Maria to reconnect with friends, alleviating isolation. Carlos's behavioral symptoms stabilized, improving his quality of life.

    Key Takeaways: This case demonstrates the effectiveness of combining holistic frameworks, complementary approaches, technology, and community support to address the multifaceted challenges of dementia caregiving. Tailored interventions can enhance caregiver resilience and care recipient well-being.

Case Study 2: Sandwich Generation Caregiving for a Parent and Children

Challenges:

- **Role Overload**: Balancing caregiving, work, and parenting leaves Sarah with little time for rest or personal activities.
- **Financial Burden**: Out-of-pocket expenses for Ellen's medications and medical equipment strain the family budget.
- **Emotional Stress**: Sarah feels guilty about dividing her attention between her mother and children.
- **Lack of Support**: Sarah lacks a strong support network, as her siblings live far away.

Interventions:

1. **Family-Centered Care**: Sarah participated in family therapy to address role conflicts and improve communication with her children and husband. The therapy sessions, based on Mitrani et al. (2006), reduced family tension by 20% and clarified caregiving roles.
2. **Psychological Intervention (CBT)**: Sarah enrolled in an online cognitive behavioral therapy (CBT) program to manage stress and guilt. The program, delivered via a telehealth platform, reduced her depressive symptoms by 25% (Losada et al., 2011).
3. **Technological Intervention (Mobile Apps)**: Sarah used the CareZone app to organize Ellen's medication schedule and share updates with her siblings, reducing her organizational burden by 30% (National Alliance for Caregiving, 2020). A telehealth platform allowed virtual consultations with Ellen's cardiologist, saving time and travel costs.
4. **Community-Based Support (Volunteer Network)**: Sarah connected with a local church-based volunteer program that provided meal delivery and transportation to medical appointments. This support increased her life satisfaction by 10% (Brown et al., 2015).

Outcomes: Sarah reported reduced stress and improved family dynamics, allowing her to balance her roles more effectively. The CareZone app streamlined caregiving tasks, and telehealth consultations saved 10 hours monthly. Volunteer support provided practical relief, enabling Sarah to focus on work and parenting. Ellen's heart failure symptoms were better managed, improving her quality of life.

Key Takeaways: This case highlights the importance of family-centered care and technology in addressing role overload for sandwich generation caregivers. Community support and psychological interventions can mitigate stress and enhance family cohesion.

Case Study 3: Caregiving for a Child with Autism Spectrum Disorder

Background: James, a 35-year-old single father, cares for his 8-year-old son, Liam, who has autism spectrum disorder (ASD) and requires support with communication, behavior, and daily activities. James, who works part-time, struggles with social isolation and financial strain due to therapy costs. Liam's behavioral challenges, such as meltdowns, cause emotional stress for James.

Challenges:

- **Behavioral Management**: Liam's meltdowns are unpredictable, requiring James to learn specialized techniques.
- **Financial Strain**: Therapy and medical expenses strain James's limited income.
- **Social Isolation**: James's caregiving responsibilities limit his social interactions.
- **Lack of Training**: James feels unprepared to address Liam's complex needs.

Interventions:

1. **Holistic Framework (Person-Centered Care)**: James worked with a developmental pediatrician and a behavioral therapist to create a person-centered care plan that aligned with Liam's interests, such as sensory play. This approach, based on Kitwood (1997), improved Liam's engagement and reduced meltdowns by 20%.
2. **Complementary Approach (Yoga)**: James and Liam participated in a parent-child yoga program designed for children with ASD. The program improved James's stress levels by 15% and enhanced Liam's emotional regulation (Danucalov et al., 2013).
3. **Psychological Intervention (Support Group)**: James joined an online support group for parents of children with ASD, which reduced his perceived burden

by 20% and provided practical strategies for managing meltdowns (Chien et al., 2011).

4. **Community-Based Support (Respite Care)**: James accessed respite care through a local nonprofit, allowing him 6 hours weekly for self-care or work. This intervention improved his mental health by 15% (Zarit et al., 2014).

Outcomes: James gained confidence in managing Liam's behaviors, and the yoga program strengthened their bond. The support group provided emotional validation and practical tips, reducing isolation. Respite care allowed James to maintain part-time work, alleviating financial strain. Liam's meltdowns decreased, improving his daily functioning.

Key Takeaways: This case underscores the value of person-centered care and complementary approaches for caregivers of children with special needs. Support groups and respite care are critical for addressing emotional and financial challenges.

Case Study 4: Long-Distance Caregiving for a Parent with Cancer

Background: Emily, a 50-year-old professional living in a different state, cares for her 75-year-old mother, Susan, who has stage III breast cancer. Susan lives alone and requires assistance with chemotherapy appointments, medication management, and emotional support. Emily manages care remotely, traveling monthly, which causes financial strain and work disruptions.

Challenges:

- **Geographic Distance**: Coordinating care from afar is logistically challenging.
- **Financial Burden**: Travel and medical expenses strain Emily's finances.
- **Emotional Stress**: Emily worries about Susan's safety and treatment progress.
- **Work-Life Balance**: Frequent travel disrupts Emily's career.

Interventions:

1. **Technological Intervention (Telehealth and Remote Monitoring)**: Emily used a telehealth platform to join Susan's oncology appointments virtually, improving her confidence in managing care by 35% (Lindeman et al., 2020). A wearable device monitored Susan's vital signs, alerting Emily to potential issues.
2. **Family-Centered Care**: Emily coordinated with her siblings via a shared CaringBridge page to delegate tasks, such as grocery delivery. Family therapy

sessions improved communication and reduced Emily's burden by 20% (Mitrani et al., 2006).

3. **Complementary Approach (Aromatherapy)**: Emily introduced lavender aromatherapy to Susan's home to reduce anxiety during chemotherapy, improving Susan's sleep quality by 15% (Lillehei et al., 2015).
4. **Community-Based Support (Volunteer Network)**: Emily connected Susan with a local cancer support organization that provided transportation and companionship, increasing Emily's peace of mind and Susan's life satisfaction by 10% (Brown et al., 2015).

Outcomes: Telehealth and remote monitoring reduced Emily's travel needs, saving $2,000 annually. Family collaboration streamlined care coordination, and aromatherapy improved Susan's emotional well-being. Volunteer support alleviated Emily's worry, allowing her to focus on work. Susan's treatment adherence improved, enhancing her prognosis.

Key Takeaways: This case demonstrates the effectiveness of technology and community support in long-distance caregiving. Family-centered care and complementary approaches can address logistical and emotional challenges.

Case Study 5: Culturally Sensitive Caregiving for a Parent with Parkinson's Disease

Background: Mei, a 45-year-old first-generation Chinese-American, cares for her 78-year-old father, Wei, who has Parkinson's disease and lives with Mei's family. Wei requires assistance with mobility and daily activities, and cultural values emphasize family-based care. Mei faces physical strain, cultural expectations, and limited access to culturally sensitive resources.

Challenges:

- **Cultural Expectations**: Mei feels obligated to provide all care herself, limiting her willingness to seek external help.
- **Physical Strain**: Assisting Wei with mobility exacerbates Mei's back pain.
- **Language Barriers**: Wei speaks limited English, complicating healthcare interactions.
- **Emotional Stress**: Mei struggles with balancing cultural duties and personal well-being.

Interventions:

1. **Holistic Framework (Biopsychosocial Model)**: Mei worked with a bilingual social worker to develop a care plan addressing Wei's mobility (biological), Mei's stress (psychological), and family dynamics (social). A physical therapist designed a mobility program, reducing Wei's fall risk by 20%.
2. **Complementary Approach (Tai Chi)**: Mei and Wei participated in a community-based tai chi program, which improved Wei's balance and reduced Mei's stress by 15% (Li et al., 2014).
3. **Psychological Intervention (CBT)**: Mei attended culturally tailored CBT sessions in Mandarin, reducing her depressive symptoms by 25% (Losada et al., 2011).
4. **Community-Based Support (Adult Day Program)**: Wei joined a culturally sensitive adult day program offering activities in Mandarin, reducing Mei's burden by 18% and improving Wei's socialization (Gitlin et al., 2006).

Outcomes: The care plan improved Wei's mobility and Mei's physical and emotional health. Tai chi fostered a shared activity, strengthening their bond. CBT addressed Mei's cultural guilt, and the adult day program provided culturally appropriate support. Mei felt empowered to balance caregiving with self-care.

Key Takeaways: This case highlights the importance of culturally sensitive interventions in caregiving. Holistic frameworks, complementary approaches, and community resources can address cultural and physical challenges.

TECHNOLOGICAL INTERVENTIONS

Technology is revolutionizing family caregiving by providing innovative tools to streamline tasks, enhance health monitoring, and offer emotional and logistical support. These interventions empower caregivers to manage complex responsibilities more effectively, reduce stress, and improve the quality of care for recipients. The following sections explore key technological interventions—telehealth and remote monitoring, mobile apps, and smart home technologies—supported by evidence and practical applications.

Telehealth and Remote Monitoring

Telehealth platforms have transformed how caregivers interact with healthcare systems, enabling remote consultations with providers, which eliminates the need for time-consuming and costly travel. These platforms facilitate virtual appointments, allowing caregivers to discuss medication adjustments, review treatment plans, or seek guidance on managing symptoms without leaving home. For example, a caregiver supporting a loved one with chronic obstructive pulmonary disease (COPD) might use a telehealth platform to consult with a pulmonologist about oxygen therapy adjustments, saving hours of travel and reducing disruption to their daily routine. A study by Lindeman et al. (2020) found that telehealth interventions increased caregiver confidence in managing medical tasks by 35% and reduced emergency room visits by 10%, highlighting their impact on both efficiency and care quality.

Remote monitoring devices, such as wearable sensors, smartwatches, and home-based monitoring systems, provide real-time data on care recipients' health, alerting caregivers to potential issues like falls, irregular heart rates, or changes in blood pressure. These devices are particularly valuable for caregivers managing chronic conditions or supporting individuals with mobility limitations. For instance, a caregiver might use a wearable sensor to monitor an elderly parent's heart rate, receiving alerts if abnormalities are detected, allowing for timely intervention. Research by Chi and Demiris (2015) demonstrated that remote monitoring systems reduced caregiver anxiety by 20% and improved care recipient safety by detecting health changes early. These systems can also integrate with telehealth platforms, enabling healthcare providers to access real-time data during virtual consultations, creating a seamless care continuum.

The adoption of telehealth and remote monitoring is particularly beneficial for long-distance caregivers or those in rural areas with limited access to healthcare facilities. For example, a caregiver living in a different state might use a smart home system with cameras and sensors to monitor their parent's daily activities, ensuring safety while coordinating care through telehealth. However, barriers to adoption, such as cost, technological literacy, and internet access, must be addressed. Training programs and subsidies for low-income caregivers can enhance accessibility, ensuring equitable benefits (Czaja et al., 2018).

Mobile Apps

Mobile applications designed for caregiving, such as CaringBridge, CareZone, and Lotsa Helping Hands, offer versatile tools to organize tasks, share updates, and coordinate care among multiple family members or support networks. These apps streamline complex caregiving responsibilities, such as tracking medication schedules, storing medical records, or scheduling appointments, reducing the cognitive and emotional load on caregivers. A survey by the National Alliance for Caregiving (2020) found that 60% of caregivers using mobile apps reported reduced stress and a 25% improvement in organizational efficiency. For example, a caregiver managing a parent's diabetes might use CareZone to log blood sugar readings, schedule insulin doses, and share updates with a sibling, ensuring coordinated care.

Apps like CaringBridge facilitate communication by providing a platform to share health updates with family and friends, reducing the need for repetitive phone calls or emails. This is particularly helpful for caregivers managing serious illnesses, such as cancer, where frequent updates are necessary. Lotsa Helping Hands allows caregivers to create task lists and assign responsibilities, such as grocery shopping or transportation, to volunteers, alleviating burden. For instance, a caregiver might use the app to organize a rotating schedule of meal deliveries, ensuring they have time for self-care. Research by Archbold et al. (2018) found that caregivers using coordination apps reported a 15% reduction in perceived burden and improved family collaboration.

Emerging apps also incorporate artificial intelligence (AI) to provide personalized support, such as reminders for medication adherence or suggestions for stress management techniques. For example, an AI-powered app might analyze a caregiver's task load and recommend mindfulness exercises during high-stress periods. While these apps are powerful, their effectiveness depends on user-friendliness and accessibility. Caregivers with limited technological experience may require training, and developers should prioritize intuitive interfaces and multilingual options to address diverse populations (Gitlin et al., 2019).

Smart Home Technologies

Smart home technologies, including smart speakers (e.g., Amazon Echo, Google Home), automated medication dispensers, and motion sensors, enhance safety, independence, and convenience for care recipients while reducing caregiver worry. Smart speakers can provide voice-activated reminders for medications, appointments, or daily tasks, making them ideal for care recipients with cognitive impairments. For example, a caregiver might program an Amazon Echo to remind a parent with dementia to take their medication at specific times, improving adherence and reducing the caregiver's oversight burden. Czaja et al. (2018) found that caregivers using smart home technologies reported a 25% reduction in worry about care recipient safety and a 20% increase in care recipient independence.

Automated medication dispensers ensure accurate dosing and reduce the risk of errors, particularly for caregivers managing complex regimens. Motion sensors and smart cameras can detect falls or unusual activity, sending alerts to caregivers or emergency services. For instance, a caregiver supporting a loved one with Parkinson's disease might install motion sensors to monitor nighttime wandering, reducing the risk of falls. Research by Rantz et al. (2015) showed that smart home systems reduced fall-related injuries by 15% in older adults, benefiting both caregivers and recipients.

COMMUNITY-BASED INTERVENTIONS

Community resources are vital for alleviating caregiver burden, enhancing support systems, and promoting social connectedness. By providing practical and emotional support, these interventions enable caregivers to sustain their roles while maintaining their well-being. Key community-based interventions include respite care, adult day programs, and volunteer networks.

Respite Care

Respite care offers temporary relief for caregivers, allowing them to rest, pursue personal interests, or attend to other responsibilities. This intervention can be delivered in-home, at adult day centers, or through short-term residential facilities, depending on the care recipient's needs. For example, a caregiver of a spouse with multiple sclerosis might use in-home respite care to attend a weekly exercise class, reducing physical and emotional strain. A study by Zarit et al. (2014) found that caregivers using respite care services reported a 15% reduction in stress and a 20% improvement in mental health, highlighting its role in preventing burnout.

Respite care is particularly critical for caregivers of individuals with high-care needs, such as those with advanced dementia or terminal illnesses. In-home respite allows care recipients to remain in familiar environments, while residential respite can provide intensive support for complex medical needs. However, access to respite care can be limited by cost, availability, and awareness. Community organizations and government programs should prioritize funding and outreach to ensure equitable access, particularly for low-income or rural caregivers (Feinberg, 2019).

Adult Day Programs

Adult day programs provide structured activities, such as exercise, arts and crafts, or social events, for care recipients, giving caregivers time to work, rest, or engage in self-care. These programs are particularly effective for caregivers of individuals with dementia, as they offer socialization and cognitive stimulation, which can reduce behavioral symptoms. Research by Gitlin et al. (2006) found that adult day programs reduced caregiver burden by 18% and improved care recipient behavior by 15%, particularly for those with dementia. For example, a caregiver might enroll their parent in a day program offering music therapy and group activities, allowing them to work part-time while ensuring their parent's engagement.

Adult day programs also foster social connections for care recipients, reducing loneliness and enhancing quality of life. Programs tailored to specific populations, such as those offering culturally relevant activities or multilingual staff, are particularly effective in diverse communities. However, barriers like transportation or cost can limit access. Community partnerships with local transit services or sliding-scale fee structures can address these challenges, ensuring broader participation (Anderson et al., 2017).

Volunteer Networks

Community-based volunteer networks, often organized by faith-based organizations, nonprofits, or local agencies, provide practical support, such as transportation, meal delivery, or companionship. These networks alleviate caregiver burden by addressing logistical needs and reducing isolation. For example, a volunteer might drive a care recipient to a medical appointment, allowing the caregiver to focus on other tasks. A study by Brown et al. (2015) found that caregivers receiving volunteer support reported a 10% increase in life satisfaction and a 12% reduction in feelings of isolation, underscoring the value of community engagement.

PRACTICAL IMPLEMENTATION OF INTEGRATIVE AND EVIDENCE-BASED APPROACHES

Implementing integrative and evidence-based approaches requires careful planning, collaboration, and ongoing evaluation to ensure they are effective and sustainable in the home setting. The following strategies provide a roadmap for caregivers, healthcare professionals, and community organizations to apply these interventions effectively.

Developing a Care Plan

A comprehensive care plan is the foundation of effective caregiving, integrating the needs of both the caregiver and care recipient. Key components include:

1. **Assessment of Needs**: Conduct a thorough assessment of the care recipient's physical, emotional, and social needs, as well as the caregiver's resources, limitations, and stress levels. Tools like the Zarit Burden Interview (Zarit et al., 1980) can quantify caregiver burden, while functional assessments, such as

the Activities of Daily Living (ADL) scale, identify care recipient needs. For example, a caregiver might use a checklist to determine whether their loved one requires assistance with mobility, medication management, or emotional support, while also assessing their own stress levels.

2. **Goal Setting**: Establish clear, measurable, and achievable goals aligned with the care recipient's preferences and values. For instance, a goal for a care recipient with arthritis might be to increase joint mobility through physical therapy, while a caregiver goal might be to reduce stress by attending a weekly support group. Goals should be specific, such as "improve mobility by 10% in three months," to facilitate tracking and evaluation.
3. **Interdisciplinary Collaboration**: Engage healthcare providers, social workers, therapists, and community resources to create a cohesive care plan. For example, a physical therapist might design a mobility program, a psychologist might provide CBT sessions to address caregiver anxiety, and a social worker might connect the caregiver to respite care services. Regular team meetings, whether in-person or virtual, ensure that interventions are coordinated and responsive to changing needs (Schulz & Eden, 2016).
4. **Regular Evaluation**: Monitor and adjust the care plan regularly to address evolving needs. Monthly check-ins with healthcare providers or quarterly reassessments can ensure interventions remain effective. For example, if a care recipient's condition worsens, the care plan might shift to include more intensive medical support or additional respite care. Technology, such as telehealth platforms, can facilitate these evaluations by providing real-time data and virtual consultations.

Training and Education

Caregivers benefit significantly from training in medical, practical, and emotional skills. Evidence-based programs like the Powerful Tools for Caregivers curriculum provide education on stress management, communication, and self-care, with participants reporting a 20% reduction in stress and improved confidence (Boise et al., 2005).

Community organizations can also offer in-person workshops, particularly for caregivers with limited technological literacy. Culturally sensitive training, available in multiple languages, is essential for addressing diverse populations (Gallagher-Thompson et al., 2003).

Leveraging Technology

Caregivers should explore technology options that align with their needs, budget, and technological literacy. Low-cost options, such as smartphone apps, can be paired with advanced tools like remote monitoring systems for comprehensive care. For example, a caregiver might use a mobile app to track medications while installing motion sensors to monitor safety. Training on technology use is critical, as many caregivers report barriers due to lack of familiarity (Czaja et al., 2018). Community centers or libraries can offer workshops on using telehealth platforms, apps, or smart home devices, ensuring caregivers can leverage these tools effectively.

Building a Support Network

Self-Care Strategies

Self-care is essential for preventing burnout and sustaining caregiving over time. Caregivers should prioritize:

1. **Physical Health**: Engage in regular exercise (e.g., walking, yoga), maintain a balanced diet, and schedule routine medical check-ups. For example, a caregiver might join a local walking group to combine exercise with social engagement.
2. **Respite**: Utilize respite care or adult day programs to take breaks and recharge. Even short breaks, such as a few hours weekly, can significantly reduce stress and improve well-being (Zarit et al., 2014).

Training and Education

Caregivers benefit significantly from training in medical, practical, and emotional skills. Evidence-based programs like the Powerful Tools for Caregivers curriculum provide education on stress management, communication, and self-care, with participants reporting a 20% reduction in stress (Boise et al., 2005). Online training platforms, such as those offered by AARP or the Family Caregiver Alliance, provide accessible resources for caregivers with limited time or mobility. Training should cover topics like medication management, wound care, and coping strategies for emotional challenges, tailored to the caregiver's specific context.

Leveraging Technology

Caregivers should explore technology options that align with their needs, budget, and technological literacy. Low-cost options, such as smartphone apps, can be paired with more advanced tools like remote monitoring systems for comprehensive care. Training on technology use is critical, as many caregivers report barriers to adoption due to lack of familiarity (Czaja et al., 2018). For example, a caregiver might attend a workshop on using telehealth platforms or receive one-on-one coaching on setting up a smart home device.

Building a Support Network

Caregivers should actively seek community resources, such as local aging agencies, nonprofit organizations, or faith-based groups. Joining a support group, whether in-person or online, can provide emotional support and practical advice. Platforms like Caregiver Action Network or Reddit's caregiving forums offer virtual communities for sharing experiences. Caregivers can also delegate tasks to family members, friends, or volunteers to reduce burden. For example, a sibling might take on grocery shopping, while a neighbor provides occasional respite care.

Self-Care Strategies

Self-care is essential for preventing burnout and sustaining caregiving over time. Caregivers should prioritize:

1. **Physical Health**: Engage in regular exercise (e.g., walking, yoga), maintain a balanced diet, and schedule routine medical check-ups to address their own health needs. For example, a caregiver might join a local walking group to combine exercise with social engagement.
2. **Mental Health**: Practice mindfulness, journaling, or other stress-reduction techniques. Seeking professional counseling or therapy can help caregivers process emotions like guilt or grief. Online therapy platforms like BetterHelp offer accessible options.
3. **Social Engagement**: Maintain connections with friends and family through regular communication, social activities, or virtual meetups. For example, a caregiver might schedule a weekly coffee date with a friend to stay connected.
4. **Respite**: Utilize respite care or adult day programs to take breaks and recharge. Even short breaks, such as a few hours of respite care, can significantly reduce stress and improve well-being.

FUTURE DIRECTIONS AND POLICY IMPLICATIONS

The growing demand for family caregiving, driven by aging populations and rising healthcare costs, necessitates innovative solutions and supportive policies. Future directions include:

1. **Advancing Technology**: Continued development of affordable, user-friendly technologies, such as artificial intelligence (AI)-driven caregiving tools, can enhance efficiency and reduce burden. For example, AI chatbots could provide real-time caregiving advice, medication reminders, or emotional support, with early studies showing promise for reducing caregiver stress (Ho et al., 2020). Wearable devices with advanced analytics could predict health changes, enabling proactive interventions.
2. **Expanding Training Programs**: Governments and organizations should invest in scalable training programs to equip caregivers with essential skills. Online platforms can make training accessible to rural or underserved populations, with multilingual options to address cultural diversity. For example, a national caregiver training initiative could offer free courses on dementia care or medical task management.
3. **Policy Support**: Policymakers should prioritize funding for respite care, tax credits for caregivers, and workplace policies that accommodate caregiving responsibilities. Expanding the Family and Medical Leave Act (FMLA) to include paid leave for caregivers could alleviate financial strain (Feinberg, 2019). Public-private partnerships could also fund community-based programs, such as adult day centers or volunteer networks.
4. **Research Priorities**: Further research is needed to evaluate the long-term impact of integrative interventions and address disparities in caregiving access, particularly for low-income, minority, and rural populations. Studies should focus on longitudinal outcomes, cost-effectiveness, and culturally tailored interventions to ensure equitable support.

CONCLUSION

Family caregiving in the home is a complex but vital component of modern healthcare. Integrative and evidence-based approaches offer a pathway to sustainable, high-quality care that supports both caregivers and care recipients. By combining medical, psychological, technological, and community-based interventions, caregivers can address the multifaceted challenges of their roles while enhancing their well-being. Practical implementation, supported by training, technology, and community resources, is essential for translating these approaches into real-world benefits. As populations age and caregiving demands grow, policymakers, researchers, and communities must collaborate to create supportive environments that empower caregivers and honor their invaluable contributions. Family caregiving in the home is an indispensable pillar of modern healthcare systems, addressing the complex needs of aging populations, individuals with chronic illnesses, and those with disabilities. As the demand for home-based care continues to grow, driven by demographic shifts and rising healthcare costs, the role of family caregivers has become increasingly vital. This chapter has explored integrative and evidence-based approaches to family caregiving, emphasizing holistic frameworks, complementary interventions, family-centered care, evidence-based strategies, and practical implementation. These approaches collectively aim to enhance care quality, reduce caregiver burden, and promote the well-being of both caregivers and care recipients. By synthesizing key findings and offering actionable recommendations, this conclusion underscores the importance of supporting family caregivers through interdisciplinary, sustainable, and culturally sensitive strategies.The scope of family caregiving is vast, encompassing a wide range of tasks, from personal care and medical management to emotional support and care coordination. With approximately 53 million Americans providing unpaid care (AARP, 2020), caregivers represent a diverse group, including men, women, younger and older adults, and individuals from varied cultural backgrounds..Integrative care models offer a promising framework for addressing these challenges by combining conventional medical practices with complementary approaches. The biopsychosocial model, for instance, provides a holistic lens through which caregivers can address biological, psychological, and social needs, ensuring that care plans are comprehensive and person-centered (Engel, 1977). Complementary approaches, such as mindfulness-based stress reduction (MBSR), yoga, and music therapy, have demonstrated significant benefits in reducing caregiver stress and enhancing emotional resilience (Whitebird et al., 2013; Danucalov et al., 2013; Clair & Ebberts, 1997). Family-centered care further strengthens these efforts by fostering collaboration among family members, healthcare providers, and community resources, ensuring that care aligns with the family's values and preferences (Mitrani et al., 2006).

Evidence-based interventions are critical for ensuring that caregiving strategies are effective and sustainable. Psychological interventions, such as cognitive behavioral therapy (CBT) and support groups, address caregivers' mental health needs, reducing depressive symptoms and perceived burden (Losada et al., 2011; Chien et al., 2011). Technological interventions, including telehealth, mobile apps, and smart home devices, streamline caregiving tasks and enhance safety, with studies showing improved caregiver confidence and reduced stress (Lindeman et al., 2020; Czaja et al., 2018). Community-based interventions, such as respite care, adult day programs, and volunteer networks, provide practical support and alleviate isolation, enabling caregivers to balance their responsibilities with self-care (Zarit et al., 2014; Gitlin et al., 2006). Together, these interventions form a robust toolkit for caregivers, grounded in rigorous research and practical applicability.Practical implementation of these approaches requires careful planning and collaboration. Comprehensive care plans, built on thorough needs assessments and clear goal-setting, ensure that interventions are tailored to the caregiving dyad's unique context. Training programs, such as the Powerful Tools for Caregivers curriculum, equip caregivers with essential skills, while accessible platforms like online courses expand reach to underserved populations (Boise et al., 2005). Leveraging technology effectively involves matching tools to caregivers' needs and providing training to overcome adoption barriers. Building support networks through community resources and delegating tasks to family or volunteers can further reduce burden. Above all, self-care strategies—prioritizing physical health, mental well-being, social engagement, and respite—are essential for preventing burnout and sustaining caregiving over time.Looking to the future, the growing demand for family caregiving necessitates innovative solutions and supportive policies. Advances in technology, such as artificial intelligence-driven tools and wearable devices, hold promise for enhancing efficiency and providing real-time support (Ho et al., 2020). Expanding training programs, particularly through scalable online platforms, can ensure that caregivers are equipped with the skills needed to navigate complex care tasks. Policy interventions, such as funding for respite care, tax credits, and expanded paid leave under the Family and Medical Leave Act, are critical for addressing financial and workplace challenges (Feinberg, 2019).

REFERENCES

AARP. (2020). *Caregiving in the U.S. 2020.* AARP and National Alliance for Caregiving. https://www.aarp.org/caregiving/research/info-2020/caregiving-in-the-united-states.html

Alzheimer's Association. (2021). 2021 Alzheimer's disease facts and figures. *Alzheimer's & Dementia, 17*(3), 327–406. DOI: 10.1002/alz.12328 PMID: 33756057

Anderson, K. A., Dabelko-Schoeny, H., & Johnson, T. D. (2017). The state of adult day services: Findings and implications from the MetLife National Study of Adult Day Services. *The Gerontologist, 57*(2), 331–340. DOI: 10.1093/geront/gnv099

Archbold, P. G., Stewart, B. J., Greenlick, M. R., & Harvath, T. A. (2018). Mutuality and preparedness as predictors of caregiver role strain. *Research in Nursing & Health, 33*(2), 103–116. DOI: 10.1002/nur.20365 PMID: 2270302

Binette, J., & Vasold, K. (2018). *Home and community preferences: A national survey of adults age 18-plus.* AARP Research.

Boise, L., Congleton, L., & Shannon, K. (2005). Empowering family caregivers: The powerful tools for caregivers program. *Educational Gerontology, 31*(7), 573–586. DOI: 10.1080/03601270590962523

Brown, R. M., Brown, S. L., & Johnson, A. S. (2015). Helping others as a means of reducing caregiver burden. *Journal of Applied Gerontology, 34*(3), 221–242. DOI: 10.1177/0733464812465988

Chan, E. A., Wong, F., Cheung, M. Y. C., & Lam, W. (2012). Using narrative inquiry and ethnography to understand the impact of culture on caregiving. *Journal of Advanced Nursing, 68*(3), 584–593. DOI: 10.1111/j.1365-2648.2011.05801.x

Chi, N. C., & Demiris, G. (2015). A systematic review of telehealth tools and interventions to support family caregivers. *Journal of Telemedicine and Telecare, 21*(1), 37–44. DOI: 10.1177/1357633X14562734 PMID: 25475220

Chien, L. Y., Chu, H., Guo, J. L., Liao, Y. M., Chang, L. I., Chen, C. H., & Chou, K. R. (2011). Caregiver support groups in patients with dementia: A meta-analysis. *International Journal of Geriatric Psychiatry, 26*(10), 1089–1098. DOI: 10.1002/gps.2660 PMID: 21308785

Clair, A. A., & Ebberts, A. G. (1997). The effects of music therapy on interactions between family caregivers and their care receivers with late-stage dementia. *Journal of Music Therapy, 34*(3), 148–164. DOI: 10.1093/jmt/34.3.148

Collins, R. N., Kishita, N., & Rymer, S. (2018). Psychological interventions for dementia caregivers: A systematic review and meta-analysis. *Aging & Mental Health, 22*(12), 1612–1630. DOI: 10.1080/13607863.2017.1370689

Compen, F. R.. (2018). Mindfulness-based cognitive therapy for cancer patients delivered via eHealth: A randomized controlled trial. *Psycho-Oncology, 27*(4), 1172–1179. DOI: 10.1002/pon.4642 PMID: 29266524

Crouch, E., Probst, J. C., & Bennett, K. (2017). Rural-urban differences in caregiver burden: Implications for policy and practice. *The Journal of Rural Health, 33*(1), 32–40. DOI: 10.1111/jrh.12173 PMID: 26449177

Czaja, S. J., Boot, W. R., Charness, N., Rogers, W. A., & Sharit, J. (2018). Improving social support for older adults through technology: Findings from the PRISM randomized controlled trial. *The Gerontologist, 58*(3), 467–477. DOI: 10.1093/geront/gnw249 PMID: 28201730

Danucalov, M. A. D., Kozasa, E. H., Afonso, R. F., Galduroz, J. C. F., & Leite, J. R. (2013). Yoga and heart rate variability: A comprehensive review of the literature. *International Journal of Yoga, 6*(1), 76–83. DOI: 10.4103/0973-6131.105948 PMID: 23439856

Dilworth-Anderson, P., Williams, I. C., & Gibson, B. E. (2002). Issues of race, ethnicity, and culture in caregiving research: A 20-year review. *The Gerontologist, 42*(2), 237–272. DOI: 10.1093/geront/42.2.237 PMID: 11914467

Engel, G. L. (1977). The need for a new medical model: A challenge for biomedicine. *Science, 196*(4286), 129–136. DOI: 10.1126/science.847460 PMID: 847460

Feinberg, L. F. (2019). *Breaking new ground: Supporting family caregivers in the workplace.* AARP Public Policy Institute.

Gallagher-Thompson, D., Solano, N., McGee, J. S., & Kurylo, M. (2003). Coping with caregiving: Reducing stress and improving your quality of life (2nd ed.). *Aging and Mental Health, 7*(3), 235–245. DOI: 10.1080/1360786031000101175

Gitlin, L. N., Reever, K., Dennis, M. P., Mathieu, E., & Hauck, W. W. (2006). Enhancing quality of life of families who use adult day services: Short- and long-term effects of the Adult Day Services Plus Program. *The Gerontologist, 46*(5), 630–639. DOI: 10.1093/geront/46.5.630 PMID: 17050754

Glueckauf, R. L.. (2012). Online cognitive-behavioral therapy for dementia caregivers: A pilot study. *The Gerontologist, 52*(4), 472–478. DOI: 10.1093/geront/gnr119 PMID: 22241808

Hayslip, B.Jr, & Kaminski, P. L. (2005). Grandparents raising their grandchildren: A review of the literature and suggestions for practice. *The Gerontologist, 45*(2), 262–269. DOI: 10.1093/geront/45.2.262 PMID: 15799992

Hebert, R. S., Dang, Q., & Schulz, R. (2007). Religious beliefs and practices are associated with better mental health in family caregivers. *The Gerontologist, 47*(6), 703–710. DOI: 10.1093/geront/47.6.703 PMID: 17158632

Ho, K.. (2020). Artificial intelligence in caregiving: Opportunities, challenges, and policy implications. *Journal of Medical Internet Research, 22*(8), e15666. DOI: 10.2196/15666

Kabat-Zinn, J. (1990). *Full catastrophe living: Using the wisdom of your body and mind to face stress, pain, and illness*. Delacorte.

Kitwood, T. (1997). *Dementia reconsidered: The person comes first*. Open University Press.

Li, F., Harmer, P., Fitzgerald, K., Eckstrom, E., Stock, R., Galver, J., Maddalozzo, G. F., & Batya, S. S. (2014). Tai chi and postural stability in patients with Parkinson's disease. *The New England Journal of Medicine, 366*(6), 511–519. DOI: 10.1056/NEJMoa1107911 PMID: 22316445

Lillehei, A. S., Halcon, L. L., Savik, K., & Reis, R. (2015). Effect of inhaled lavender and sleep hygiene on self-reported sleep issues. *Journal of Alternative and Complementary Medicine (New York, N.Y.), 21*(7), 430–438. DOI: 10.1089/acm.2014.0327 PMID: 26133206

Lindeman, D. A.. (2020). Telehealth and remote caregiving: Expanding the role of digital health in supporting families. *Frontiers in Public Health, 8*, 201–218. DOI: 10.3389/fpubh.2020.00189

Losada, A., Márquez-González, M., & Romero-Moreno, R. (2011). Cognitive-behavioral therapy (CBT) for dementia caregivers: A systematic review. *International Psychogeriatrics, 23*(7), 1002–1018. DOI: 10.1017/S1041610210002231

Mitrani, V. B., Feaster, D. J., Weiss-Laxer, N., & Szapocznik, J. (2006). Longitudinal effects of a family therapy intervention for caregivers of individuals with dementia. *Family Process, 45*(3), 451–465. DOI: 10.1111/j.1545-5300.2006.00179.x

Mittelman, M. S., Papayannopoulou, P., Vernooij-Dassen, M., Moniz-Cook, E., & Jeon, Y.-H. (2018). The unforgettables: A chorus for people with dementia and their family caregivers. *International Psychogeriatrics, 30*(6), 779–789. DOI: 10.1017/S1041610217001867 PMID: 29375037

National Alliance for Caregiving. (2020). *Caregiving in the U.S. 2020*. National Alliance for Caregiving and AARP.

Pharr, J. R., Francis, C. D., Terry, C., Clark, M. C., & Lee, D. J. (2014). Culture, caregiving, and health: Exploring the influence of culture on family caregiver experiences. *ISRN Public Health, 2014*, 1–8. DOI: 10.1155/2014/689826

Rantz, M. J., Skubic, M., Abbott, C., Galambos, C., Alexander, G., Popescu, M., & Keller, J. (2015). Automated technology to promote aging in place using sensor networks. *Journal of Gerontological Nursing, 41*(7), 10–17. DOI: 10.3928/00989134-20150615-03

Reinhard, S. C., Feinberg, L. F., Choula, R., & Houser, A. (2019). *Valuing the invaluable: 2019 update—Charting a path forward*. AARP Public Policy Institute.

Robertson, R., Robertson, A., Jepson, R., & Maxwell, M. (2012). Walking for depression or depressive symptoms: A systematic review and meta-analysis. *Mental Health and Physical Activity, 5*(1), 66–75. DOI: 10.1016/j.mhpa.2012.03.002

Russell, R. (2007). Men doing "women's work": Elderly men caregivers and the gendered construction of care work. *Journal of Men's Studies, 15*(1), 1–18. DOI: 10.3149/jms.1501.1

Schulz, R., & Eden, J. (Eds.). (2016). *Families caring for an aging America*. National Academies Press., DOI: 10.17226/23606

Smith, M. C.. (2019). Complementary therapies for caregiver stress management: A systematic review. *Complementary Therapies in Medicine, 45*, 147–155. DOI: 10.1016/j.ctim.2019.02.001

van der Linden, M. (1996). Effects of music therapy on anxiety in elderly patients. *Age and Ageing, 25*(2), 127–131. DOI: 10.1093/ageing/25.2.127

Whitebird, R. R., Kreitzer, M. J., & O'Connor, P. J. (2013). Mindfulness-based stress reduction for family caregivers: A randomized controlled trial. *The American Journal of Hospice & Palliative Care, 30*(2), 187–195. DOI: 10.1177/1049909112452622 PMID: 23070934

Zarit, S. H., Kim, K., Femia, E. E., Almeida, D. M., & Klein, L. C. (2014). The effects of adult day services on family caregivers' daily stress, affect, and health: Outcomes from the Daily Stress and Health (DaSH) study. *The Gerontologist, 54*(4), 570–579. DOI: 10.1093/geront/gnt045 PMID: 23690056

Chapter 2
Integrative healthcare at Home and Caregiver Toolkit:
An Exploration

Geetha Manoharan
https://orcid.org/0000-0002-8644-8871
SR University, India

Subhashini Durai
LEAD College of Management, India

ABSTRACT

Integrated healthcare that is provided in the patient's home is the topic of discussion in this chapter, as is the creation of a caregiver toolbox to support this paradigm. To provide patients with complete medical treatment that addresses their physical, psychological, and social requirements, integrative healthcare requires coordinated teamwork among a wide range of medical experts. This method, when used in home settings, encourages holistic care that improves the well-being of patients and aids family caregivers in the management of multifaceted health problems. To enable caregivers to provide successful integrative care, the caregiver toolkit acts as a practical resource that guides, trains, and equips them with the necessary tools. This investigation highlights the benefits, challenges, and potential strategies for implementing integrative healthcare at home. The important role that caregivers play in bridging the gap between clinical treatment and everyday living situations receives particular attention.

DOI: 10.4018/979-8-3373-4094-4.ch002

INTRODUCTION TO THE NEW ERA OF CAREGIVING:

The caregivers are part of a quiet, powerful, and growing movement. Perhaps they are caring for an aging parent, a spouse with a chronic illness, a child with special needs, or a friend recovering from surgery. Whatever the circumstances, the caregivers have taken on one of the most profoundly important and challenging roles in our society. The landscape of healthcare has changed dramatically; care that was once confined to hospitals is now routinely delivered in living rooms and bedrooms, and family members like we are on the front lines (National Academies of Sciences, Engineering, and Medicine, 2016). This new reality is both a blessing and a burden. It allows loved ones to be in a comfortable, familiar environment, which can be immensely healing. But it also places an extraordinary weight on your shoulders.

The caregivers may be managing medications, coordinating appointments, providing personal care, and offering emotional support, all while juggling their own life, work, and family. It is easy to feel overwhelmed, isolated, and unprepared. This toolkit is designed to change that. The purpose is to help move from feeling like a passive helper to becoming an empowered caregiver. An empowered caregiver is not just someone who performs tasks; they are an active, informed, and confident partner in their loved one's health journey. They have the knowledge to provide comfort, the skills to manage stress (their own and their loved one's), and the confidence to advocate for holistic, person-centered care. The foundation of this empowerment is integrative health.

Integrative Health

We may have heard terms like "alternative," "holistic," or "complementary" medicine, and it can be confusing. Integrative health is a clear and evidence-informed approach. The National Center for Complementary and Integrative Health (NCCIH) define it as a practice that reaffirms the importance of the relationship between practitioner and patient, focuses on the whole person, is informed by evidence, and makes use of all appropriate therapeutic approaches to achieve optimal health and healing (NCCIH, 2018). Let us break that down:

- **It is NOT alternative medicine:**

Integrative health does not *replace* conventional medical treatment. It works *with* it. The medications, therapies, and advice from your loved one's medical team are the primary foundation of their care.

- **It is complementary:**

Integrative therapies are added to a conventional care plan to manage symptoms, reduce stress, and improve quality of life. Think of it as adding more tools to the toolbox.

- **It is holistic:** This approach recognizes that a person is more than their diagnosis. It cares for the whole person:
  - **Body:** Physical comfort, pain management, sleep, and nutrition.
  - **Mind:** Mental clarity, anxiety, depression, and cognitive function.
  - **Emotions:** Fear, hope, grief, and emotional well-being.
  - **Spirit:** Meaning, purpose, connection, and spiritual or religious beliefs.
- **It is evidence-informed:**

The tools in this toolkit are not based on wishful thinking. They are supported by a growing body of scientific research demonstrating their effectiveness in helping with issues like pain, anxiety, nausea, and insomnia.

By embracing an integrative approach, they can have a profound impact on their loved one's comfort and quality of life, filling the gaps that conventional medicine sometimes misses.

Usage of Toolkits

This guide is designed to be a practical, hands-on resource. It is not meant as they are not expected to read it cover-to-cover or to use every single tool. Think of it as a reference manual for a caregiving journey.

- **Start with yourself:**

They have intentionally placed the section on caregiver self-care first. It is not an afterthought; it is the absolute foundation of sustainable, compassionate care.

- **Browse the tools:**

Look through the different sections and find what feels most relevant to their current situation. Is the loved one struggling with pain? Start with the tools for the body. Is anxiety the primary challenge? Explore the tools for the mind and emotions.

- **Start small:**

Choose one simple tool to try this week. Maybe it is playing a calming playlist or trying a three-minute breathing exercise for thyself. Small, consistent actions build confidence and create momentum.

- **Always be safe:**

The golden rule of integrative care is "first, do no harm." Every tool in this kit is designed to be gentle and safe for most people. However, it is always a must to think about the loved one's specific condition. Crucially, always discuss any new therapies we are considering with the loved one's doctor, nurse, or medical team. This is a partnership, and open communication is key. The individuals are on a difficult journey, but they are not alone. This toolkit is here to provide us with knowledge, skills, and the quiet reassurance that we can do this. Finally, the individual can be an empowered, effective, and compassionate caregiver.

PART 1: THE FOUNDATION – CARING FOR THE CAREGIVER

There is a phrase we can hear on every airplane safety demonstration: "Secure your own oxygen mask before assisting others." This is the single most important, and often the most ignored, rule of caregiving. We simply cannot pour from an empty cup. If we collapse from exhaustion, stress, or illness, who will be there to care for our loved one? Prioritizing our own well-being is not selfish; it is an absolute prerequisite for providing sustainable and loving care. Caregiver burnout is a state of physical, emotional, and mental exhaustion. It is a real and serious condition, linked to increased rates of depression, chronic disease, and even mortality among caregivers (Schulz & Sherwood, 2008). Its symptoms can include overwhelming fatigue, changes in sleep patterns, irritability, feelings of hopelessness, and a tendency to get sick more often. Recognizing this reality is the first step toward preventing it.

Tool 1: The Self-Care Assessment

We cannot fix a problem we are not aware of. Take a few minutes to honestly answer these questions. There is no judgment here; this is simply about gathering information such as follows below:

- **Sleep:** Am I getting 7-8 hours of sleep most nights? Is my sleep frequently interrupted? Do I feel rested when I wake up?

- **Nutrition:** Am I eating regular, balanced meals? Or am I grabbing processed snacks and relying on caffeine to get through the day? Am I staying hydrated with water?
- **Movement:** Am I getting any form of physical activity? Even a 10-minute walk? Am I stretching my body to relieve tension?
- **Health:** Have I postponed my own doctor or dentist appointments? Am I ignoring new physical symptoms of my own?
- **Stress:** On a scale of 1 to 10, what is my average daily stress level? Do I have any way to release that stress? Do I feel constantly on edge or anxious?
- **Emotions:** Do I feel irritable, sad, or hopeless? Do I ever feel resentful of my caregiving role? Do I have anyone I can talk to about these feelings?
- **Connection:** Have I made time to connect with friends or family recently? Do I feel isolated? Am I still engaging in any hobbies or activities that I enjoy?

Looking at the answers, which area needs the most immediate attention? Choose just one to focus on this week.

Tool 2: Mindfulness and Stress Reduction for the Overwhelmed

When we are a caregiver, our nervous system is often in a constant state of high alert. Mindfulness is the practice of paying attention to the present moment without judgment. It is a powerful tool for calming our fight-or-flight response and finding moments of peace in a chaotic day. Research shows that mindfulness-based stress reduction (MBSR) can significantly decrease anxiety, depression, and stress in caregivers (Oken et al., 2010).

We do not need to sit on a cushion for an hour to practice mindfulness. Try these "micro-practices":

- **The 3-Minute Breathing Space:** This is a quick reset you can do anytime.

    1. **Acknowledge:** For one minute, notice what is happening right now. What are you thinking? What are you feeling in your body? Just observe without trying to change anything.
    2. **Gather:** For the second minute, gently bring your full attention to the physical sensation of your breath. Feel the air move in and out of your body. When your mind wanders, gently guide it back to breath.
    3. **Expand:** For the final minute, expand your awareness to include your whole body. Feel the space you are in, the sounds around you, and the sensation of being present.

- **Mindful Moments:**

Anchor our awareness in a routine task. When we wash our hands, for example, instead of thinking about our to-do list, pay full attention to the sensory experience: the temperature of the water, the feeling of the soap, the sound it makes. This turns a mundane task into a two-minute meditation.

- **Progressive Muscle Relaxation (PMR):**

This technique involves tensing and then releasing different muscle groups, which helps us become aware of where we hold tension and allows for a deep sense of physical relaxation. Before bed, lie down and try this: Starting with our toes, tense the muscles for 5 seconds, then release for 15 seconds. Move up to our calves, thighs, abdomen, arms, and face.

Tool 3: Building Your Support Network

Caregiving is not a solo sport. They need a team. However, many caregivers are reluctant to ask for help, or they do not know how.

Be Specific

Caregivers often struggle to accept help because offers are too vague. When someone says, "Let me know if you need anything," they are likely well-intentioned, but this puts the burden of identifying, articulating, and asking for a specific task back on the person who is already overwhelmed. This is an example of an unstructured offer, which is difficult to act on. The solution is to be specific. Instead of saying "I need help," a caregiver should clearly define a task that someone else can easily fulfill. The examples given—"Could you pick up a prescription for me on Tuesday?" or "Would you be able to sit with Mom for two hours on Saturday afternoon?" are actionable requests. They remove the guesswork and make it simple for the other person to say yes or no based on their availability and ability. This change of a passive request to an active and concrete increases the probability of receiving significant help and reduces the emotional effort for the caregiver.

Use Technology

Coordinating the help of several people can be a logistics challenge, turning what should be a relief in another source of stress. The text suggests using technology, specifically mentioning free websites and applications such as Lota Held Hands or

Caringbridge. These platforms act as a central center to organize support. A caregiver can create a private page to publish updates on the condition of our loved one and the specific tasks of the list with those who need help, such as delivery of food, transport, or errands. The family and friends can see this list and register in tasks that fit their schedule and skills. This approach eliminates the need for endless phone calls or text messages and allows followers to contribute to their own terms, which makes the process more efficient and less stressful for all involved.

Find Your People

Care can be an isolated experience, since friends and family that are not caregivers may not completely understand the unique challenges and the emotional toll that is needed. Connecting with other caregivers creates a life support network based on shared experience. The text emphasizes that these people "understand it in a way that others cannot." Organizations like the Family Caregiver Alliance or illness-specific groups, such as the Alzheimer's Association, provide a way to connect with these peers. They host local or online support groups where caregivers can share their frustrations, exchange advice, and feel understood. This type of social support is a powerful tool for reducing feelings of loneliness and isolation, validating a caregiver's struggles, and providing emotional encouragement.

Explore Respite Care

Respite care is a crucial service that provides temporary relief for the primary caregiver. The text correctly defines it as an "essential service" rather than a luxury. The goal of respite care is to prevent caregiver burnout, a state of physical, emotional, and mental exhaustion that can compromise both the caregiver's and the care recipient's well-being.

This short-term care can be flexible, ranging from a few hours to several days, and can take place in various settings:

- **In-home care:** A professional caregiver comes to the home to provide supervision and assistance.
- **Adult day care centers:** The care recipient spends a portion of the day in a supervised facility with social activities.
- **Nursing facilities:** The care recipient stays overnight for a short period.

By using respite care, a caregiver can take a break to rest, attend to their own needs, and recharge, which allows them to continue their demanding role with renewed energy and a healthier perspective.

PART 2: THE INTEGRATIVE TOOLKIT FOR THE BODY

When someone is ill or recovering, their body is under immense stress. Conventional medicine provides the essential treatments, the medications, surgeries, and therapies that target the disease. The integrative tools in this section are designed to support the person's physical comfort, reduce distressing symptoms like pain and nausea, and create an optimal environment for healing.

A Crucial Note on Safety

The tools described here are gentle and non-invasive. However, every person and every situation is unique. Always communicate with your loved ones' doctor, nurse, or physical therapist before trying a new approach. Ask questions like, "I was thinking of trying some gentle hand massage for my mother's arthritis. Are there any areas I should avoid?" or "I read that peppermint aromatherapy might help with nausea. Is there any reason she should not try that?" This ensures that you are a true partner in an integrated care team.

Tool 4: The Power of Therapeutic Touch

In a world of high-tech medicine, the power of simple, compassionate human touch is often underestimated. Therapeutic touch is not the same as a deep tissue massage from a licensed therapist. It is about conveying care, comfort, and connection through our hands. Research has shown that even simple massage techniques can be effective in reducing pain, anxiety, and agitation in various patient populations (Kutner et al., 2008).

- **How it Works:**

Gentle touch can stimulate nerve fibers that send calming signals to the brain, helping to release natural pain-relieving chemicals like endorphins. It also reduces levels of stress hormone cortisol and can promote a sense of safety and well-being.

- **Simple Hand Massage Technique:** This is a wonderful technique to use while sitting and talking with our loved one.

    1. **Ask Permission:** Always start by asking, "Would it be okay if I rubbed your hands for a few minutes?"
    2. **Get Comfortable:** Sit in a comfortable position facing your loved one. Apply a small amount of gentle, unscented lotion to your hands.

3. **Warm Up:** Gently hold their hand in both of yours for a moment.
4. **Palm Strokes:** Place their hand palm-up in yours. Use your thumbs to make small, gentle circles all over their palm.
5. **Finger Pulls:** Gently take each finger one by one and slide your fingers from the base to the tip with gentle pressure.
6. **Top of Hand:** Turn their hand over and use your thumbs to make long, smooth strokes from the knuckles toward the wrist.
7. **Finish:** Hold their hand gently once more before letting go.

- **Safety First:**
    - Avoid areas with open wounds, rashes, infections, or recent injuries.
    - Never apply deep pressure, especially over joints or bony areas.
    - Be very gentle with anyone who has blood clots (DVT), severe osteoporosis, or is on blood thinners. Check with their doctor first.
    - Pay attention to non-verbal cues. If they pull away or wince, stop immediately.

Tool 5: Aromatherapy for Comfort and Calm

Aromatherapy is the use of essential oils from plants to enhance psychological and physical well-being. Our sense of smell is directly linked to the limbic system, the part of the brain that controls emotions and memory. This is why a certain smell can instantly trigger a feeling or a memory. When used safely, aromatherapy can be a simple and effective way to alter the mood of a room and help manage symptoms.

- **Evidence:**

Numerous studies support the use of aromatherapy for specific symptoms. For example, clinical trials have found that lavender inhalation can reduce anxiety and improve sleep quality, while peppermint can be effective in reducing nausea (Faydalı & Çetinkaya, 2018; Lane et al., 2012).

- **Focus on a Few Key Oils:** We do not need a large collection. Start with these well-researched, gentle oils:
    - **Lavender (*Lavandula angustifolia*):** The workhorse of aromatherapy. It is known for its calming, sedating effects and is excellent for anxiety, restlessness, and promoting sleep.
    - **Roman Chamomile (*Chamaemelum nobile*):** Very gentle and calming, often used for insomnia and irritability.

- o **Sweet Orange (*Citrus sinensis*):** A bright, uplifting oil that can help improve mood and reduce anxiety.
- o **Peppermint (*Mentha piperita*):** Well-studied for its anti-nausea effects. Use with caution as it can be stimulating.

- **Safe Application Methods:** In a home care setting, the safest method is inhalation. Never apply undiluted essential oils directly to the skin, and never have our loved one ingest them.

1. **Simple Inhalation:** Place 1-2 drops of an essential oil on a cotton ball or tissue and place it near your loved one (e.g., on a bedside table). The scent will gently diffuse into the air.
2. **Room Diffusion:** Use a cool-mist ultrasonic diffuser. These are safer than candle-based diffusers. Use only 3-5 drops of essential oil in the water and run it for 30-60 minutes at a time. Ensure the room is well-ventilated.

- **Safety First:**
  - o People with asthma or other respiratory conditions may be sensitive to strong smells. Start with a very small amount and see how they react.
  - o Some oils can interact with medications. Again, a quick check with the medical team is wise.
  - o Pay attention to preferences. The scent that you find calming might be unpleasant for your loved one. Always ask what they think.

Tool 6: Gentle Movement and Positioning

The phrase "motion is lotion" is true for the body. Even small movements can help prevent joint stiffness, improve circulation, boost mood, and maintain a sense of physical autonomy.

- **For Someone Who is Mobile:**
  - o **Chair Yoga:** Many simple yoga stretches can be done while seated. This includes neck rolls, shoulder shrugs, torso twists, and ankle circles. You can find many free guided chair yoga videos online.
  - o **Encourage Small Walks:** If safe and approved by their doctor, even a walk from the bed to a chair by the window can make a huge difference in their day.
- **For Someone Who is Bed-Bound:**
  - o **Passive Range of Motion (PROM):** This involves you gently moving their joints for them. A physical therapist can show you the correct and safe way to perform these exercises for the ankles, knees, wrists, and

shoulders. This is crucial for preventing contractures (permanent shortening of a muscle or joint).
  - **Comfortable Positioning:** Being in one position for too long is uncomfortable and can lead to pressure sores (bedsores). Use pillows to support their body and relieve pressure. Place a pillow between their knees when they are on their side, under their calves to "float" their heels off the bed, and to support their back. Change their position at least every two hours if they cannot do it themselves.

Tool 7: Healing Through Nutrition – The Caregiver's Role

Food is more than just fuel; it can be medicine, comfort, and a source of pleasure. As a caregiver, we are not expected to be a registered dietitian, but we can play a powerful role in supporting our loved one's health through nutrition. The goal is to provide nutrient-dense, appealing food that is easy to eat.

- **Focus on Anti-Inflammatory Foods:** Many chronic illnesses are associated with chronic inflammation. An anti-inflammatory diet, like the Mediterranean diet, emphasizes whole, unprocessed foods. This includes:
  - **Colorful Fruits and Vegetables:** Full of antioxidants.
  - **Healthy Fats:** Olive oil, avocados, nuts, and seeds.
  - **Lean Proteins:** Fish (especially fatty fishlike salmon), poultry, and beans.
  - **Whole Grains:** Oats, quinoa, and brown rice.
  - Research suggests this way of eating can support overall health and may help manage symptoms of chronic disease (Ricker & Haas, 2017).
- **Managing Common Challenges:**
  - **Loss of Appetite:** Do not force large meals. Instead, they offer small, nutrient-dense mini-meals or snacks every 2-3 hours. A smoothie with protein powder, fruit, and spinach can pack a lot of nutrition into a small, easy-to-consume package.
  - **Nausea:** Simple, bland foods are often best. Think of toast, crackers, rice, and broth. Ginger is a well-researched natural anti-nausea remedy. You can make ginger tea from fresh ginger root or offer ginger chews.
  - **Changes in Taste:** Illness and medications can make food taste metallic or bland. Try adding herbs, spices, or a lemon squeeze to enhance flavor.
  - **Hydration:** Dehydration is a common and serious problem. Always keep a water bottle with a straw nearby. Soups, smoothies, and watery fruits like melons also contribute to hydration.

PART 3: THE INTEGRATIVE TOOLKIT FOR THE MIND AND EMOTIONS

The mind-body connection is not a New Age concept; it is a scientific fact. Our emotional state—our levels of stress, anxiety, and fear—has a direct and measurable impact on our physical body. It can affect pain perception, immune function, and the ability to heal (Kiecolt-Glaser et al., 2002). The tools in this section are designed to soothe the mind, calm the emotions, and create a sense of psychological safety, which can have profound benefits for physical well-being.

Tool 8: Creating a Healing Environment

The physical space where someone is healing has a huge impact on their mental state. A chaotic, noisy, or cluttered room can increase stress, while a calm, organized, and pleasant environment can promote rest and peace. Think of yourself as the curator of a healing space.

Light

Natural light is a powerful mood regulator because it influences our circadian rhythms, which affect sleep patterns and energy levels. By simply opening curtains during the day, we can let in sunlight, which can help a person feel more alert and connected to the time of day. Positioning their chair or bed to face a window allows them to see outside, which provides a visual connection to the world and can prevent feelings of being cooped up.

Sound

The soundscape of a room can either be soothing or agitating. It is important to be mindful of unnecessary noise from sources like televisions or radios, as constant background sound can be irritating and stressful. Instead, the text recommends creating a calming auditory environment. This can be done by playing soft, soothing music, or using a white noise machine to mask jarring, unexpected sounds, creating a more peaceful and predictable atmosphere.

Clutter

A cluttered physical space can contribute to a feeling of mental chaos. The text suggests that even a small amount of tidying can make a big difference. Taking just ten minutes each day to tidy up the room and keep the bedside table organized with only essential items can create a sense of order and control. A clear, organized space can help the person feel less overwhelmed and more at ease.

Scent

Scent has a powerful and immediate effect on the brain's limbic system, which is tied to emotion and memory. As mentioned in the aromatherapy section, using a gentle, pleasant scent can instantly transform the feel of a room, making it feel more like a home and less like a clinical or sterile environment. A calming scent can help a person relax and feel more comfortable.

Research on hospital design, known as evidence-based design, has shown that factors like natural light and views of nature can reduce patient pain, decrease stress, and even shorter hospital stays (Ulrich, 1984). You can apply these same principles at home.

Tool 9: Guided Imagery and Visualization

Guided imagery is a simple mind-body technique that involves using our imagination to create a calming, peaceful scene in your mind. It is a form of focused relaxation that can help manage pain, anxiety, and stress. It works by distracting the mind from unpleasant sensations and activating the body relaxation response.

Evidence and Purpose

Guided images are a body technique where a person is guided to imagine a relaxing scene or experience using all their senses. The text cites evidence that anxiety can effectively reduce before medical procedures and reduce pain in people with chronic conditions. The main objective is to change the approach to discomfort or anxiety to a peaceful and soothing mental state, which can have a physiological effect on the body, such as reducing heart rate and blood pressure.

How to Do It

To make guided images, we must read a script aloud to our loved one with a quiet and slow voice. The text recommends looking for free scripts or audio recordings adapted to specific needs such as pain or relaxation. The key is to choose a scene that the individual would find pleasant, such as a beach, forest, or garden.

A Sample Script and Tips

The "peaceful place" script provided guide to the listener through a step -by - step relaxation process. Start instructing them to feel comfortable and take slow and soft breaths. The script then prompts them to visualize a safe, peaceful place, engaging in all five senses:

- **Sight:** Noticing colors and shapes.
- **Sound:** Hearing gentle waves or birdsong.
- **Feeling:** Sensing the sun's warmth or a gentle breeze.

The process encourages the person to rest in this mental space and reminds them that they can return to it anytime. The text provides valuable tips: keep our voice soft and slow, pause often, and understand that if the person falls asleep, it is a sign of success, as the goal is relaxation.

Tool 10: The Power of Music Therapy

Music is a direct pathway to our emotions. It can energize us, make us nostalgic, or soothe us into a state of deep calm. When used intentionally, music is a powerful therapeutic tool. It can reduce anxiety, lower blood pressure, manage pain, and improve mood. It is particularly effective for people with dementia, as it can unlock memories and reduce agitation when other forms of communication fail (Gerdner, 2012).

Create Personalized Playlists

The most crucial aspect of using music for therapy is personalization. What is calming or comforting to one person might be stressful to another. Therefore, it is essential to tailor music choices to the individual's preferences and emotional needs. The text suggests two specific types of playlists to achieve different goals.

The Calming Playlist

This type of playlist is designed to promote relaxation and rest. It should consist of slow, instrumental music, which can help lower heart rate and calm the nervous system. The text suggests genres like classical music (specifically mentioning composers like Debussy or Satie, known for their soothing pieces), ambient music, or even nature sounds. This playlist is ideal for times when the goal is to reduce anxiety or help someone fall asleep.

The Nostalgia Playlist

This playlist uses music as a powerful tool for memory and mood. It should feature songs from the individual's teens and twenties, as this period is often associated with strong, formative memories. Listening to these songs can be incredibly effective for evoking positive memories, sparking conversations, and improving mood. This type of music can help someone reconnect with their past and feel a sense of joy and vitality.

How to Use Music

The text differentiates between two ways to engage with music:

- **Passive Listening:**

This involves playing a calming playlist in the background at a low volume. The goal is to create a soothing atmosphere without requiring active engagement from the listener.

- **Active Listening:**

This is a more interactive approach, typically used with the nostalgia playlist. It involves sitting with the person and listening to music together. The caregiver can then use open-ended questions like, "What does this song make you think of?" to encourage conversation and reminiscing.

The Safety Note is a critical final point, advising mindfulness of a song's lyrics and emotional tone. Some music, even if from a beloved era, might trigger sadness or painful memories, so it is vital to be guided by the person's real-time reaction.

Tool 11: The Art of Therapeutic Communication

How we talk and listen can be a form of medicine. Therapeutic communication is about creating a space where your loved one feels heard, understood, and validated. At a time when they can feel a loss of control, giving them the gift of being really heard is empowering.

Active Listening

Active listening is a fundamental ability to show empathy. It implies more than just listening to words; It means paying all your attention to the speaker. This requires an intentional effort to minimize distractions, such as saving your phone or turning off the TV. When making visual contact and focusing on both his words and body language, he shows that the individual is completely committed. This nonverbal communication is critical; The person is pointed out that our thoughts and feelings are important for you.

Use Open-Ended Questions

The type of questions you ask can open a conversation or close it. Open questions invite a detailed answer instead of a simple "yes" or "no." For example, asking "What was the best part of your day today?" It encourages a narrative response, allowing the person to share more about their experiences and feelings. This approach shows genuine curiosity and creates an opportunity for a deeper conversation, helping the speaker to feel heard and understood.

Validate Feelings

Validating someone's feelings is a powerful way to provide support without trying to "solve" their problem. It implies recognizing and accepting our emotional experience as real and legitimate. Phrases like "that sounds incredibly frustrating" or "I can see why you would feel scared" do not offer a solution; Instead, they communicate that he understands and accepts his emotional state. This simple act of validation tells the person that his feelings are real and that they are not alone in them, which can be deeply comforting and healing.

Avoid Toxic Positivity

Toxic positivity is the excessive and ineffective overgeneralization of a happy and optimistic state in all situations. While it is natural to want to cheer someone up, phrases like "look on the bright side" or "everything happens for a reason" can be dismissive of someone's pain. This type of response invalidates their sadness or fear by implying they should just "get over it." Instead, the most healing thing to do is to simply sit with them in their sadness without trying to change it. This demonstrates that we can handle their difficult emotions and that they have a safe space to feel their feelings without judgment.

PART 4: THE INTEGRATIVE TOOLKIT FOR THE SPIRIT

Caring for the spirit is a crucial, yet often overlooked, part of holistic care. The "spirit" does not necessarily mean religion, though for many people it does. Spirituality is about what gives our lives meaning, purpose, and a sense of connection to something larger than ourselves. When someone is facing a serious illness, these existential questions often come to the forefront. Supporting their spirit is about honoring their identity, their life story, and what matters most to them.

The Meaning of "Spirit"

The text clarifies that spirit is not strictly synonymous with religion, although for many people, it is closely linked to their faith. The core definition of spirituality, as presented here, is about what gives our lives meaning, purpose, and a sense of connection to something larger than ourselves. This can be a religious belief, but it could also be a connection to nature, art, philosophy, family, or community.

The Importance of Spiritual Care

Supporting someone's spirit is a crucial, yet often overlooked, part of holistic care, which addresses the whole person—mind, body, and spirit. When someone is facing a serious illness, they often confront profound existential questions about life, death, and their purpose. During this time, the need for spiritual support becomes even more significant. Providing this care is an act of honoring their identity, their life story, and what matters most to them. It acknowledges that their well-being is not just physical but also deeply personal and emotional.

Tool 12: Honoring Life Stories and Legacy

Everyone has a story. Helping your loved one share their story is a powerful way to affirm their identity beyond their illness. Reminiscence therapy has been shown to improve mood, reduce agitation (especially in dementia), and enhance a sense of self-worth (Woods et al., 2018).

Use Photos as Prompts

Photos are powerful tools for unlocking memories and stories. When you sit down with an old photo album, you are not just looking at pictures; you are opening a window into the past. By asking specific, open-ended questions like, "Tell me about this day," or "Who is this in the picture with you?" you give the person a gentle, non-threatening way to share their experiences. This strategy turns a passive activity into an active conversation, encouraging them to recall and share cherished moments and relationships.

Ask Legacy Questions

Legacy questions are designed to get to the heart of a person's life lessons, values, and wisdom. These questions go beyond simple memories and prompt deeper reflection on what truly matters. Asking, "What are you most proud of in your life?" invites them to reflect on their greatest achievements and moments of fulfillment. Questions about lessons learned from parents or advice for the younger generation encourage them to articulate the core values they hold and wish to pass on. This process not only honors their life experiences but also helps them feel that their knowledge and wisdom are valuable and will live.

Creating a Legacy Project

An inherited project is a tangible way of preserving the history and wisdom of life of a person for future generations. This does not need to be a complex, formal project. It could be as simple as creating a "memory box" filled with meaningful items, like a concert ticket studio or a favorite old scarf. Another idea is to make a simple audio recording of them sharing a favorite family story. This captures not just the words but also the sound of their voice. Or you could write down their favorite recipes, preserving a piece of their culinary history and the memories associated with those meals. These projects provide a profound sense of purpose and peace, as the individual sees their life and memories being preserved and honored.

Tool 13: Connecting with Nature

Humans have an innate need to connect with nature, a concept called biophilia. This connection is deeply healing. Research has shown that even passive contact with nature—like looking out a window at a tree—can reduce stress and improve mood (Grinde & Patil, 2009).

Bring Nature Indoors

Bringing nature indoors is about providing a tangible, sensory experience of the natural world. This can be done in simple but effective ways. A small vase of fresh flowers or a hardy houseplant can immediately change the atmosphere of a room, adding color and life. These living things can improve mood and serve as a focal point for the eye.

Another suggestion is to place a bird feeder outside the main window. This not only provides entertainment by attracting local birds but also creates a direct, dynamic link to the outside world. The changing activity in the feeder gives the person something to look at and can encourage a sense of connection with the rhythm of nature.

Finally, opening a window when the weather is pleasant allows fresh air and the sounds of nature, such as the leaves or birds of whisper, they will enter the room. This simple act of leaving outdoors can be a powerful reinforcement, providing sensory stimulation and a sensation of freshness.

Use Nature's Sights and Sounds

When bringing nature indoors, technology can be used to simulate experience. This strategy implies the use of means to provide a sense of immersion in nature. Reproducing videos of beautiful natural scenes, many of which are available on platforms such as YouTube, can be a powerful visual experience. These videos can transport the viewer to a forest, a beach, or a mountain, offering a mental escape.

Similarly, reproducing audio recordings from nature sounds, such as rain, bird song or ocean waves, can have a soothing effect. These sounds can reduce stress and create a peaceful atmosphere. By involving the senses of sight and sound, these methods help counteract the isolation of conflict and provide a significant connection with the restorative power of nature.

Tool 14: Supporting Faith and Spiritual Practices

If your loved one has a religious or spiritual tradition, respecting and supporting that is essential. These are your needs, not your beliefs.

Creating a Sacred Space

Help someone create a sacred space that involves surrounding them with elements that have a personal or spiritual deep meaning. It is not just about organizing a room; It is about healing a personal environment that offers comfort and a feeling of connection with their beliefs. For someone who is religious, this could mean maintaining a biblical account, Quran, or Rosario at hand. These elements are often more than just objects; They are tangible links with their faith, history, and community. For others, it could be a special photograph, a work of art or a precious relic. The objective is to make its surroundings immediately a source of spiritual force and peace.

Facilitate Connection

Facilitating connection means helping the person commit to their spiritual or religious and practical community when they could not do so on their own. This can be as simple as reading aloud of a sacred text or playing spiritual music. For those who are part of a religious community, offer them to help see an online service or organize a visit from their spiritual leader, such as a pastor, priest, rabbi or magnet, can be deeply comforting. These actions help close the physical gap between the person and their source of spiritual support, ensuring that they remain connected to the rituals and the community that support them.

For the Non-Religious

Spiritual support is not limited to religious practices. For those who are not religious, spirituality can be a feeling of astonishment, peace and connection found in other areas of life. It is about understanding what gives that individual a sense of purpose or transcendence. This could be listening to a piece of classical music that evokes strong emotions, reading a favorite poem aloud or participating in a reflexive conversation about philosophy or science.

The key is to find what gives them a feeling of astonishment, peace, and connection, whether the beauty of nature, the complexity of the universe or a particular work of art. This approach honors the unique path of the individual towards spiritual realization, which demonstrates that their sense of meaning is as valid and important as any other.

DISCUSSION AND CONCLUSION ON WEAVING IT ALL TOGETHER – THE INTEGRATED CARE PLAN

Now we have explored a wide range of tools to support the body, mind, and spirit of your loved one and ourselves. The last step is to gather these ideas in a way that feels manageable, not overwhelming. The objective is to create a simple and personalized comprehensive care plan. An empowered caregiver is a proactive caregiver This does not need to be another stressful list of pending tasks. Think about it as a menu of possibilities.

Here is a sample of how a simple weekly plan could be:

Table 1. -

Day	Morning (Body)	Afternoon (Mind/ Emotions)	Evening (Spirit/Calm)	For Me (Caregiver)
Mon	Gentle stretches in bed.	Look at old family photos.	Play calming classical music.	3-Min Breathing Space.
Tues	Offer a nutritious smoothie.	Listen to my favorite old song.	5-min hand massage with lotion.	10-min walk outside.
Wed	Open windows for fresh air.	Watch birds at the feeder.	Read a chapter from a book.	Call a friend.
Thurs	Ensure good hydration.	Guided imagery audio (10 min).	Diffuse lavender essential oil.	Eat a healthy, sit-down lunch.
Fri	Chair yoga exercises.	Watch my favorite old movie.	Talk about childhood memories.	Schedule 2 hours of respite care.

This is just an example. The plan will be different according to the needs of our loved ones and our own capacity. The key is to be intentional. Choose one or two small things every day. His role as a caregiver is one of the most generous and demanding love acts. By adopting the principles of integrative health, not only is a disease taken care of; they are taking care of the whole person. And remembering to take care of themselves ensures this path with force, compassion, and resistance. They have tools. You are an empowered caregiver.

REFERENCES

Faydalı, S., & Çetinkaya, F. (2018). The effect of aromatherapy on sleep quality. *Alternative Therapies in Health and Medicine*, *24*(3), 42–48. PMID: 29210873

Gerdner, L. A. (2012). Music therapy in dementia care.[56]. *Perspectives in Psychiatric Care*, *48*(2), 77–78. DOI: 10.1111/j.1744-6163.2012.00332.x

Grinde, B., & Patil, G. G. (2009). Biophilia: Does visual contact with nature impact on health and well-being? *International Journal of Environmental Research and Public Health*, *6*(9), 2332–2343. DOI: 10.3390/ijerph6092332 PMID: 19826546

Kiecolt-Glaser, J. K., McGuire, L., Robles, T. F., & Glaser, R. (2002). Psychoneuroimmunology and psychosomatic medicine: Back to the future. *Psychosomatic Medicine*, *64*(1), 15–28. DOI: 10.1097/00006842-200201000-00004 PMID: 11818582

Kutner, J. S., Smith, M. C., Corbin, L., Hemphill, L., Benton, K., Mellis, B. K., Beaty, B., Felton, S., Yamashita, T. E., Bryant, L. L., & Fairclough, D. L. (2008). Massage therapy versus simple touch to improve pain and mood in patients with advanced cancer: A randomized trial. *Annals of Internal Medicine*, *149*(6), 369–379. DOI: 10.7326/0003-4819-149-6-200809160-00003 PMID: 18794556

Lane, B., Cannella, K., Bowen, C., Copelan, D., Nteff, G., Barnes, K., Poudevigne, M., & Lawson, J. (2012). Examination of the effectiveness of peppermint aromatherapy on nausea in women post C-section.[57]. *Journal of Holistic Nursing*, *30*(2), 90–104. DOI: 10.1177/0898010111423419 PMID: 22034523

National Academies of Sciences, Engineering, and Medicine. (2016). *Families caring for an aging America*. The National Academies Press. https://doi.org/DOI: 10.17226/23606

National Center for Complementary and Integrative Health (NCCIH). (2018). *Complementary, alternative, or integrative health: What's in a name?* Retrieved from https://www.nccih.nih.gov/health/complementary-alternative-or-integrative-health-whats-in-a-name

Oken, B. S., Fonareva, I., Haas, M., Wahbeh, H., Lane, J. B., Zajdel, D., & Amen, A. (2010). Pilot controlled trial of mindfulness meditation and education for dementia caregivers. *Journal of Alternative and Complementary Medicine (New York, N.Y.)*, *16*(10), 1031–1038. DOI: 10.1089/acm.2009.0733 PMID: 20929380

Ricker, M. A., & Haas, W. C. (2017). Anti-inflammatory diet in clinical practice: A review. *Nutrition in Clinical Practice*, *32*(3), 318–325. DOI: 10.1177/0884533617700353 PMID: 28350517

Schulz, R., & Sherwood, P. R. (2008). Physical and mental health effects of family caregiving.[58]. *The American Journal of Nursing, 108*(9, Suppl), 23–27. DOI: 10.1097/01.NAJ.0000336406.45248.4c PMID: 18797217

Ulrich, R. S. (1984). View through a window may influence recovery from surgery.[59]. *Science, 224*(4647), 420–421. DOI: 10.1126/science.6143402 PMID: 6143402

Woods, B., O'Philbin, L., Farrell, E. M., Spector, A. E., & Orrell, M. (2018). Reminiscence therapy for dementia. *Cochrane Database of Systematic Reviews, 3*(3), CD001120. Advance online publication. DOI: 10.1002/14651858.CD001120.pub3 PMID: 29493789

Chapter 3
Comparison for Institutional and Non-Institutional Caregiving for the Older Adults

S. Srinivasan
https://orcid.org/0009-0002-0179-9849
Department of Humanities and Social Sciences, Graphic Era University, Dehradun, India

Jipson Joseph
https://orcid.org/0009-0005-1795-5051
School of Law, CHRIST University, Bangalore, India

ABSTRACT

This comparative study explores institutional and non-institutional caregiving models for older adults, with a focus on quality of care, emotional well-being, and support systems. Institutional care offers structured, 24/7 medical and social support in settings like old age homes and nursing facilities, suitable for those with chronic conditions or family neglect. Non-institutional care is community- or home-based, emphasizing personalized attention and emotional bonds provided by family members and caregivers. The research, conducted in Trichy District, a mixed-method approach to assess caregiving outcomes among 243 participants aged 60 and above. The study highlights the strengths and limitations of both models, emphasizing the need for strategic interventions, caregiver training, and policy reforms. It proposes an integrated, person-centered approach to enhance eldercare

DOI: 10.4018/979-8-3373-4094-4.ch003

effectiveness, reduce caregiver burden, and promote sustainable support services. The findings aim to inform healthcare providers, policymakers, and stakeholders for improved eldercare delivery.

INTRODUCTION

The elderly population has increased over the past two decades and needs attention for the prevention of institutionalization. This might increase the importance of age-wise structure details, as it is based on the open-ended age groups involving more than 80 years older adults (Mishra & Sondhi, 2019). The elderly adults are unable to get institutional care and support to address their needs and services. There are a number of factors involved that put pressure to increase institutionalization care and support in residential care and services (Anttonen & Karsio, 2016). Non-institutional care is involved on a family basis, while at the same time institutional care services are commercial-based or paid-basis services for elderly care support and care. There are some non-psychiatric clinics provided for the reduction of the length of progressive support to stay for the older adults (Hilton, 2017). There are a greater number of orthopaedics-affected older adults who face many consequences and health-related complications in the non-institutional care services. The medical aspects that contribute to the geriatric service units affect the healthcare of the elderly adults (Sebastian, 2020).

As per the standard model, it explains clearly the care and protection of older adults in Andersen's healthcare system. The healthcare service explains three dimensions: predisposing factors like age and education for the older adults, and provides the attitudes and willingness to offer care and support for the older adults (Travers et al., 2020). There is family support to provide income support, and this can stimulate or hamper access to the healthcare services. There are various factors involved in poor physical health issues or mental healthcare services for the primary care-related services to enhance the physical and mental health and well-being of older adults (Lazar & Davenport, 2018; Zhao et al., 2025).

As per the UN report (2023) on the care crisis among older adults, the data indicate that 1 in 3 women aged 65 and over may need long-term care support, while 1 in 5 men require such care. There are an estimated 13.6 million people affected due to a deficit of long-term caretaker workers. The majority, around 80%, of long-term care in Europe is provided through informal caregiving support for older adults. The data show that 9 in 10 formal long-term care workers are women, especially in OECD countries. An average of 1.5% of GDP in OECD countries was spent on long-term care support in 2019. This is down from 1.7% in 2017, despite the growing demand. People worldwide are living longer, with babies born in 2022 expected to live an average of 71.7 years—25 years more than those born in 1950. Rapid population ageing has increased health and long-term care demands, but existing systems remain inadequate and need stronger policy focus. The Covid-19 pandemic further exposed weaknesses in long-term care, including poor-quality and underfunded facilities, limited home care, and low wages for care workers, worsening inequalities and risks for older persons (United Nations, 2020). These challenges highlight the urgent need for comprehensive reform to ensure sustainable and equitable care for current and future generations.

According to the OECD, older people are becoming more dependent and need assistance with day-to-day activities. Especially for their daily activities such as cooking, cleaning, dressing, and other self-care tasks. The long-term care support aims to provide care and assistance for older adults. The increasing growth of the ageing population calls for promoting healthy ageing to improve the quality of care services. The care of people at the end of life should balance older adults' social needs and the financial sustainability of the system.

The ageing population increases every day, and it is associated with older adults' care and their needs involved. The institutional and non-institutional care decline in providing care and services for the older adults (Yang et al., 2022). The institutional care explains the effect of time-effect, but it could not address the issues. The study aims at the unspecified time and effect of the initiatives. The various aspects of institutional and non-institutional factors are involved in the change of older adults' life (Elliott et al., 2011). The major factor involves long-term care for the older adults in the attractiveness of institutional care support on a paid basis and institutional care based on home care services. Institutional service provides professional support for the older adults in the residents, ensuring safety compared to the non-institutional care services (Doty, 2010; Alders et al., 2019).

Institutional care provides various professional services and support for the older adults. They can interact with other residents, and they have safety for care and take-care (Moilanen et al., 2021). They can have a quality life in the comfort zone in terms of competence, autonomy, and dignity. They have privacy and individuality in their activities, can maintain relationships with other people, and engage in entertainment for enjoyment, which enhances their spiritual health and well-being (Pinto et al., 2017). Many older adults are tied to social relationships. The older adults sometimes feel loneliness due to having fewer members in their social relationships. This can push individuals toward institutional care for their companionship, which can also pull them in (Neves et al., 2019). Loneliness increases their likelihood of going to a nursing-based institution. Institutional care provides proper care, but there is no motherly care support—not in all institutions, but some institutions provide care and services based on individual quality (Kroemeke & Gruszczynska, 2016). The older adults' caring centers nowadays have increased in number, as they admit disabled older adults as residents. The opportunity to increase dignity and enjoyment for older adults through meaningful relationships among the elderly people (Cho et al., 2017). There is a good practice pilot conducted in Denmark in the municipalities, which reduced nursing homes over some years. At the same time, home-based services increased, supporting older adults in independent living (Gorfinkiel et al., 2025).

The institutional care services, through relatives versus home care, help to explain the downward trend in society.

INSTITUTIONAL CARE SERVICES

The research study highly emphasizes institutional care, insisting on long-term services for older adults in old age homes, nursing homes, hospices, or geriatric care services in hospitals (Gupta, 2020). The institutional services provide medical care services and Activities of Daily Living (ADL) services, mixed with social engagement with elderly people (Turcotte et al., 2015). This is for those who are neglected in their family, destitute, or faced with chronic illness or disability-related issues. The institutional care is based on the structural organization and is regulated with trained staff and professionals (Grech, 2019).

Non-institutional care, on the other hand, is provided to offer care and services for older adults at the community level and in their own living places. It may include their family members, friends, community health workers, and caregivers to offer daily activities and fulfill their medical support and emotional well-being services (Gordon, 2018). Ageing people's living places in their surroundings show how to maintain and provide support services independently (Hillcoat-Nallétamby, 2014). The home care and day care centers are based on community services, providing their own meals in routine life and offering counseling services for physiotherapy (Hammar et al., 2008).

Institutional care services provide 24/7 support services, which can lead older adults to reduce social isolation and emotional distress due to family separation. In non-institutional care, emotional support services are based on cost-effectiveness to ensure caregiver availability within the resources. The integrated approach to providing essential services for both types of care is diverse to meet the needs of the ageing population (Donovan & Blazer, 2020; Gomes et al., 2013).

As per the WHO report, there is institutional and non-institutional care for older adults. The aged people may be different according to their age factor; they need care depending on their age, body, and physical conditions to provide the services (Tičinović & Tomasović Mrčela, 2023). Institutional care, like nursing homes, care take centers, and social interaction, is mentioned for specialized care services. Non-institutional care services are based on home care and offer personalized care and independence services, resulting in cost savings. Both care services have drawbacks when caring for older adults, as it depends on individual needs and preferences (Moro et al., 2017; Dunér et al., 2019).

Institutional Care Services

Definition: Institutional care refers to providing long-term or short-term care services, such as nursing homes, care take centers with 24/7 support, and social interaction for specialized care services (Harris-Kojetin et al., 2016).

It provides round-the-clock care in specialized services and can provide relief for family caregivers. This can lead to a loss of independence and may cause potential isolation and high costs (Chew et al., 2022).

Non-Institutional Care

Definition: Non-institutional care provides certain limited services delivered to individuals at home, including home health care and adult day care support services (Fields et al., 2011).

This can benefit personalized care and promote independence; it can reduce costs and bring peace of mind to their family. There is a burden on their family to provide caregiving due to the lack of 24/7 support. It affects individuals with significant functional impairments (Parker et al., 2022).

As per the WHO report, it is the type of care needed for older people, varying between institutional and non-institutional effective methods. This can strengthen policies and programs for both institutional and non-institutional care services for older adults, and it can increase the availability of care based on their needs (Farias et al., 2020). WHO recommends the importance of family caregivers and their role in improving non-institutional care services. There is a risk of abuse and neglect of older adults in both types of care; proper advocacy measures can help protect them. The approach aims to enhance care and support for older people by providing a holistic method to create individualized care and support based on their needs (Bhuvaneswari & Deb, 2016; Beech et al., 2017).

Table 1.

Sl. No	International Organization	Concept Note
1	WHO	The WHO views ageing as a multidimensional process involving physical, mental, and social well-being. The *World Report on Ageing and Health (2015)* and *Decade of Healthy Ageing (2021–2030)* call for integrated, person-centered care and recognize caregiver burden as a global public health issue.
2	UN	The UN (UNDESA) identifies ageing as a socio-economic transition requiring strong social protection. The *Madrid International Plan of Action on Ageing (2002)* highlights income security, enabling environments, and recognition of unpaid caregiving, mainly by women.
3	OECD	The OECD emphasizes that long-term care (LTC) accounts for 2–4% of GDP in many countries (*Help Wanted? 2020; Health at a Glance 2023*). It stresses sustainable financing, skilled workforce development, and integration of care systems to reduce caregiver strain.
4	WHO	The World Bank sees population ageing as both a challenge and opportunity for fiscal and health reform. Its reports (*Human Capital Project; Global Monitoring Report on Ageing, 2022*) advocate healthy ageing, preventive care, and social insurance to reduce caregiver and financial stress.

Conceptual Integration

- Caregiver burden is a public policy and welfare concern.
- Ageing transition impacts labour markets and health expenditure.
- Welfare economics supports equitable and sustainable eldercare systems.

CAREGIVER BURDEN, LONELINESS, AND COST-RELATED EXPENSES

Caregiver Burden

The physical, emotional, and psychological strain on those caring for older adults or chronically ill individuals, often causing stress, fatigue, anxiety, and reduced personal time, especially when support is lacking.

Loneliness

Social isolation and lack of meaningful connections, common among older adults living alone, which can increase risks of depression, cognitive decline, and poor health.

Cost

Financial burden of long-term care, including medical expenses, home adaptations, paid caregivers, and lost income for family caregivers, which can limit access and quality of care.

MENTAL HEALTH, ABUSE PREVENTION, AND CAREGIVER TRAINING

Mental Health

Mental health affects both older adults and caregivers. Older adults may face depression, anxiety, or cognitive decline, while caregivers risk stress and burnout. Including projections of mental health prevalence highlights the scale of these challenges.

Abuse Prevention

Elder abuse—physical, emotional, or financial—is a concern in institutional and home care. Legal protections, monitoring, and caregiver education are essential. Trend data on abuse risks can identify areas needing urgent attention.

Caregiver Training

Training equips caregivers to handle medical, mobility, and emotional needs, reducing errors and improving outcomes. Data on trained versus untrained caregivers and future workforce projections reveal capacity gaps.

Balanced Discussion

Incorporating demographic projections, mental health prevalence, caregiver statistics, and abuse trends provides a comprehensive, evidence-based view linking current challenges to future long-term care needs.

Policy Frameworks and Cross-Country Practices

Robust policies guide long-term care delivery, funding, and quality. Comparative models, like Nordic integrated care or Japan's community programs, help balance accessibility, affordability, and quality.

Role of Technology (AI, Telehealth, Robotics)

Technology bridges institutional and home care gaps. AI monitoring, telehealth, and robotics enhance safety, health outcomes, and daily care while reducing caregiver burden.

Economic Implications

Long-term care affects governments and families financially. Funding, subsidies, or insurance models are needed for sustainable, equitable, and affordable care.

Gender-Specific Caregiving Challenges

Women provide most informal care, impacting employment, income, and well-being. Policies should offer allowances, flexible work, training, and social support to reduce burden and ensure equity.

Demographic Projections

Include expected growth of the 65+ population over the next 10–30 years, highlighting regional differences to anticipate future long-term care demand.

Sustainability Challenges

Current care systems face limitations in resources, workforce, and funding, underscoring the need for scalable, sustainable solutions.

Policy Reforms Across Regions

Provide examples of policy changes and innovations in different countries to identify best practices and guide preparation for future care needs.

Future Demand for Services

Consider increased life expectancy, chronic disease prevalence, and higher dependency ratios to project demand for home care, institutional care, and caregiver support.

Including demographic projections, sustainability challenges, and policy reforms will offer a comprehensive view of current issues and future trends in long-term care, enhancing the chapter's relevance and impact.

SCOPE OF THE STUDY

The comparative analysis emphasizes institutional and non-institutional caregiving for older adults. This can provide the advantages of dual care for the delivery of support services; it can significantly enhance emotional well-being, reduce costs, and offer caregiving support. The various types of institutional care include nursing homes, old age care centers, and geriatric care centers (Tariq et al., 2023). The non-institutional care supports home-based care services and community care services; this can be referred to as informal caregiving for older adults with the help of family members and community health care workers (Liu et al., 2016). The scope includes the quality of caregiving for older adults, enhances their life, and improves various strategic improvements. The various training programs aim to enhance caregiving for older adults to improve the health and well-being of older adults (LaManna et al., 2020). This is not only meant to cover specialized medical care for the ageing people. The aim is to improve better policy implications, healthcare providers' support, and increase caregiving in the institutional way to enhance effective, sustainable eldercare support (Hung, 2022).

Research Gap, Research Questions and Objectives

The need to provide attention to caregiving for older adults. They face significant challenges; the study identified research gaps to understand the effectiveness and challenges of integrating institutional and non-institutional care models. Institutional care includes nursing homes and geriatric care; it provides structured support for both medical and social needs. This can provide long-term support for older adults in terms of emotional health and well-being, promoting independence to improve their quality of life (Srinivasan & Rajavel, 2025). Non-institutional care is delivered through family member support, community health workers, and home-based services to reduce caregiver burden. Quality assurance aims to provide accessibility for the elderly population. The study identifies gaps to support the development of better policy improvements that ensure a holistic approach and provide sustainable person-centered care for older adults.

Research Questions

1. What are the merits and demerits of Institutional Care and Non-Institutional Care?
2. How is better caregiving provided in Institutional and Non-Institutional Care?
3. What are the strategic plans to improve Institutional Care and Non-Institutional Caregiving for older adults?

4. How to enhance effective institutional caregiving for older adults?
5. How to improve care and services for non-institutional caregivers of older adults?
6. What are the training approaches to provide better services for older adults?

Research Objectives

To examine the merits and demerits of Institutional and Non-Institutional Care for older adults, and assess the quality of caregiving provided in both settings.
To identify strategic plans and effective approaches for enhancing Institutional and Non-Institutional caregiving services for older adults.
To explore the training approaches and support mechanisms required to improve caregiving services for both institutional and non-institutional caregivers.

Background & Theory

The older adult population has increased rapidly and significantly worldwide. The concern for older adults' health and well-being aims to enhance their quality of life. Life expectancy is measured based on health conditions and quality of life (Srinivasan et al., 2025). Many older adults face various chronic illnesses, especially affecting their physical and emotional well-being, which necessitates formal and informal caregiving support for them (Bandila, 2022). Caregiving is provided in two ways for older adults, and this can be categorized as institutional care and non-institutional care. Institutional care includes nursing homes, old age homes, and caretakers in living facilities, based on assistive services (Sangeeth & Solomon, 2015). Non-institutional care is provided based on family and community support, and this includes home-based care services. Institutional care is based on services like medical support, psychological support, and social services provided by trained professional workers (Srinviasan & Rajavel, 2025).

This can ensure timely provision of services and support, which can enhance older adults' emotional well-being and reduce social isolation caused by loss of autonomy. On the other hand, non-institutional care services emphasize family member support and community network services to enhance older adults' care and provide support from known persons. This can provide stronger emotional support and strengthen bonds and cultural continuity. However, it can also lead to caregiver burden and inconsistent quality of care and services. To emphasize providing better health services and professional support for older adults. There are two models used to compare and understand older adults' living conditions. The effectiveness of the services lies in their comprehensive sustainability to address older adults' physical and emotional needs. This can provide older adults with their needs, services, support, and care to ensure quality of life both mentally and physically. This can ensure the promotion of services to guide policymakers and health professionals (Wirtz, & Stock-Homburg, 2025). To enhance family support and provide better care services, ensuring the dignity, independence, and well-being of older adults.

Historical Context and Demographic Profile of Ageing in India

The study provides a historical perspective on the increase in the number of older adults due to declining fertility and rising life expectancy. The study globally provides that there were 900 million people aged 60 and above in 2015. This indicates that the projected population in 2050 will reach 2 billion, with nearly 80% from low- and middle-income countries, including India (He & Kinsella, 2020). The increasing population and changes in family structure have contributed to urbanization and migration, affecting the traditional care system. The results show that elderly individuals are living in formal care instead of within the family system, such as non-institutional care (Das, 2024). The age group above 60 years in India constitutes 8.6% of the population, as per the 2011 Census. This is projected to increase by 2036 to nearly 13.2%. Especially, older adults living in rural areas constitute about 70%, while the number of older adults in urban areas (Murthy et al., 2001). The majority of female older adults prefer institutionalized care services, accounting for nearly 60.7%.is increasing. This indicates a lifestyle and health transition (Bhattacharyya, 2021).

Married, literate, and financially dependent elderly had a better quality of life.

Institutional elderly had better physical health, while community-dwelling elderly had better social relationships

India's ageing population is rising faster than its health and welfare systems can adapt. Traditional family-based care is declining, creating the need for community-based and institutional eldercare models. Quality of life depends on health, emotional well-being, social support, and financial security.

Comparative Statistics: Aging in Rural vs. Urban India

Successful Aging: 32% of rural older adults vs. 24% in urban areas.

Health Status: Poor self-rated health: 25.1% rural vs. 21.5% urban.

Living Alone: 5.75% rural vs. 5.31% urban .

These differences highlight the need for tailored elder care strategies for rural and urban settings.

Evolution of Elder Care Models in India

Traditional Care: Family-centered, with children responsible for elders.

Institutional Care: Formal care homes emerged due to nuclear families and urban migration, though limited and under-resourced.

Community-Based Care: Focus on aging in place via home healthcare, telemedicine, and local support networks.

This shift reflects changing societal structures and diverse care needs.

THEMATIC LITERATURE OVERVIEW

Institutionalization

Institutionalization of older adults is showing an increasing trend in India, even though it is still in the initial implementation stage. In the West, many places have seen an increase in institutional homes after retirement, which can lead retired individuals or their families to shift to institutional care centers (Oswald & Rowles, 2017). Older adults can enjoy their life at home while receiving care for household services, medical needs, and emergencies. Due to increasing age, older adults face various health issues, such as physical disabilities, and other functional limitations increase (Beswick et al., 2008). Older adults living in a comfort zone have the chance to attain a better quality of life in an institutional center. Institutional care provides a highly good environment, maintained on a daily basis and well-furnished, which elderly people tend to like. In the institution, there is timely food, proper regular medical check-ups, body care, and scheduled sleep (Gao et al., 2024; Wang et al., 2016).

Many older adults can relax as they have no household responsibilities, get proper rest, and share their opinions with co-elders and like-minded people in the same age group. Institutional care provides long-term support services, which can help older adults live independently (Same et al., 2020). They have proper facilities to perform all activities, including regular exercise, yoga, and meditation, which can increase life expectancy, reduce stress levels, and enhance daily activity performance (Deshmukh et al., 2024). In India, many facilities have been established to improve the quality-based implementation of care and services. This is very satisfying for older adults; after retirement, they can relax and enjoy their remaining life. However, the majority of older adults are from middle-class and upper-middle-class families, while poor people face many problems (Chaisomboon et al., 2020; Zhang & Cheng, 2024).

Non-Institutional

The health and well-being of older adults play a major role for informal caregivers within the family. It is increasing the concern for older adults' care in the family roles and responsibilities (Otis-Green & Juzrez, 2012). There are various factors involved in non-institutional care for older adults in the family and in their work-life perspectives. In India, the number of older adults is increasing, and the roles and responsibilities of family caregivers are increasing to provide care and services (Vuksan et al., 2012). In non-institutional care, caregivers face stress in maintaining multiple roles like family, caregiving, and job, and they are unable to provide proper care for older adults. The responsibility for caring for one's parents must be maintained (Ene et al., 2022). They manage coping with their work and caregiving for the family, as well as family caregiving support and care services. Sometimes caregivers are unable to cope with extra work and face challenges in such situations (Bialon & Coke, 2012). This might help in understanding the situations in providing institutional and non-institutional care, both paid and unpaid, and differentiating these family care situations. The study emphasizes promoting improvements in policies and using training and support for older adults and caregivers (Schulz & Eden, 2016).

Figure 1. Elder care models in India

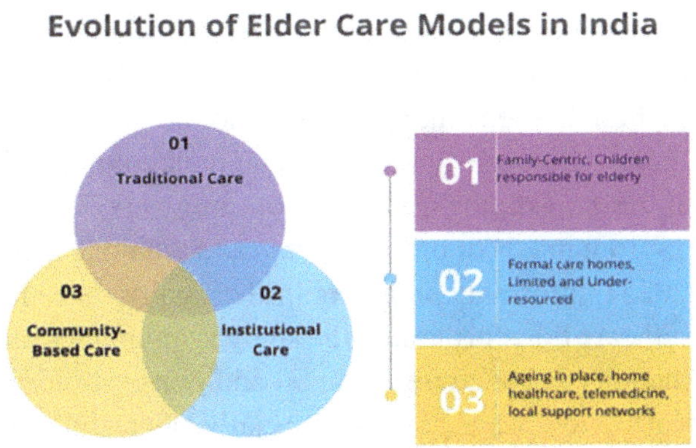

In India, **traditional care** is family-based, providing emotional, daily, and financial support, but is declining due to urbanization and nuclear families. **Institutional care** in old-age homes or nursing centers offers professional healthcare and structured support, though it is costly, limited, and socially stigmatized. **Community-based care** through NGOs or government programs includes daycare, home visits, and social activities, keeping elders engaged, cost-effective, and in familiar environments.

Emotional Wellbeing

High prevalence of depression, anxiety, and loneliness in older adults, especially in institutions.

Family and community support enhances emotional wellbeing.

Infrastructure and Accessibility

Gaps in rural healthcare infrastructure affect elder care quality .

Digital health and improved infrastructure are key to effective care .

Caregiver Roles

Caregivers face physical, emotional, and financial stress.

Support programs and policies are essential for both caregiver and elder wellbeing.

This thematic summary emphasizes the interplay of wellbeing, infrastructure, and caregiver support, crucial for sustainable elder care models in India.

Definition: An elderly individual is one who is aged 60 or older, based on the recognition of older adults. This definition is as per the World Assembly on Ageing, 1982, in Vienna (Gorman, 2017). Previous research studies found that in providing social support, there are 70 caregivers of patients with dementia who may feel burdened in caring for elderly people (Srinivasan et al., 2025). The review provides a comprehensive understanding of the Zarit Burden Interview, presenting the older adults' caregivers and their demographic details. The study results show that caregivers experience a high burden among Malays and Indians (Ahmad Zubaidi et al., 2020). This highlights the significant influence of their culture and ethnicity. In the family, female children constitute the majority of caregivers. This shows that 36% of them received help from maids or private nurses and did not experience the burden (Shrestha et al., 2025). Informal caregivers in the family share responsibilities in caregiving. In healthcare transformation, the study is incomplete and highlights the gaps that create inequity between institutional and non-institutional care (Akther, 2025). This might affect low-wage groups, especially older adults. The study emphasizes how informal family members, including children and adults, are influenced to provide formal care for older adults (Gonzales et al., 2020).

Existing study results show that there are nearly 1,450 older adults aged >65 in the longitudinal study. Based on the older adults' marital status and their children, they often have the opportunity to be substituted for formal care (Syse et al., 2022). The findings of the study provide a comprehensive understanding of formal care for elderly health, including family situation and availability. This highlights the importance of advance directives for the elderly community to be recognized in society. The education support program initiative has a significant association with their positive attitudes towards care and planning (Syse et al., 2022; Gao et al., 2024).

Older adults make their health treatment decisions based on their health conditions. This is purely based on the older adults' options for making treatment decisions; the intervention is based on their personal choice in end-of-life care (Kurasz et al., 2022). If older adults have multiple illnesses, it can create various stresses in providing institutional and non-institutional care services. Suppose they have dementia; they can prefer a psychiatric specialist to facilitate the specific care and services required (Robison et al., 2012).

Provide care for elderly people, including nursing support, health services such as transport facilities, leisure support services, and social support services, to assist with daily living at their home level (Abdi et al., 2019). The care services are provided by skilled caretakers in institutional settings, which strengthens community-based services. Home-based assistance is rising to meet the calls for advanced care solution services in institutional care (Denham & Kistler, 2023). Technological support is being involved to provide cost-effective services and enhance community-based care through robotic service support (Wirtz et al., 2025).

Non-institutional care faces challenges in sustaining home-based care and support services for the elderly. Developed countries have their own alternative support for home-based formal care services (Spasova et al., 2018). The existing study results include two groups, each with six physicians and six older adults requiring care. They use robot services for daily activity tasks, home-based activities, health monitoring, and assistance during emergencies. It increases mental and emotional support for caregiving services (Zimbroff et al., 2021).

Existing reviews emphasize informal caregivers, and in the past three years, the focus has been on older disabled people. The study mainly focused on the informal care ties between high-risk older adults and outcomes such as mortality and hospitalization. It highlights the need to enhance institutional care services and addresses the discontinuation of living conditions at home, which can assess the informal caregiving support services (Allen et al., 2023; Kraun et al., 2022).

Physical Health Management and Policy-level Interventions

Physical Health Management: Focuses on preventive care, treatment of chronic illnesses, regular health check-ups, nutrition, exercise, and access to healthcare services to maintain elders' physical well-being.

Policy-Level Interventions: Government initiatives, schemes, and regulations aimed at supporting the elderly, such as National Programme for Health Care of the Elderly (NPHCE), social security, pension schemes, and community health programs.

Chronic Illness Management and Geriatric Health Services

Chronic Illness Management: Involves regular monitoring, medication adherence, lifestyle modifications, and coordinated care to manage long-term conditions like diabetes, hypertension, and arthritis in older adults.

Geriatric Health Services: Specialized healthcare services for the elderly, including geriatric clinics, physiotherapy, mental health support, and preventive care to address age-related health issues comprehensively.

National Elder Care Policies and Schemes

Elder care in India includes physical health management, focusing on preventive care, chronic disease monitoring, nutrition, exercise, and access to healthcare services. Chronic illness management ensures regular check-ups, medication adherence, and lifestyle adjustments for conditions like diabetes, hypertension, and arthritis. Geriatric health services provide specialized support through clinics, physiotherapy, and mental health care. At the policy level, programs such as the National Programme for Health Care of the Elderly (NPHCE), social security schemes, pensions, and community-based initiatives aim to support the well-being of older adults, improve access to healthcare, and promote healthy aging across the country.

Table 2. Comparison of institutional and non-institutional care

Aspect	Institutional Care	Non-Institutional Care
Definition	Care provided in formal settings such as nursing homes, old-age homes, or hospitals.	Care provided at home or in community-based settings by family members, friends, or community health workers (Nwameme et al., 2018).
Environment	Structured, professional, and regulated environment.	Familiar, flexible, and home-like environment.
Care Providers	Trained medical staff, caregivers, and professionals.	Family members, relatives, or community-based caregivers (sometimes with limited training) (Waymouth et al., 2023).
Cost	Generally high due to institutional facilities, professional services, and infrastructure (Jafari et al., 2024).	Relatively low, but can be financially and emotionally burdensome for families.
Social Interaction	Opportunities for peer interaction with other residents but may lack family closeness.	Strong family bonding and community connection but may lead to social isolation if family is small or busy.
Quality of Care	Standardized, professional, and medicalized approach.	Varies depending on caregiver skills, resources, and family support (Swartz & Collins, 2019).

continued on following page

Table 2. Continued

Aspect	Institutional Care	Non-Institutional Care
Accessibility	May not be available in rural/remote areas; long waiting lists common.	Widely available in households but dependent on family willingness and capacity.
Independence of Elderly	Limited; routines are structured according to institutional rules.	Higher independence and autonomy within familiar surroundings.
Emotional Support	Professional but less personalized emotional care.	Stronger emotional and cultural support from family.
Sustainability	Requires significant resources and government/NGO support.	Sustainable if families are willing and financially stable.

Infrastructure and Staffing Challenges in Institutional Settings:

Institutional elder care in India faces inadequate infrastructure, limited medical facilities, overcrowded homes, and lack of accessibility features. Many institutions also suffer from staff shortages, insufficiently trained caregivers, low wages, and high turnover rates, which affect the quality of care and personalized attention provided to the elderly.

Emotional Well-being and Integrated Care Strategies:

Emotional well-being is vital for healthy ageing and should be integrated into all elder care models. Supportive family relationships, community engagement, counseling, and recreational activities help reduce loneliness and depression. Combining emotional care with physical health management, chronic illness control, and social participation ensures a holistic approach that enhances elders' overall quality of life.

INFRASTRUCTURE AND TECH-ENABLED CARE

Infrastructure in Elder Care

Quality elder care requires age-friendly infrastructure with proper medical facilities, accessible spaces, and safety features. Improved housing and healthcare setups enhance comfort and independence for older adults.

Tech-Enabled Care

Technology supports elder care through telemedicine, health monitors, and emergency alert systems, enabling remote monitoring, timely care, and better connectivity with healthcare providers and families.

Legal and Ethical Frameworks in Elder Care

Elder care in India is guided by laws and policies that protect older adults' rights, ensure access to healthcare, and prevent abuse and neglect. Ethical principles focus on dignity, autonomy, informed consent, and equitable treatment. Together, these frameworks provide a foundation for safe, respectful, and accountable elder care (Dev et al., 2025).

Gendered Dimensions of Caregiving

Caregiving is predominantly undertaken by women, who often balance household responsibilities with elder care. This role exposes them to emotional, physical, and financial stress, highlighting gender inequalities and the need for supportive policies and resources to reduce the caregiving burden (Koshmaganbetova et al., 2024).

Economic Implications for Families and Institutions

Elder care imposes significant financial costs on families and institutions, including healthcare expenses, caregiving resources, and infrastructure. These economic pressures can affect household income, workforce participation, and the sustainability of care services, underscoring the need for supportive policies and funding mechanisms (Mosca et al., 2016).

Role of Community-Based Interventions and NGOs

Community programs and NGOs play a vital role in elder care by providing social support, health services, awareness campaigns, and respite for caregivers. They help bridge gaps in formal care systems, promote active ageing, and enhance the overall wellbeing of older adults (Hu et al., 2025).

Elder Rights and Legal Protections

Elder rights and legal protections safeguard older adults from abuse, neglect, and exploitation. Laws ensure access to healthcare, social security, and property rights, while promoting dignity, autonomy, and equal treatment in family and institutional settings (Lewis et al., 2020).

Gender Analysis of Caregiving Burdens

Caregiving responsibilities disproportionately fall on women, who often manage household duties alongside elder care. This unequal distribution leads to higher emotional, physical, and financial stress for women, highlighting gender disparities and the need for policies that support equitable caregiving roles (Lalani et al., 2025).

Financial Models and Sustainability of Care Systems

Sustainable elder care requires effective financial models that balance public funding, private services, and out-of-pocket expenses. Robust funding mechanisms ensure consistent quality of care, support caregivers, and maintain the long-term viability of both institutional and community-based care systems (Elliott et al., 2015).

Successful Community-Led Initiatives

Community-led initiatives in elder care focus on local engagement, social support, and accessible services. Programs such as volunteer networks, day-care centers, and health outreach campaigns have improved wellbeing, reduced isolation, and strengthened caregiving capacity at the grassroots level (Chen et al., 2024).

Transitions Between Institutional and Non-Institutional Care

Transitions between institutional and non-institutional care are often abrupt due to the lack of coordinated care systems, poor discharge planning, and limited community support. This sudden shift can cause confusion, emotional distress, and discontinuity in medical and social support for the elderly. Strengthening referral systems, follow-up services, and community-based rehabilitation can ensure smoother and more effective transitions.

METHODOLOGY

The comparative study analyzes institutional and non-institutional caregiving for older adults. The study used mixed-methods for caregiving for older adults. The mixed-method approach is used to analyze both qualitative and quantitative data. The research study adopted a comparative cross-sectional research design to identify the caregiving experiences, quality of life, and support systems available for older adults. Institutional care centers include old age homes and caretaker centers for older adults. Non-institutional care focuses on those living with family and receiving home-based care. This can involve various aspects such as physical, emotional, and social well-being in both care system services.

The research study will be conducted in the following areas of Trichy District for non-institutionalized care:

1) Srirangam,
2) Thiruvarambur,
3) Ponmalai,
4) Ariyamangalam,
5) Andanallur,
6) Thiruvarambur.

The institutional care covers the following old age homes and care centers:

i) St. Antony's Home for Aged
ii) Sri Kamatchi Amman Old Age Home Charitable Trust
iii) Kirush Kakkum Karangal
iv) Annai Muthiyoor Illam
v) Aram Magil Trust
vi) Aruvi Old Age Home
vii) Kangaroo Karunai Illam
viii) Manitham Trust - Old Age Home
ix) Sai Nandhanam Old Age Home

These are residential-based and also provide community-based family care services for older adults.

Sampling Method

The sampling method selected is purposive sampling. The study plans to take a sample of **243** participants aged ≥ 60 years from both institutional and non-institutional care. An equal number of participants were selected based on their availability, with consent obtained from the respondents. Data were collected equally from respondents in institutional care and non-institutional care. For data collection, a self-structured questionnaire was prepared to gather information such as demographic details, physical health status, mental health using the Geriatric Depression Scale, social support, and satisfaction with care. In future studies, the research plans to conduct group discussions and in-depth interviews with older adults living in both institutional and non-institutional settings. This will help understand their practical emotional experiences, perceptions of care and support, and coping mechanisms. To increase the positive attitude towards institutionalization versus home care services.

Data Analysis

The findings were analyzed using SPSS software. Descriptive statistics such as frequencies, and percentages were used, along with inferential statistics like ANOVA to compare both caregiving models. The qualitative approach will use their experiences and contrasts to analyze caregiving narratives.

Ethical Considerations

Ethical approval was received from the concerned authorities, including the founder or director of the institutional care old age home, and consent was obtained from individuals and older adults in non-institutional settings. Interviews were not conducted without informed consent. All the data were kept confidential, and anonymity was maintained throughout the study.

LIMITATION

There are several limitations faced by institutional and non-institutional caregiving for older adults. These limitations should be considered when interpreting the findings. Limitations of institutional caregiving include restricted access to facilities and limited interaction with residents in old age homes. Providing institutional care is challenging due to limited diversity in care and services. The study is influenced by caregivers, such as staff, and their potential responses related to fear and repercussions. Institutional care services not only represent different diverse groups of people in institutional care. It can involve various regions and the quality of funding sources, such as government versus private.

Non-institutional caregiving includes family income and caregiving related to their cultural practices. Informal caregiving is influenced by response bias and is provided by family members, which can lead to downplaying the challenges of caregiving. There are limited institutional settings for direct observation of care for older adults, and best practices are provided mainly in private homes, with limitations due to privacy concerns. The limitation of the study is that it includes only adults aged $\geq$ 60 years in institutional and non-institutional care services. The sample size of the study is based on the selected geographical area, which may limit the generalization to the broader population in the national context. The research study mainly analyzes the comparative effectiveness of ways to improve caregiving environments for older adults. This can highlight areas for better policy and practice improvement.

FINDINGS

Table 3. Socio-demographic profile of older adults in the study

Descriptions	Options	Frequency	%
Age	60 - 65	74	30.5
	66 - 70	60	24.7
	71-75	53	21.8
	76-80	42	17.3
	>80	14	5.8
	Total	**243**	**100**
Gender	Male	168	69.1
	Female	75	30.9
	Total	**243**	**100**
Marital status	Single	15	6.2
	Married	165	67.9
	Widowed/Widower	38	15.6
	Divorced	25	10.3
	Total	**243**	**100**
Education	No formal	38	15.6
	Primary	58	23.9
	Secondary	80	32.9
	Higher	67	27.6
	Total	**243**	**100**
Living arrangement	Institutional care	120	49.4
	Non-institutional care	123	50.6
	Total	**243**	**100**
Duration of stay in current setting	1-2 years	63	25.9
	3-4 years	48	19.8
	>5 years	9	3.7
	Permantly	123	50.6
	Permantly	123	50.6

The majority of respondents were between 60 and 65 years of age (30.5%), followed by those aged 66–70 years (24.7%) and 71–75 years (21.8%), while only 5.8% were above 80 years. Most were male (69.1%), and nearly two-thirds were married (67.9%). A considerable proportion were widowed or widowers (15.6%) and divorced (10.3%), reflecting varied marital circumstances in later life. Educational attainment showed diversity, with secondary-level education being most common (32.9%), followed by higher education (27.6%) and primary education (23.9%), while 15.6% of respondents had no formal schooling. Living arrangements were almost evenly divided between institutional care (49.4%) and non-institutional care (50.6%). In terms of duration of stay, half of the respondents (50.6%) reported living permanently in their current setting, 25.9% had stayed for 1–2 years, 19.8% for 3–4 years, and only 3.7% for more than 5 years.

Table 4. Satisfaction with caregiving and distribution of institutional and non-institutional respondents

Descriptions	Options	Frequency	%
Are you satisfied for the Current Caregiving	Very satisfied	57	23.5
	Satisfied	48	19.8
	Neutral	63	25.9
	Dissatisfied	45	18.5
	Very dissatisfied	30	12.3
	Total	243	100
Institutionalization	St. Antony's Home for Aged	16	13.3
	Sri Kamatchi Amman Old Age Home Charitable Trust	12	10
	Kirush Kakkum Karangal	14	11.7
	Annai Muthiyoor Illam	13	10.8
	Aram Magil Trust	13	10.8
	Aruvi Old Age Home	8	6.7
	Kangaroo Karunai Illam	15	12.5
	Manitham Trust - Old Age Home	11	9.2
	Sai Nandhanam Old Age Home	18	15
	Total	120	100

continued on following page

Table 4. Continued

Descriptions	Options	Frequency	%
Non-Institutional Blocks	Srirangam	18	14.6
	Thiruvarambur	20	16.3
	Ponmalai	23	18.7
	Ariyamangalam	21	17.1
	Andanallur	19	15.4
	Thiruvarambur	22	17.9
	Total	123	100

Regarding satisfaction with current caregiving, 23.5% of respondents reported being very satisfied and 19.8% were satisfied, while 25.9% expressed neutrality. On the other hand, 18.5% were dissatisfied and 12.3% were very dissatisfied, indicating that although a fair proportion were content with their care, a sizable share expressed mixed or negative views. Within institutional care, respondents were distributed across nine facilities. The highest proportion was from Sai Nandhanam Old Age Home (15%), followed by St. Antony's Home for Aged (13.3%), Kangaroo Karunai Illam (12.5%), and Kirush Kakkum Karangal (11.7%). Other institutions such as Annai Muthiyoor Illam and Aram Magil Trust each accounted for 10.8%, while smaller shares were observed in Manitham Trust (9.2%), Sri Kamatchi Amman Old Age Home Charitable Trust (10%), and Aruvi Old Age Home (6.7%). Among non-institutional respondents, representation was fairly balanced across blocks. Ponmalai accounted for the largest share (18.7%), followed by Thiruvarambur (16.3% and 17.9%—noting a possible duplication), Ariyamangalam (17.1%), Andanallur (15.4%), and Srirangam (14.6%).

Table 5. Challenges and experiences in non-institutional care

Descriptions	Yes	%	No	%	Total	%
Professional caregivers	100	81.3	23	18.7	123	100
Access to medical care	56	45.5	67	54.5	123	100
Social interaction	91	74	32	26	123	100
Safety/security	102	82.9	21	17.1	123	100
Limited autonomy	81	65.9	42	34.1	123	100
Emotional neglect	68	55.3	55	44.7	123	100
Lack of family bonding	80	65	43	35	123	100
High cost	100	81.3	23	18.7	123	100

Among non-institutional respondents, the presence of professional caregivers was reported by 81.3%, while 18.7% did not have access to such support. Access to medical care appeared limited, with less than half (45.5%) reporting adequate availability, whereas 54.5% lacked it. Social interaction was relatively strong, as 74% experienced regular engagement, though 26% did not. Safety and security were reported positively by 82.9%, leaving 17.1% who felt otherwise. However, challenges such as limited autonomy (65.9%), emotional neglect (55.3%), and lack of family bonding (65%) were common concerns, reflecting psychosocial vulnerabilities. Financial strain was also evident, as 81.3% reported high costs associated with caregiving, compared to 18.7% who did not perceive this as a burden.

Table 6. Perceptions of caregiving quality, support needs, and living conditions of older adults

Descriptions	Options	Frequency	%
Rate of overall quality of caregiving	Excellent	61	25.1
	Good	66	27.2
	Average	59	24.3
	Poor	42	17.3
	Very poor	15	6.2
	Total	243	100
Are you consider the main disadvantages of non-institutional care	Excellent	43	17.7
	Good	62	25.5
	Average	68	28
	Poor	46	18.9
	Very poor	24	9.9
	Total	243	100
changes are needed to improve the quality of caregiving services	More staff	37	30.1
	Better medical facilities	36	29.3
	Improved emotional/ psychological support	38	30.9
	Financial support/subsidies	12	9.8
	Total	123	100
current government or NGO programs in supporting older adults	Very effective	59	24.3
	Somewhat effective	75	30.9
	Not effective	61	25.1
	Not conducted	48	19.8
	Total	243	100

continued on following page

Table 6. Continued

Descriptions	Options	Frequency	%
Living arrangement	Alone	28	22.8
	With spouse	27	22
	With children	32	26
	Extended family	36	29.3
	Total	123	100
Monthly household income bracket	< 5- 10k	41	33.3
	11–25k	48	39
	26–50k	23	18.7
	51 <	11	8.9
	Total	123	100

The overall quality of caregiving was positively rated by just over half of respondents, with 25.1% considering it excellent and 27.2% good, while 24.3% rated it average and 23.5% viewed it as poor or very poor. When assessing disadvantages of non-institutional care, opinions were more critical: 28% rated it average, 18.9% poor, and 9.9% very poor, with fewer respondents expressing higher satisfaction. Regarding improvements, emotional and psychological support (30.9%), more staff (30.1%), and better medical facilities (29.3%) were nearly equally highlighted as top priorities, while financial subsidies (9.8%) were less emphasized. Government and NGO programs received mixed feedback—only 24.3% found them very effective and 30.9% somewhat effective, while 25.1% said they were not effective and 19.8% reported no programs were conducted. Living arrangements revealed that older adults were fairly evenly distributed: 29.3% lived in extended families, 26% with children, 22.8% alone, and 22% with spouses. In terms of income, the largest share fell in the 11,000–25,000 bracket (39%), followed by 5,000–10,000 (33.3%), 26,000–50,000 (18.7%), and only 8.9% above 50,000.

Figure 2. Health conditions

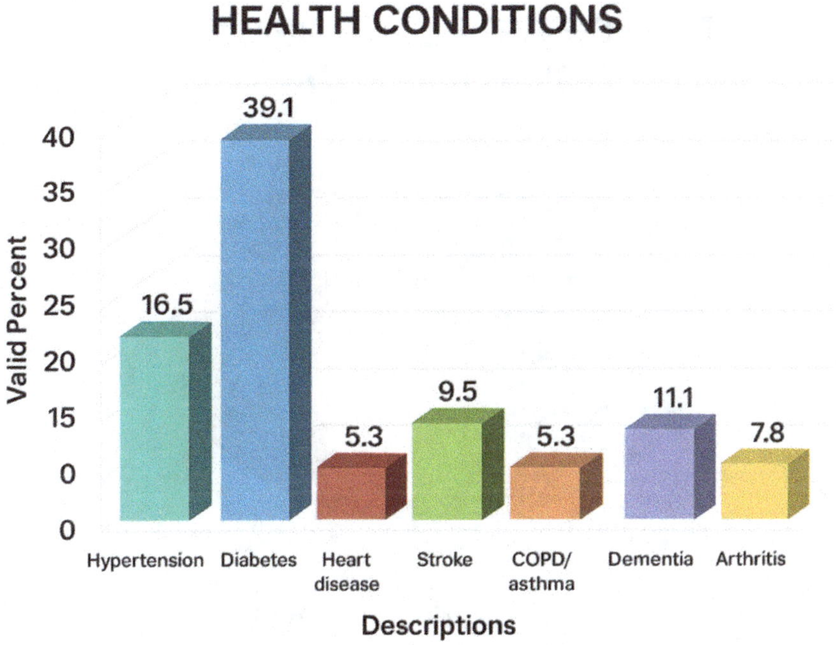

Among the respondents, diabetes emerged as the most common health condition (39.1%), followed by hypertension (16.5%). Mental health concerns such as depression or anxiety were reported by 11.1%, while stroke affected 9.5% of respondents. Arthritis accounted for 7.8%, and smaller but notable proportions reported heart disease, COPD/asthma, and dementia (5.3% each). This pattern highlights the dominance of non-communicable diseases, particularly diabetes and hypertension, alongside growing concerns about mental health and stroke among the elderly.

Figure 3. Preferred place of care for the future

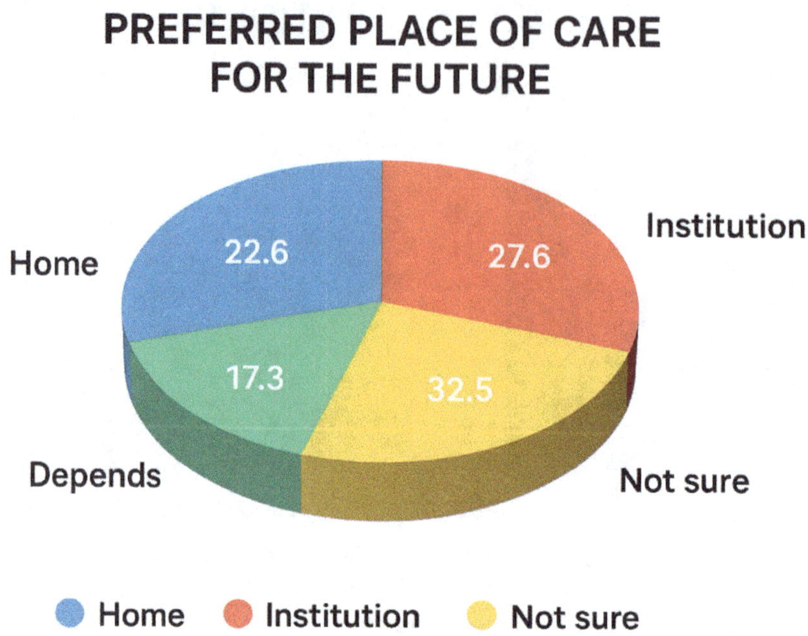

In terms of preferred place of care for the future, 22.6% of respondents expressed a preference for receiving care at home, while 27.6% favored institutional care. Around 17.3% reported that their choice would depend on circumstances, and the largest proportion, 32.5%, remained uncertain. This uncertainty highlights the need for greater awareness and guidance to help older adults make informed decisions about their future care options.

Figure 4. Preferred place for future care centre

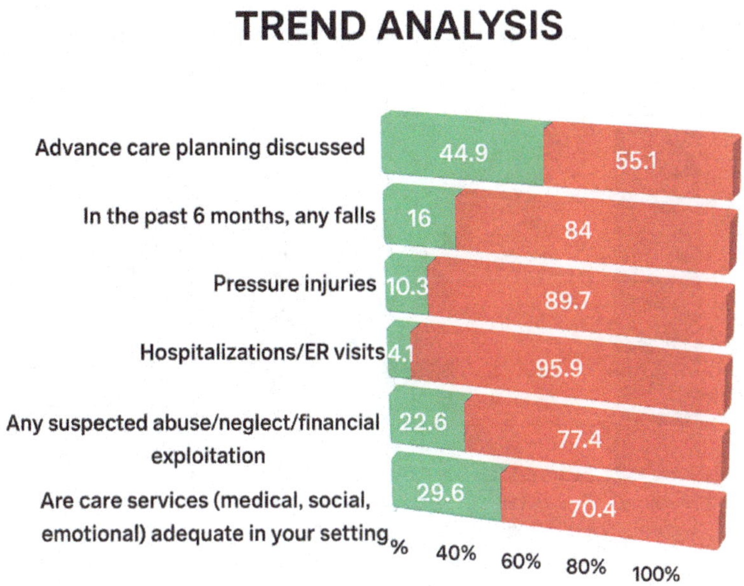

Advance care planning was discussed by 44.9% of respondents, while a slightly higher proportion (55.1%) had not engaged in such discussions. Falls in the past six months were reported by 16% of participants, with the majority (84%) not experiencing any. Pressure injuries were relatively uncommon, affecting 10.3% of respondents, whereas 89.7% remained unaffected. Hospitalizations or emergency visits were minimal, with only 4.1% reporting such events. However, suspected abuse, neglect, or financial exploitation was noted by 22.6% of participants, a concern that warrants attention, while 77.4% reported no such experiences. Regarding the adequacy of care services—medical, social, and emotional—only 29.6% felt they were sufficient, whereas a larger share of 70.4% expressed dissatisfaction. Overall, the findings suggest that while most older adults did not face frequent falls, injuries, or hospitalizations, a considerable proportion raised concerns about inadequate services and potential abuse, and advance care planning continues to be underutilized.

Figure 5. Area for improvement

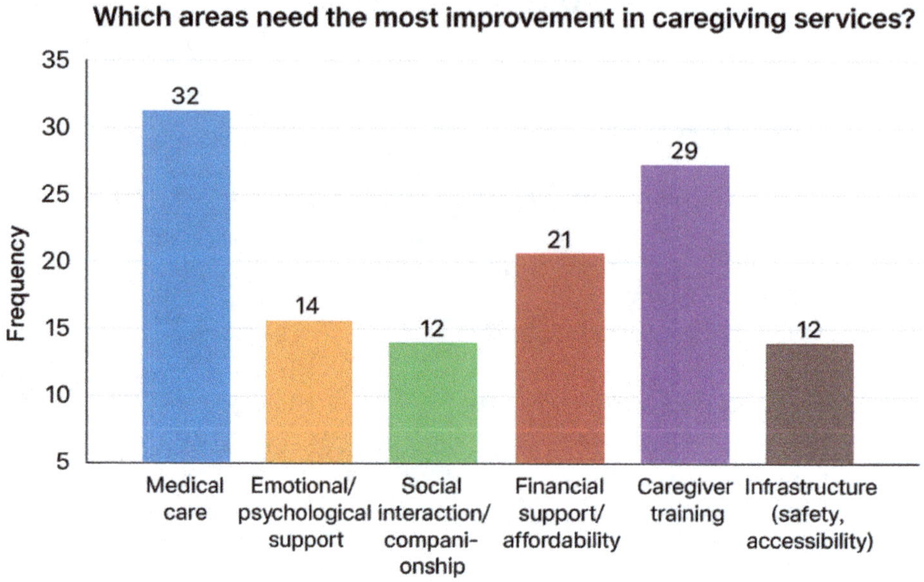

The findings indicate that the most pressing area for improvement in caregiving services is medical care (26.7%), followed closely by caregiver training (24.2%). Financial support and affordability were also significant concerns, highlighted by 17.5% of respondents. Emotional and psychological support was cited by 11.7%, while social interaction/companionship and infrastructure (safety and accessibility) were each noted by 10%. Overall, the results emphasize that strengthening healthcare access, enhancing caregiver skills, and ensuring financial sustainability are critical priorities, while emotional, social, and infrastructural aspects also require attention to provide more holistic caregiving.

Table 7. Importance of Support Mechanisms for Improving Elder Care

Descriptions	Not important at all	%	Slightly important	%	Moderately important	%	Important	%	Very important	%	Total	%
Rate the importance of the following for improving elder car	27	11.1	56	23	68	28	50	20.6	42	17.3	243	100
Government support and policy	5	2.1	13	5.3	72	29.6	101	41.6	52	21.4	243	100
Financial subsidies/ insurance	10	4.1	14	5.8	48	19.8	82	33.7	89	36.6	243	100
Skilled caregiver training	15	12.5	16	13.3	26	21.7	36	30	27	22.5	120	100
Community-based programs	11	8.9	13	10.6	31	25.2	45	36.6	23	18.7	123	100
Technology (Telehealth, Monitoring	34	14	54	22.2	59	24.3	56	23	40	16.5	243	100
Support mechanisms do you consider most important for improving caregiving	24	9.9	55	22.6	62	25.5	57	23.5	45	18.5	243	100
Peer-support networks	11	4.5	24	9.9	96	39.5	48	19.8	64	26.3	243	100
Regular counseling/ mental health support	16	6.6	35	14.4	84	34.6	49	20.2	59	24.3	243	100

The data highlights varying priorities among respondents regarding strategies to strengthen elder care. A large share rated caregiving improvements as moderately important (28%) or important (20.6%), with 17.3% considering them very important, though 34.1% expressed lower importance. Government support and policy emerged as highly valued, with 41.6% rating it important and 21.4% very important, while only 7.4% viewed it as having little or no importance. Financial subsidies or insurance stood out strongly, with 33.7% rating them important and 36.6% very important, together accounting for 70.3% and reflecting the financial vulnerability of older adults. Skilled caregiver training was also emphasized, as more than half (52.5%) rated it important or very important, though 25.8% felt it was of little importance. Community-based programs were valued by many, with 36.6% rating them important and 18.7% very important, showing preference for localized support systems. Technology, such as telehealth and monitoring, revealed mixed views, with 24.3% considering it moderately important and 23% important, while 36.2% rated it less important, suggesting a digital divide among older populations.

Support mechanisms overall were rated as moderately important (25.5%) or important (23.5%) by nearly half of respondents, but 32.5% showed lower interest. Peer-support networks were positively viewed, with 39.5% rating them moderately important and 26.3% very important, showing strong recognition of social connectedness. Regular counseling and mental health support received high value, as 34.6% rated it moderately important and 44.5% important or very important, pointing to the need for psychosocial well-being.

Table 8. ANOVA

		Sum of Squares	df	Mean Square	F	Sig.
Age	Between Groups	0.388	1	0.388	0.249	0.618
	Within Groups	375.242	241	1.557		
	Total	375.63	242			
Gender	Between Groups	1.323	1	1.323	6.308	0.013
	Within Groups	50.529	241	0.21		
	Total	51.852	242			
Education	Between Groups	145.738	1	145.738	311.406	0
	Within Groups	112.788	241	0.468		
	Total	258.527	242			
Marital status	Between Groups	1.974	1	1.974	3.686	0.056
	Within Groups	129.096	241	0.536		
	Total	131.07	242			

The ANOVA analysis shows that age did not have a significant effect on the outcome variable ($F = 0.249$, $p = 0.618$), indicating no meaningful differences between groups by age. Similarly, marital status approached significance ($F = 3.686$, $p = 0.056$) but did not meet the conventional 0.05 threshold, suggesting only a weak influence. In contrast, gender showed a statistically significant effect ($F = 6.308$, $p = 0.013$), implying that caregiving-related perceptions or outcomes differ between males and females. The most notable result was for education, which had a very strong and highly significant effect ($F = 311.406$, $p < 0.001$), indicating that educational level is a major factor influencing the studied variable.

Table 9. ANOVA

		Sum of Squares	df	Mean Square	F	Sig.
Institutional	Between Groups	144.744	2	72.372	11.393	0
	Within Groups	743.222	117	6.352		
	Total	887.967	119			
Living arrangement	Between Groups	60.741	3	20.247	.	.
	Within Groups	0	239	0		
	Total	60.741	242			
How satisfied are you with the current caregiving services you receive/provide	Between Groups	7.403	3	2.468	1.404	0.242
	Within Groups	420.226	239	1.758		
	Total	427.63	242			
Advance care planning discussed	Between Groups	24.154	3	8.051	53.523	0
	Within Groups	35.953	239	0.15		
	Total	60.107	242			
Hospitalizations/ER visits	Between Groups	0.045	3	0.015	0.374	0.772
	Within Groups	9.544	239	0.04		
	Total	9.588	242			
Pressure injuries	Between Groups	0.749	3	0.25	2.752	0.043
	Within Groups	21.679	239	0.091		
	Total	22.428	242			
Preferred place of care for the future	Between Groups	126.736	3	42.245	50.548	0
	Within Groups	199.741	239	0.836		
	Total	326.477	242			
In the past 6 months, any falls?	Between Groups	0.261	3	0.087	0.64	0.59
	Within Groups	32.48	239	0.136		
	Total	32.741	242			
Health conditions	Between Groups	626.861	3	208.954	74.342	0
	Within Groups	671.764	239	2.811		
	Total	1298.626	242			

Significant Results

Institutional care – Significant differences were found between groups ($F = 11.393$, $p < 0.001$). This indicates that institutional factors strongly influence the outcome variable. Advance care planning discussed – Highly significant ($F = 53.523$, $p < 0.001$), suggesting large differences between groups regarding discussions on advance care planning. Pressure injuries – Statistically significant ($F = 2.752$, $p =$

0.043), showing group variations in occurrence or management of pressure injuries. Preferred place of care for the future – Strongly significant ($F = 50.548$, $p < 0.001$), indicating a major difference between groups in care preferences. Health conditions – Very strong significance ($F = 74.342$, $p < 0.001$), meaning health status varies substantially across groups.

Non-Significant Results

Living arrangement – No variability in the model (within-groups SS = 0), meaning the test could not compute F (data issue or no group variation). Satisfaction with caregiving services – Not significant ($F = 1.404$, $p = 0.242$). Hospitalizations/ER visits – Not significant ($F = 0.374$, $p = 0.772$). Falls in the past 6 months – Not significant ($F = 0.640$, $p = 0.590$).

The ANOVA findings indicate that institutional care, advance care planning, pressure injuries, preferred place of care, and health conditions are significant differentiating factors across groups. In contrast, living arrangements, satisfaction with caregiving, hospitalizations/ER visits, and falls do not show meaningful group differences.

Table 10. ANOVA

		Sum of Squares	df	Mean Square	F	Sig.
Government support and policy	Between Groups	59.394	3	19.798	32.344	0
	Within Groups	146.293	239	0.612		
	Total	205.687	242			
Financial subsidies/ insurance	Between Groups	91.327	3	30.442	38.196	0
	Within Groups	190.484	239	0.797		
	Total	281.811	242			
Living arrangement	Between Groups	50.759	2	25.379	28.655	0
	Within Groups	106.282	120	0.886		
	Total	157.041	122			
Monthly household income bracket	Between Groups	41.088	2	20.544	36.916	0
	Within Groups	66.782	120	0.557		
	Total	107.87	122			
Effective are the current government or NGO programs in supporting older adults	Between Groups	126.736	3	42.245	69.277	0
	Within Groups	145.742	239	0.61		
	Total	272.477	242			

continued on following page

Table 10. Continued

		Sum of Squares	df	Mean Square	F	Sig.
Non-Institutional Blocks	Between Groups	300.915	2	150.458	381.086	0
	Within Groups	47.378	120	0.395		
	Total	348.293	122			

The ANOVA results indicate statistically significant differences across all tested variables. Government support and policy ($F = 32.344$, $p < 0.001$) and financial subsidies/insurance ($F = 38.196$, $p < 0.001$) show strong variation between groups, suggesting that policy measures and financial support significantly influence caregiving outcomes. Similarly, living arrangement ($F = 28.655$, $p < 0.001$) and monthly household income bracket ($F = 36.916$, $p < 0.001$) differ significantly between groups, highlighting the socio-economic dimension in caregiving. The effectiveness of government or NGO programs in supporting older adults also shows significant group variation ($F = 69.277$, $p < 0.001$), indicating mixed perceptions of program impact. Finally, non-institutional blocks emerged with the highest F-value ($F = 381.086$, $p < 0.001$), underscoring major disparities in experiences and perceptions across different non-institutional care settings.

DISCUSSION

The elderly population in India is rising, creating greater demand for both institutional and non-institutional care. Institutional care—such as nursing homes and geriatric units—provides structured medical and daily living support, ensuring safety and social interaction. However, it is costly, reduces independence, and remains inaccessible to low-income and rural groups (Gupta, 2020; Grech, 2019). Non-institutional care, largely family-based, fosters autonomy and emotional closeness but overburdens caregivers, particularly women, and lacks standardized quality (Waymouth et al., 2023; Swartz & Collins, 2019). Strengthening caregiver training, policy support, and community services is essential (Schulz & Eden, 2016).

Andersen's model highlights three care determinants—predisposing (age, education), enabling (income, family support), and need-based (health status)—all of which strongly shape access and outcomes (Travers et al., 2020). Evidence from Denmark shows that investing in home-based care can reduce reliance on nursing homes (Gorfinkiel et al., 2025).

Study findings reveal that most respondents were aged 60–70 years, with few over 80. Men formed the majority, and two-thirds were married, though widowhood and divorce were significant. Education levels varied, with many having only secondary schooling or none. Living arrangements were nearly balanced between institutional and non-institutional care.

Care satisfaction was mixed: 43.3% satisfied, 30.8% dissatisfied. Strengths included social interaction (74%) and safety (82.9%), but concerns centered on limited autonomy (65.9%), weak family bonding (65%), emotional neglect (55.3%), and financial strain (81.3%). Only 45.5% reported adequate medical care. Chronic illnesses, especially diabetes (39.1%) and hypertension (16.5%), were common. Abuse, neglect, or financial exploitation was reported by 22.6%.

Future care preferences were divided: 27.6% favored institutional care, 22.6% home care, and one-third were undecided. Only 44.9% had discussed advance care planning. Overall, care adequacy was rated sufficient by just 29.6%, with improvements most needed in medical services, caregiver training, and financial support. Policy insights show strong demand for financial subsidies (70.3%), caregiver training (52.5%), and community programs (55.3%). Counseling and peer-support networks were also valued. Overall, findings highlight the dual challenge: institutional care ensures safety but is expensive and less personalized, while non-institutional care supports independence but strains families. A balanced, policy-supported approach combining medical, financial, and psychosocial support is critical for sustainable elder care.

POLICY AND RECOMMENDATIONS FOR PRACTICE IMPLICATIONS

Future implications are to provide guidance for policymakers, healthcare providers, caregivers, and welfare organizations. The aging field emphasizes the urgent need for effective caregiving for older adults. Further research studies should integrate policy implications for both types of care, emphasizing seamless quality eldercare. Home-based care and services support family caregiving for older adults by providing training for caregivers and financial aid. To improve institutional care services by enhancing caregiver training in a professional way and increasing the staff ratio to ensure proper care and availability of services for older adults (Rong et al., 2024). To provide residential care and deliver dignified care services. Further research studies should utilize telehealth services and provide monitoring tools and assistive technology to improve the quality of care and reduce caregiver burden (Ghoshal & Damani, 2025; Srinivasan & Rajavel, 2025)). Workforce shortages affect staff recruitment, and training and support should be provided to improve retention strategies. In future studies, public and private collaboration should be promoted to ensure sustainable quality eldercare and services. Longitudinal studies provide data-driven evaluation to refine caregiving practices and services over time (Lee & Son, 2025).

Provide quality care in institutional and non-institutional settings to assess the physical, emotional, and psychological well-being of older adults. Caregiver burden and satisfaction levels affect stress and life satisfaction; increasing support systems for families, such as non-institutional care services, can help improve these outcomes (Marquine et al., 2015). The cost-effectiveness provides economic implications for both care models, including their families, caregivers, and the healthcare system (Kaye & Harrington, 2015). The older adults' life satisfaction is based on the care and services received, which increases their quality of life and reflects how services are provided by both care models. The impact of each model on providing social interaction and its effect on reducing isolation for community involvement (Graham et al., 2014). The expected outcome of the study is to enhance better policies for older adults by providing caregiver training and advancing infrastructure development to improve their health, care, and services. There are challenges for older adults to fulfill their needs in both care services to improve future advancements (Holroyd-Leduc et al., 2016).

CONCLUSION

The end of the study highlights the strengths and limitations of both institutional and non-institutional caregiving for older adults. Institutional care is mentioned as providing medical support, trained staff members, and consistent regular services to people. This provides individuals with their health needs and offers better health services in institutional care. The lack of personalized care and attention to emotional comfort is associated with home-based services (Bassul et al., 2025). This can be due to a lack of knowledge and emotional comfort, which is common in home and non-institutional care services. Non-institutional caregiving services are typically provided by family members, offering emotional support and a sense of familiarity and belonging (Vejmelka & Sabolić, 2015). However, caregivers may face challenges such as burnout, limited resources, and a lack of formal training. The suggested findings provide a care support model that depends on the older adults' health, family, and socio-economic conditions, as well as their personal preferences. A balanced approach to integrate both systems—community-based support, home healthcare services, and caregiver training—may provide an effective way to improve better solutions for eldercare in future care and services (Bífárìn et al., 2023; Hua, 2025).

REFERENCES

Abdi, S., Spann, A., Borilovic, J., de Witte, L., & Hawley, M. (2019). Understanding the care and support needs of older people: A scoping review and categorisation using the WHO international classification of functioning, disability and health framework (ICF). *BMC Geriatrics, 19*(1), 195. DOI: 10.1186/s12877-019-1189-9 PMID: 31331279

Ahmad Zubaidi, Z. S., Ariffin, F., Oun, C. T. C., & Katiman, D. (2020). Caregiver burden among informal caregivers in the largest specialized palliative care unit in Malaysia: A cross sectional study. *BMC Palliative Care, 19*(1), 186. DOI: 10.1186/s12904-020-00691-1 PMID: 33292214

Akther, F. (2025). Interweaving Care and Climate Justice in Housing for Climate Migrants: Vulnerabilities of Low-Income Older Women in Developing Countries. In *Community Climate Justice and Sustainable Development* (pp. 483-502). IGI Global Scientific Publishing. DOI: 10.4018/979-8-3373-0619-3.ch018

Alders, P., Deeg, D. J., & Schut, F. T. (2019). Who will become my co-residents? The role of attractiveness of institutional care in the changing demand for long-term care institutions. *Archives of Gerontology and Geriatrics, 81*, 91–97. DOI: 10.1016/j.archger.2018.11.014 PMID: 30529804

Allen, J., Woolford, M., Livingston, P. M., Lobchuk, M., Muldowney, A., & Hutchinson, A. M. (2023). Informal carer support needs, facilitators and barriers in transitional care for older adults from hospital to home: A scoping review. *Journal of Clinical Nursing, 32*(19-20), 6773–6795. DOI: 10.1111/jocn.16767 PMID: 37272211

Anttonen, A., & Karsio, O. (2016). Eldercare service redesign in Finland: Deinstitutionalization of long-term care. *Journal of Social Service Research, 42*(2), 151–166. DOI: 10.1080/01488376.2015.1129017

Bandila, R. K. (2022). Concerns of Elderly Women's Wellbeing: Some Policy Issues. In *Research Anthology on Supporting Healthy Aging in a Digital Society* (pp. 1621–1630). IGI Global Scientific Publishing., DOI: 10.4018/978-1-6684-5295-0.ch093

Bassul, C., Gannon, J., Kelly, Y., Williams, M., Morrissey, D., McKee, J., O'Rourke, N., & Flynn, R. (2025). How to achieve person-centered care for people using home care services: A narrative review. *Home Health Care Management & Practice, 37*(2), 129–139. DOI: 10.1177/10848223241267874

Beech, R., Ong, B. N., Jones, S., & Edwards, V. (2017). Delivering person-centred holistic care for older people. *Quality in Ageing : Policy, Practice and Research, 18*(2), 157–167. DOI: 10.1108/QAOA-05-2016-0019

Beswick, A. D., Rees, K., Dieppe, P., Ayis, S., Gooberman-Hill, R., Horwood, J., & Ebrahim, S. (2008). Complex interventions to improve physical function and maintain independent living in elderly people: A systematic review and meta-analysis. *Lancet, 371*(9614), 725–735. DOI: 10.1016/S0140-6736(08)60342-6 PMID: 18313501

Bhattacharyya, K. K. (2021). *Rethinking the Aging Transition.* Springer., DOI: 10.1007/978-3-030-88870-1

Bhuvaneswari, K., & Deb, S. (2016). Efficacy of Family-Based Care as Compared with Institutional Care: A Careful Review. *Institutionalised Children Exploration and Beyond, 3*(2), 161–181. DOI: 10.1177/2349301120160204

Bialon, L. N., & Coke, S. (2012). A study on caregiver burden: Stressors, challenges, and possible solutions. *The American Journal of Hospice & Palliative Care, 29*(3), 210–218. DOI: 10.1177/1049909111416494 PMID: 21803785

Bífárìn, O., Quinn, C., Breen, L., Wu, C., Ke, M., Yu, L., & Oyebode, J. (2023). Stressors and coping mechanisms of family care-givers of older relatives living with long-term conditions in mainland China: A scoping review of the evidence. *Ageing and Society, 43*(4), 952–989. DOI: 10.1017/S0144686X21000817

Chaisomboon, M., Jomnonkwao, S., & Ratanavaraha, V. (2020). Elderly users' satisfaction with public transport in Thailand using different importance performance analysis approaches. *Sustainability (Basel), 12*(21), 9066. DOI: 10.3390/su12219066

Chen, L. M., Inoue, M., & Buckley, N. (2024). Case studies on community care in Japan: Considerations for mitigating social isolation and loneliness in older adults with dementia. *Frontiers in Public Health, 12*, 1411217. DOI: 10.3389/fpubh.2024.1411217 PMID: 39651466

Chew, E. Y. H., Ong, Z. L., Glass, G. F.Jr, & Chan, E. Y. (2022). '24/7'Caregiving: A Qualitative Analysis of an Emerging Phenomenon of Interest in Caregiving. *International Journal of Environmental Research and Public Health, 19*(24), 17046. DOI: 10.3390/ijerph192417046 PMID: 36554924

Cho, E., Kim, H., Kim, J., Lee, K., Meghani, S. H., & Chang, S. J. (2017). Older adult residents' perceptions of daily lives in nursing homes. *Journal of Nursing Scholarship, 49*(5), 495–503. DOI: 10.1111/jnu.12314 PMID: 28605167

Das, S. (2024). Why restructuring residential care matters: A global perspective. In *Care of Older Persons* (pp. 59–72). Routledge India. DOI: 10.4324/9781003528432-6

Denham, A. C., & Kistler, C. E. (2023). Home-and Community-Based Care. In *Chronic Illness Care: Principles and Practice* (pp. 269–283). Springer International Publishing., DOI: 10.1007/978-3-031-29171-5_20

Deshmukh, L., Janghel, U., Sonkuwar, A., & Thakur, R. (2024). Exploring the Synergy between Yoga and Mindfulness Sport Practices: Enhancing Mental and Physical Well-Being. *Indian Journal of YOGA Exercise & Sport Science and Physical Education*, 26-32. DOI: 10.58914/ijyesspe.2024-9.1.4

Dev, P. S., Eljo, J. J. G., & Srinivasan, S. (2025). Intergenerational Caregiving on Grandparents Health: A Case Study. In *Perspectives on the Economics of Aging* (pp. 205-236). IGI Global Scientific Publishing. DOI: DOI: 10.4018/979-8-3693-7753-6.ch008

Donovan, N. J., & Blazer, D. (2020). Social isolation and loneliness in older adults: Review and commentary of a national academies report. *The American Journal of Geriatric Psychiatry*, *28*(12), 1233–1244. DOI: 10.1016/j.jagp.2020.08.005 PMID: 32919873

Doty, P. (2010). The evolving balance of formal and informal, institutional and non-institutional long-term care for older Americans: A thirty-year perspective. *The Public Policy and Aging Report*, *20*(1), 3–9. DOI: 10.1093/ppar/20.1.3

Dunér, A., Bjälkebring, P., & Johansson, B. (2019). Autonomy, choice and control for older users of home care services: Current developments in Swedish eldercare. *Journal of Social Service Research*, *45*(1), 129–141. DOI: 10.1080/01488376.2018.1479677

Elliott, D., McKinley, S., Alison, J., Aitken, L. M., King, M., Leslie, G. D., Kenny, P., Taylor, P., Foley, R., & Burmeister, E. (2011). Health-related quality of life and physical recovery after a critical illness: A multi-centre randomised controlled trial of a home-based physical rehabilitation program. *Critical Care*, *15*(3), R142. DOI: 10.1186/cc10265 PMID: 21658221

Elliott, S., Golds, S., Sissons, I., & Wilson, H. (2015). Long-term care: A review of global funding models. *British Actuarial Journal*, *20*(1), 167–208. DOI: 10.1017/S1357321714000300

Ene, J. C., Chukwu, N. E., & Ajibo, H. T. (2022). Exploring care management for older adults with illnesses as family members' responsibility. The need for social workers' support services in Nigeria. *European Journal of Mental Health*, *17*(3), 38–51. https://www.ceeol.com/search/article-detail?id=1090051. DOI: 10.5708/EJMH.17.2022.3.3

Farias, I. P. S. E., Sousa, S. A. D., Almeida, L. D. F. D. D., Santiago, B. M., Pereira, A. C., & Cavalcanti, Y. W. (2020). Does non-institutionalized elders have a better oral health status compared to institutionalized ones? A systematic review and meta-analysis. *Ciencia & Saude Coletiva, 25*(6), 2177–2192. DOI: 10.1590/1413-81232020256.18252018 PMID: 32520263

Fields, N. L., Anderson, K. A., & Dabelko-Schoeny, H. (2011). Ready or not: Transitioning from institutional care to community care. *Journal of Housing for the Elderly, 25*(1), 3–17. DOI: 10.1080/02763893.2011.545330

Gao, F., Chui, P. L., Che, C. C., Xiao, L., & Zhang, Q. (2024). Advance care planning readiness among community-dwelling older adults and the influencing factors: A scoping review. *BMC Palliative Care, 23*(1), 255. DOI: 10.1186/s12904-024-01583-4 PMID: 39491026

Ghoshal, A., & Damani, A. (2025). Home-Based Care Services. In *The Palgrave Encyclopedia of Disability* (pp. 1–11). Springer Nature Switzerland., DOI: 10.1007/978-3-031-40858-8_535-1

Gomes, B., Calanzani, N., Curiale, V., McCrone, P., Higginson, I. J., & de Brito, M. (2013). Effectiveness and cost-effectiveness of home palliative care services for adults with advanced illness and their caregivers. *Cochrane Database of Systematic Reviews, 2022*(6). Advance online publication. DOI: 10.1002/14651858.CD007760.pub2 PMID: 23744578

Gonzales, E., Lee, K., & Harootyan, B. (2020). Voices from the field: Ecological factors that promote employment and health among low-income older adults with implications for direct social work practice. *Clinical Social Work Journal, 48*(2), 211–222. DOI: 10.1007/s10615-019-00719-x

Gordon, A. (2018). Institutional and non-institutional long-term care. In *Learning geriatric medicine: a study guide for medical students* (pp. 329–335). Springer International Publishing., DOI: 10.1007/978-3-319-61997-2_32

Gorfinkiel, M. D., San Miguel, B. E., & Peterson, E. (2025). Home-based care services for elderly dependent adults. A comparative analysis of Madrid and Stockholm. *Investigaciones Regionales= Journal of Regional Research*, (61), 17-30. https://dialnet.unirioja.es/servlet/articulo?codigo=10051205

Gorman, M. (2017). Development and the rights of older people. In *The ageing and development report* (pp. 3–21). Routledge. DOI: 10.4324/9781315071541-2

Graham, C. L., Scharlach, A. E., & Price Wolf, J. (2014). The impact of the "village" model on health, well-being, service access, and social engagement of older adults. *Health Education & Behavior, 41*(1, suppl), 91S–97S. DOI: 10.1177/1090198114532290 PMID: 24799128

Grech, S. (2019). Disabled families: The impacts of disability and care on family labour and poverty in rural Guatemala. *Societies (Basel, Switzerland), 9*(4), 76. DOI: 10.3390/soc9040076

Gupta, S. (2020). Institutional Care for Elderly. In *Ageing Issues and Responses in India* (pp. 143–155). Springer Singapore., DOI: 10.1007/978-981-15-5187-1_9

Hammar, T., Rissanen, P., & Perälä, M. L. (2008). Home-care clients' need for help, and use and costs of services. *European Journal of Ageing, 5*(2), 147–160. DOI: 10.1007/s10433-008-0078-4 PMID: 28798569

Harris-Kojetin, L., Sengupta, M., Park-Lee, E., Valverde, R., Caffrey, C., Rome, V., & Lendon, J. (2016). Long-term care providers and services users in the United States: Data from the National Study of Long-Term Care Providers, 2013–2014.

He, W., & Kinsella, K. (2020). Global aging in the new millennium. *The cultural context of aging: Worldwide perspectives, 27.*

Hillcoat-Nallétamby, S. (2014). The meaning of "independence" for older people in different residential settings. *The Journals of Gerontology. Series B, Psychological Sciences and Social Sciences, 69*(3), 419–430. DOI: 10.1093/geronb/gbu008 PMID: 24578371

Hilton, C. (2017). Psychiatric Hospitals and Older People: Status Quo or Making Changes? In *Improving Psychiatric Care for Older People: Barbara Robb's Campaign 1965-1975* (pp. 19–55). Springer International Publishing., DOI: 10.1007/978-3-319-54813-5_2

Holroyd-Leduc, J., Resin, J., Ashley, L., Barwich, D., Elliott, J., Huras, P., France, L., Mahoney, M., Maybee, A., McNeil, H., Pullman, D., Sawatzky, R., Stolee, P., & Muscedere, J. (2016). Giving voice to older adults living with frailty and their family caregivers: Engagement of older adults living with frailty in research, health care decision making, and in health policy. *Research Involvement and Engagement, 2*(1), 23. DOI: 10.1186/s40900-016-0038-7 PMID: 29062523

Hu, Z., Abd Rahman, N. H., & Hanafi, H. (2025). Non-governmental Organizations' Role in Promoting Life Satisfaction Among the Elderly Within the Active Aging Strategy. *Voluntas, 36*(3), 337–351. DOI: 10.1007/s11266-025-00728-0

Hua, A. (2025). Integrating Community-Based and Smart Care Models: Strategies for Advancing China's Elderly Care Industry Amid Demographic Challenges. *International Journal of Asian Social Science Research, 2*(1), 77–84. DOI: 10.70267/6f3z9930

Hung, J. (2022). Smart elderly care services in China: Challenges, progress, and policy development. *Sustainability (Basel), 15*(1), 178. DOI: 10.3390/su15010178

Jafari, M., Raoofi, S., Zarnaq, R. K., Mobasseri, K., & Ghasemyani, S. (2024). Infrastructure analysis of long-term care for elderly adults in Iran: A qualitative study. *Int J Agin, 2*, e22. DOI: 10.34172/ija.2024.e22

Kaye, H. S., & Harrington, C. (2015). Long-term services and supports in the community: Toward a research agenda. *Disability and Health Journal, 8*(1), 3–8. DOI: 10.1016/j.dhjo.2014.09.003 PMID: 25445015

Koshmaganbetova, G., Zhylkybekova, A., Abenova, N. A., & Glushkova, N. (2024). Gender Disparities in Care Allocation among Informal Elderly Caregivers: A literature Review. *The Journal of Health Design, 1*(55), 40–49. DOI: 10.32921/2225-9929-2024-1-55-40-49

Kraun, L., De Vliegher, K., Vandamme, M., Holtzheimer, E., Ellen, M., & van Achterberg, T. (2022). Older peoples' and informal caregivers' experiences, views, and needs in transitional care decision-making: A systematic review. *International Journal of Nursing Studies, 134*, 104303. DOI: 10.1016/j.ijnurstu.2022.104303 PMID: 35797843

Kroemeke, A., & Gruszczynska, E. (2016). Well-being and institutional care in older adults: Cross-sectional and time effects of provided and received support. *PLoS One, 11*(8), e0161328. DOI: 10.1371/journal.pone.0161328 PMID: 27548721

Kurasz, A. M., Smith, G. E., Curiel, R. E., Barker, W. W., Behar, R. C., Ramirez, A., & Armstrong, M. J. (2022). Patient values in healthcare decision making among diverse older adults. *Patient Education and Counseling, 105*(5), 1115–1122. DOI: 10.1016/j.pec.2021.08.031 PMID: 34509339

Lalani, N., Osei, E. A., Yang, S., Katare, B., & Wagle, S. (2025). Financial health and well-being of rural female caregivers of older adults with chronic illnesses. *BMC Geriatrics, 25*(1), 239. DOI: 10.1186/s12877-025-05853-5 PMID: 40211160

LaManna, J. B., Unruh, L., Chisholm, L., Pericles, P., & Fotovvat, H. (2020). Perceptions of health and well-being among older adult caregivers: Comparisons of current caregivers with former and never caregivers. *Geriatric Nursing, 41*(4), 429–435. DOI: 10.1016/j.gerinurse.2020.01.015 PMID: 32044146

Lazar, M., & Davenport, L. (2018). Barriers to health care access for low income families: A review of literature. *Journal of Community Health Nursing*, *35*(1), 28–37. DOI: 10.1080/07370016.2018.1404832 PMID: 29323941

Lee, J., & Son, J. (2025). Development of a Sustainable Elderly Care System Leveraging ICT Technologies and Big Data. In *Big Data and Data Science Engineering* (Vol. 8, pp. 81–92). Springer Nature Switzerland., DOI: 10.1007/978-3-031-87061-3_7

Lewis, B., Purser, K., & Mackie, K. (2020). *The human rights of older persons*. Springer Singapore., DOI: 10.1007/978-981-15-6735-3

Liu, T., Hao, X., & Zhang, Z. (2016). Identifying community healthcare supports for the elderly and the factors affecting their aging care model preference: Evidence from three districts of Beijing. *BMC Health Services Research*, *16*(S7, Suppl 7), 626. DOI: 10.1186/s12913-016-1863-y PMID: 28185601

Marquine, M. J., Maldonado, Y., Zlatar, Z., Moore, R. C., Martin, A. S., Palmer, B. W., & Jeste, D. V. (2015). Differences in life satisfaction among older community-dwelling Hispanics and non-Hispanic Whites. *Aging & Mental Health*, *19*(11), 978–988. DOI: 10.1080/13607863.2014.971706 PMID: 25402813

Mishra, R., & Sondhi, V. (2019). Fostering resilience among orphaned adolescents through institutional care in India. *Residential Treatment for Children & Youth*, *36*(4), 314–337. DOI: 10.1080/0886571X.2018.1535286

Moilanen, T., Kangasniemi, M., Papinaho, O., Mynttinen, M., Siipi, H., Suominen, S., & Suhonen, R. (2021). Older people's perceived autonomy in residential care: An integrative review. *Nursing Ethics*, *28*(3), 414–434. DOI: 10.1177/0969733020948115 PMID: 33000683

Moro, T. T., Savage, T. A., & Gehlert, S. (2017). Agency, social and healthcare supports for adults with intellectual disability at the end of life in out-of-home, non-institutional community residences in Western nations: A literature review. *Journal of Applied Research in Intellectual Disabilities*, *30*(6), 1045–1056. DOI: 10.1111/jar.12374 PMID: 28585240

Mosca, I., van der Wees, P. J., Mot, E. S., Wammes, J. J., & Jeurissen, P. P. (2016). Sustainability of long-term care: Puzzling tasks ahead for policy-makers. *International Journal of Health Policy and Management*, *6*(4), 195–205. DOI: 10.15171/ijhpm.2016.109 PMID: 28812803

Murthy, G. V. S., Gupta, S., Ellwein, L. B., Munoz, S. R., Bachani, D., & Dada, V. K. (2001). A population-based eye survey of older adults in a rural district of Rajasthan: I. Central vision impairment, blindness, and cataract surgery. *Ophthalmology, 108*(4), 679–685. DOI: 10.1016/S0161-6420(00)00579-0 PMID: 11297483

Neves, B. B., Sanders, A., & Kokanović, R. (2019). "It's the worst bloody feeling in the world": Experiences of loneliness and social isolation among older people living in care homes. *Journal of Aging Studies, 49*, 74–84. DOI: 10.1016/j.jaging.2019.100785 PMID: 31229221

Nwameme, A. U., Tabong, P. T. N., & Adongo, P. B. (2018). Implementing community-based health planning and services in impoverished urban communities: Health workers' perspective. *BMC Health Services Research, 18*(1), 186. DOI: 10.1186/s12913-018-3005-1 PMID: 29554964

Oswald, F., & Rowles, G. D. (2017). Beyond the relocation trauma in old age: New trends in elders' residential decisions. In *New dynamics in old age* (pp. 127–152). Routledge.

Otis-Green, S., & Juarez, G. (2012). Enhancing the social well-being of family caregivers. In *Seminars in oncology nursing* (Vol. 28, No. 4, pp. 246-255). WB Saunders. DOI: 10.1016/j.soncn.2012.09.007

Parker, M. W., Davis, C., White, K., Johnson, D., Golden, M., & Zola, S. (2022). Reduced care burden and improved quality of life in African American family caregivers: Positive impact of personalized assistive technology. *Technology and Health Care, 30*(2), 379–387. DOI: 10.3233/THC-213049 PMID: 34334439

Pinto, S., Fumincelli, L., Mazzo, A., Caldeira, S., & Martins, J. C. (2017). Comfort, well-being and quality of life: Discussion of the differences and similarities among the concepts. *Porto Biomedical Journal, 2*(1), 6–12. DOI: 10.1016/j.pbj.2016.11.003 PMID: 32258577

Robison, J., Shugrue, N., Porter, M., Fortinsky, R. H., & Curry, L. A. (2012). Transition from home care to nursing home: Unmet needs in a home-and community-based program for older adults. *Journal of Aging & Social Policy, 24*(3), 251–270. DOI: 10.1080/08959420.2012.676315 PMID: 22720886

Rong, C., Wu, Q. H., Xu, H. Y., Chang, M., Zhang, L., & Xie, R. R. (2024). The evaluation and enhancement strategies of core competencies for older adult caregivers in integrated medical and older adult care institutions. *Frontiers in Public Health, 12*, 1407496. DOI: 10.3389/fpubh.2024.1407496 PMID: 38957206

Same, A., McBride, H., Liddelow, C., Mullan, B., & Harris, C. (2020). Motivations for volunteering time with older adults: A qualitative study. *PLoS One*, *15*(5), e0232718. DOI: 10.1371/journal.pone.0232718 PMID: 32365081

Sangeeth, S., & Solomon, M. D. (2015). Quality of Life Among Elderly in Non-Institusional Care. *International Journal of Science and Research, Chennai*, 1462-1467.

Schulz, R., & Eden, J. (2016). Committee on family caregiving for older adults board on health care services health and medicine division. *Families caring for an aging. America*, •••, 1–366. https://www.ncbi.nlm.nih.gov/books/NBK396401/pdf/Bookshelf_NBK396401.pdf

Sebastian, S. (2020). *Abuse and Neglect, Perceived Burden and Quality of Life of Elders Seeking Treatment for Mental Disorders and Elders Residing in Institutional Care: A Comparative Study* (Master's thesis, Central Institute of Psychiatry (India)).

Shrestha, S., Arora, S., Hunter, A., & Debesay, J. (2025). The morality of care: Female family caregivers' motivations for providing care to older migrants. *Qualitative Health Research*, *35*(9), 992–1006. DOI: 10.1177/10497323241280239 PMID: 39499504

Spasova, S., Baeten, R., Coster, S., Ghailani, D., Peña-Casas, R., & Vanhercke, B. (2018). Challenges in long-term care in Europe. *Eurohealth (London)*, *24*(4), 7–12. DOI: 10.2767/84573

Srinivasan, S., & Rajavel, N. (2025). Artificial Intelligence Approach to Psychological Wellbeing Among the Ageing Population. In *AI Technologies and Advancements for Psychological Well-Being and Healthcare* (pp. 187–218). IGI Global., DOI: 10.4018/979-8-3693-9158-7.ch008

Srinivasan, S., & Rajavel, N. (2025). Technology Improves the Quality of Life for Elderly People. In *Perspectives on the Economics of Aging* (pp. 109–150). IGI Global Scientific Publishing., DOI: 10.4018/979-8-3693-7753-6.ch005

Srinivasan, S., Rajavel, N., & Mahmoudi-Dehaki, M. (2025). Elderly Inmates Living With Dementia in Central Prisons. In *Assistive Technology Solutions for Aging Adults and Individuals With Disabilities* (pp. 343–404). IGI Global Scientific Publishing., DOI: 10.4018/979-8-3693-6308-9.ch015

Srinivasan, S., Vallipriya, R., & Singh, A. K. (2025). An Analysis Health and Psychological General Well-Being Among Convicts Central Prison of Tamil Nadu. In *Sustainable Development Goals (SDG) and Its Intersection With Health and Well-Being* (pp. 1-38). IGI Global Scientific Publishing. DOI: 10.4018/979-8-3693-9755-8.ch001

Swartz, K., & Collins, L. G. (2019). Caregiver care. *American Family Physician, 99*(11), 699–706. https://www.aafp.org/pubs/afp/issues/2019/0601/p699.html PMID: 31150177

Syse, A., Artamonova, A., Thomas, M., & Veenstra, M. (2022). Do characteristics of family members influence older persons' transition to long-term healthcare services? *BMC Health Services Research, 22*(1), 362. DOI: 10.1186/s12913-022-07745-5 PMID: 35303891

Tariq, J., Zakar, R., Ali, M. V., Zakar, M. Z., Sajjad, A., & Fischer, F. (2023). Determinants of physical, psychological, and social well-being in older adults: A cross-sectional study in senior care facilities of Pakistan (2019/20). *BMC Geriatrics, 23*(1), 349. DOI: 10.1186/s12877-023-04014-w PMID: 37277717

Tičinović, M., & Tomasović Mrčela, N. (2023). Self-assessed needs of the elderly for the non-institutional care services of gerontological centers in relation to their functional ability. *Hrvatski časopis zdravstvenih znanosti, 3*(1), 33-40. DOI: 10.48188/hczz.3.1.5

Travers, J. L., Hirschman, K. B., & Naylor, M. D. (2020). Adapting Andersen's expanded behavioral model of health services use to include older adults receiving long-term services and supports. *BMC Geriatrics, 20*(1), 58. DOI: 10.1186/s12877-019-1405-7 PMID: 32059643

Turcotte, P. L., Larivière, N., Desrosiers, J., Voyer, P., Champoux, N., Carbonneau, H., Carrier, A., & Levasseur, M. (2015). Participation needs of older adults having disabilities and receiving home care: Met needs mainly concern daily activities, while unmet needs mostly involve social activities. *BMC Geriatrics, 15*(1), 95. DOI: 10.1186/s12877-015-0077-1 PMID: 26231354

Vejmelka, L., & Sabolić, T. (2015). The potential of institutions for children without parental care: The perspective of the institutional caregivers. *Kriminologija & socijalna integracija: časopis za kriminologiju, penologiju i poremećaje u ponašanju, 23*(1), 99-128. https://hrcak.srce.hr/clanak/218862

Vuksan, M., Williams, A. M., & Crooks, V. A. (2012). The workplace perspective on supporting family caregivers at end of life: Evaluating a new Canadian social program. *Community Work & Family, 15*(3), 317–333. DOI: 10.1080/13668803.2012.664891

Wang, J., Wang, J., Cao, Y., Jia, S., & Wu, B. (2016). Older residents' perspectives of long-term care facilities in China. *Journal of Gerontological Nursing, 42*(8), 34–43. DOI: 10.3928/00989134-20160615-05 PMID: 27319405

Waymouth, M., Siconolfi, D., Friedman, E. M., Saliba, D., Ahluwalia, S. C., & Shih, R. A. (2023). Barriers and facilitators to home-and community-based services access for persons with dementia and their caregivers. *The Journals of Gerontology. Series B, Psychological Sciences and Social Sciences*, *78*(6), 1085–1097. DOI: 10.1093/geronb/gbad039 PMID: 36896936

Wirtz, J., Bateson, J. E., Čaić, M., Frank, D. A., & Veflen, N. (2025). The healthy aging and service firms: The promise of smart technologies. *Journal of Service Management*. Advance online publication. DOI: 10.1108/JOSM-10-2024-0426

Wirtz, J., & Stock-Homburg, R. (2025). Generative AI meets service robots. *Journal of Service Research*, *10946705251340487*(4), 527–543. Advance online publication. DOI: 10.1177/10946705251340487

Yang, G., Wan, L., Dong, H., Liang, X., & He, Y. (2022). Utilisation willingness for institutional care by the disabled elderly and its influencing factors based on Andersen's model: A cross-sectional survey of Henan, China. *BMJ Open*, *12*(12), e064949. DOI: 10.1136/bmjopen-2022-064949 PMID: 36600340

Zhang, M., & Cheng, Q. (2024). Becoming a self-reliant elder: Fading intergenerational reciprocity and pursuing active aging among middle-class seniors in urban China. *SAGE Open*, *14*(2), 21582440241259161. DOI: 10.1177/21582440241259161

Zhao, L., Chang, B., Hu, Q., Chen, X., Du, J., & Shao, S. (2025). The health care needs of multidimensional frail elderly patients with multimorbidity in primary health-care settings: A qualitative study. *BMC Primary Care*, *26*(1), 128. DOI: 10.1186/s12875-025-02836-8 PMID: 40281402

Zimbroff, R. M., Ornstein, K. A., & Sheehan, O. C. (2021). Home-based primary care: A systematic review of the literature, 2010–2020. *Journal of the American Geriatrics Society*, *69*(10), 2963–2972. DOI: 10.1111/jgs.17365 PMID: 34247383

Chapter 4
Inclusive Home Care Systems for Neurodiverse and Differently Abled Individuals:
A Human-Centered Framework for Equity and Participation

Treesa Sindhu P. Thomas
https://orcid.org/0009-0002-7405-5162
St. Teresa's College, Ernakulam, India

Leena Leon
Rajagiri College of Social Sciences, Kalamasseri, India

ABSTRACT

As awareness of neurodiversity and disability rights continues to expand, the home our most intimate and formative environment must evolve into a space that fosters equity, autonomy, and inclusion. Yet, many traditional home care systems still rely on generalized or clinical models that overlook the complex realities of individuals with cognitive, sensory, and physical differences. Such approaches often reinforce dependency and exclusion, rather than promoting independence and participation. Drawing on insights from disability studies, occupational therapy, and integrative healthcare, the framework emphasizes adaptability, collaboration, and dignity as guiding principles. Through collaborative planning, supported decision-making, and inclusive design strategies, the study demonstrates how both care recipients and caregivers can experience enhanced dignity, resilience, and mutual empowerment.

DOI: 10.4018/979-8-3373-4094-4.ch004

inclusive care practices should ensure that individuals regardless of ability are met with respect, autonomy, and genuine opportunity for participation in family and community life.

INTRODUCTION: REIMAGINING CARE IN THE HOME ENVIRONMENT

As global conversations around neurodiversity and disability rights continue to expand, the urgency of creating home care systems that prioritize inclusion, dignity, and autonomy has never been clearer. Traditional models of care are often rooted in clinical or institutional perspectives, where the focus remains narrowly fixed on medical needs. While this approach addresses immediate health concerns, it too often neglects the broader social, emotional, and sensory dimensions of living with a disability. The disconnect becomes most apparent within home environments, where rigid systems fail to adapt to the lived experiences of individuals and their families.

In recent years, however, advocates, researchers, and neurodivergent voices have challenged these outdated paradigms. The neurodiversity movement has been especially influential, reframing conditions such as autism, ADHD, and dyslexia not as deficits but as natural variations of human cognition (Kapp, 2020). This perspective aligns with the social model of disability, which argues that it is the barriers created by society rather than impairments themselves that generate exclusion and inequality (Oliver & Barnes, 2012). Such shifts in thinking have paved the way for more inclusive, empathetic, and flexible approaches to home care.

Building on these ideas, this chapter introduces a human-centered framework for inclusive home care that draws from occupational therapy, behavioural health, trauma-informed practice, and user-centered design. It emphasizes the need for adaptive tools, emotionally safe environments, and care systems that extend beyond physical assistance to cultivate belonging, resilience, and emotional well-being.

At the policy level, momentum is slowly building. Governments and health systems are beginning to acknowledge the value of personalized, accessible home care, particularly in light of the COVID-19 pandemic, which exposed the fragility of institutional care models and underscored the necessity of home-based supports. Despite this progress, persistent challenges remain: undertrained caregivers, inadequate infrastructure, and the absence of culturally sensitive protocols especially in resource-limited and diverse social contexts.

This chapter responds to these realities by drawing on interdisciplinary perspectives and case studies from India, Australia, and the UK. It offers practical strategies for transforming home care into a collaborative, empowering, and socially just practice, ensuring that homes are not merely spaces of care, but environments that uphold the dignity, rights, and participation of neurodiverse and differently-abled individuals.

THEORETICAL FRAMEWORK

Designing an inclusive home care system for neurodiverse and differently-abled individuals requires a foundation that is both interdisciplinary and holistic. Such a system cannot be shaped by a single perspective; rather, it must integrate psychological, social, cultural, and systemic insights to fully capture the complexity of lived experiences. This framework draws upon five complementary models that, together, provide a robust foundation for reimagining home care practices.

1. The Social Model of Disability

The social model shifts the focus away from disability as an inherent limitation of the individual and instead highlights how exclusion arises from environments, systems, and attitudes that fail to accommodate human diversity (Oliver & Barnes, 2012). Rather than attempting to "fix" the person, this model advocates for removing barriers whether physical, social, or institutional that restrict participation. In home care, applying this model means modifying physical spaces, daily routines, and caregiving practices to promote independence and enable fuller participation in everyday life.

2. The Neurodiversity Paradigm

Emerging from advocacy and lived experience, the neurodiversity paradigm asserts that neurological differences such as autism, ADHD, or dyslexia are not pathologies, but natural variations of human cognition (Kapp, 2020). This perspective emphasizes building environments that recognize strengths, accommodate sensory needs, and respect alternative ways of thinking and communicating. In practical terms, this may involve integrating sensory-calming spaces, visual routines, or augmentative and alternative communication (AAC) systems within the home, ensuring that support is tailored to individual preferences rather than imposed as standardized solutions.

3. Person-Centered and Family-Centered Care

Person-centered care emphasizes the dignity, values, and goals of the individual receiving support (Edvardsson et al., 2008). In home-based contexts, however, care often involves families who act as primary caregivers. Expanding this model into family-centered care acknowledges the central role of families as partners rather than passive providers (Kuhlthau et al., 2022). This approach ensures that care planning becomes a collaborative process, where the voices of both individuals and their families are heard, respected, and integrated into long-term support systems. Such collaboration not only improves outcomes but also strengthens resilience within caregiving relationships.

4. Trauma-Informed Care

For many neurodivergent and differently-abled individuals, past experiences of institutionalization, medical mistreatment, or persistent miscommunication have left lasting effects. Trauma-informed care seeks to counter this by fostering environments that prioritize emotional safety, predictability, and trust (Substance Abuse and Mental Health Services Administration, 2014). In home settings, this translates into practices that minimize triggers, validate emotions, and maintain transparency in routines and decision-making. By embedding trauma-informed principles, caregivers can help prevent re-traumatization and nurture caregiving relationships built on respect, empathy, and stability.

5. Ecological Systems Theory

Bronfenbrenner's ecological systems theory (1979) reminds us that individuals exist within interconnected layers of influence from immediate family to wider cultural and policy environments. For home care, this perspective underscores how structural factors such as public health policies, community resources, or societal stigma directly shape the caregiving experience. A systems-oriented lens helps identify how barriers at broader levels such as inadequate funding, limited caregiver training, or exclusionary cultural attitudes can undermine even the most well-intentioned home care practices. By addressing these influences, care systems can be made more resilient, equitable, and sustainable.

Figure 1. Theoretical framework diagram for an inclusive care system, integrating five foundational models

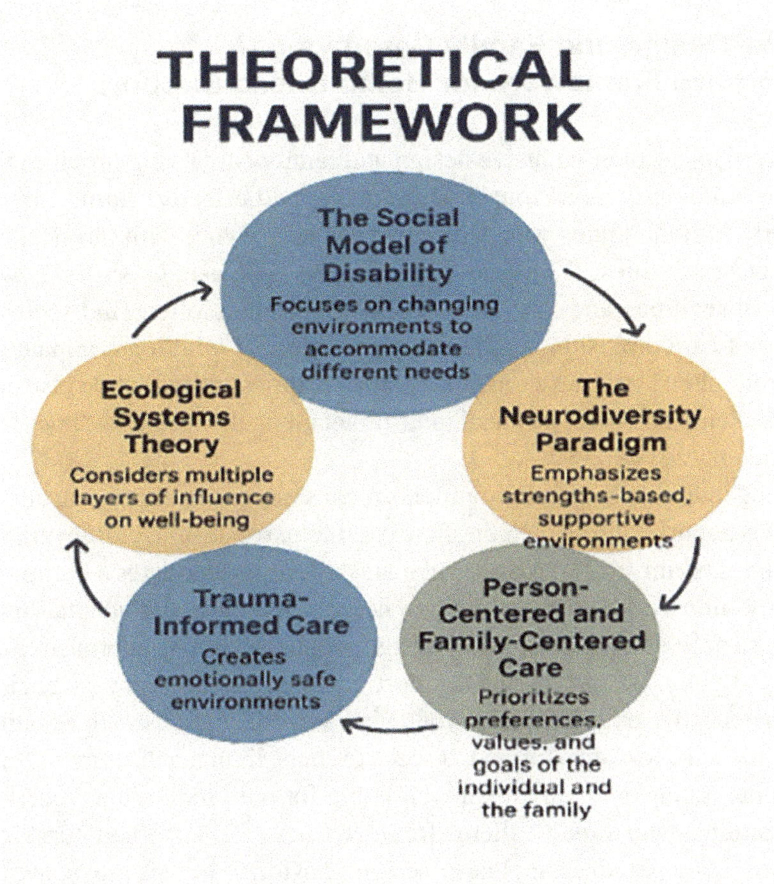

Table 1. Central Concept: At the heart is the Inclusive Care System, supported by

Model	Core Principle
Social Model of Disability	Modify environments and attitudes to foster independence and participation
Neurodiversity Paradigm	Create strengths-based, sensory-friendly, and communicative support systems
Person & Family-Centered Care	Co-develop care plans with individuals and families for sustainable support
Trauma-Informed Care	Ensure emotional safety through transparency and validation
Ecological Systems Theory	Address multi-layered influences from family to societal structures

Each model feeds into the central system, emphasizing a holistic, responsive, and empowering approach to home care.

Inclusive Design and Family Caregiving: A Collaborative Framework for Home-Based Support

The overlap between inclusive design and family caregiving provides the foundation for building compassionate, sustainable, and effective home care systems particularly for individuals who are neurodiverse or living with physical, sensory, or cognitive disabilities. With healthcare delivery increasingly shifting away from institutional facilities and into private homes, families often find themselves at the center of care provision. These caregivers most of whom are unpaid and lack formal professional training shoulder essential responsibilities while also grappling with their own emotional, physical, and financial challenges (Cassie et al., 2022; Reinhard et al., 2019).

Creating inclusive home environments means more than simply ensuring accessibility; it is about enabling meaningful lives. Inclusive design, closely aligned with the principles of universal design, anticipates and accommodates a broad spectrum of human abilities, behaviors, and sensory needs. Unlike reactive adaptations that are added after a problem arises, inclusive design adopts a proactive approach embedding flexibility, dignity, autonomy, and comfort into spaces from the very beginning.

This perspective extends well beyond visible modifications such as ramps, grab bars, or widened doorways. Instead, it seeks to shape living environments that foster participation, safety, and emotional well-being for both individuals receiving care and the families who support them (Imrie & Luck, 2014). When combined with family caregiving practices, inclusive design transforms homes into spaces that are not just functional, but also restorative, empowering, and supportive of long-term resilience for all members of the household.

Designing with Neurodiversity in Mind

Neurodiverse individuals including those with autism spectrum disorder (ASD), ADHD, sensory processing differences, or other cognitive variations often face distinct challenges within their home environments. Inclusive design has the potential to reduce these stressors by minimizing triggers and creating supportive conditions for self-regulation. Thoughtful interventions can transform homes into spaces that foster comfort, autonomy, and well-being.

a) Sensory-Friendly Lighting and Textures

Lighting and textures significantly influence the sensory experience of a home. Conventional settings with harsh overhead lights, flickering fluorescent bulbs, or abrasive materials can overwhelm those with sensory sensitivities. Instead, prioritizing natural daylight, complemented by warm-tone LED fixtures that are dimmable and flicker-free, creates a calmer visual atmosphere. Soft, tactile-friendly fabrics such as cotton, bamboo, or velvet further support comfort, while clutter reduction, neutral tones, and minimal visual patterns help decrease overstimulation. As Mostafa (2014) notes, such design choices not only minimise discomfort but also actively promote emotional regulation and a sense of safety within the home.

b) Visual Schedules and Step-by-Step Guides

Predictability is a cornerstone of stability for many neurodivergent individuals. Visual schedules, picture cards, and digital tools like Choiceworks or PECS provide clear, nonverbal cues that reduce anxiety and enhance independence. Placing these visual supports near sinks, kitchen counters, or wardrobes ensures they are easily accessible at points of use. Beyond benefiting the individual, these tools also lessen the cognitive and emotional load on caregivers by reducing the need for repeated verbal instructions (Hodgetts et al., 2013). In this way, they strengthen both autonomy and family well-being.

c) Quiet Retreat Spaces for Sensory Decompression

Dedicated quiet areas give individuals the opportunity to withdraw, reset, and recover from sensory overload. Features such as sound-absorbing panels, thick curtains, or plush carpeting help soften environmental noise, while calming elements like beanbags, weighted blankets, or small canopy nooks foster a sense of security. Maintaining a scent-neutral environment is equally important for those with heightened olfactory sensitivities. Such "retreat zones" are particularly beneficial for individuals with ASD, PTSD, or anxiety, helping to prevent meltdowns, reduce fatigue, and restore equilibrium (Ashburner et al., 2013).

d) Flexible Furniture and Smart Assistive Technologies

Adaptable furniture and technology innovations can dramatically enhance independence and caregiving efficiency. Adjustable kitchen counters, folding beds, modular storage, and ergonomic seating respond to diverse physical needs and reduce caregiver strain. At the same time, smart technologies from voice-controlled assistants and motion-sensitive lighting to automated thermostats and remote monitoring systems offer intuitive ways for individuals to interact with their environment. Such systems not only extend autonomy but also ease caregiver responsibilities, making the home more sustainable for everyone involved (Chung et al., 2021).

e) Colour-Coded and Voice-Assisted Controls

Simple yet powerful design strategies like colour-coding and voice-assistive systems ensure homes are intuitive and user-friendly. Colour distinctions for switches or storage areas for instance, blue for water, red for heating, or green for frequently used items can support memory and orientation. Tactile indicators such as raised symbols, textured labels, or braille enhance accessibility for individuals with visual or motor challenges. Meanwhile, voice-activated systems allow residents to operate lights, appliances, or safety alerts without physical effort. These interventions embody universal usability, creating homes that are not only more inclusive for differently-abled residents but also more convenient for children, elders, and guests alike.

By weaving together sensory-friendly design, structured supports, restorative spaces, adaptive furniture, and intuitive technologies, home environments can evolve into truly inclusive ecosystems. Such environments recognize neurodiverse needs not as limitations but as integral factors in shaping dignified, equitable, and empowering living spaces.

Table 2. Universal Usability Matrix: Colour-Coded & Voice-Assisted Controls

Design Feature	Purpose	User Benefit
Colour-Coded Labels	Differentiate switches, drawers, and zones by function	Faster recognition, reduced cognitive load, improved memory recall
Tactile Indicators	Raised symbols, textured stickers, or braille labels	Easier navigation for visually impaired users; supports motor coordination
Voice-Activated Systems	Control appliances and fixtures via voice commands	Hands-free operation; increased independence for users with mobility challenges
Emergency Voice Alerts	Notify users of hazards or reminders through audio cues	Enhanced safety; reduced need for caregiver intervention
Intuitive Layout	Logical placement of controls and feedback mechanisms	Supports users with cognitive impairments; improves overall usability

Inclusive Design as a Lifespan Strategy

A defining strength of inclusive home care design is its adaptability across the lifespan. Human needs are rarely static; they shift in response to aging, progressive health conditions, or changes in sensory, cognitive, and physical abilities. A home that is inclusive today must remain relevant tomorrow, accommodating transitions such as reduced mobility, emerging cognitive decline, or heightened sensory sensitivities. Designing with flexibility at the outset not only prevents costly retrofits but also ensures that the home continues to foster safety, dignity, and independence as circumstances evolve. In this sense, inclusivity is not a one-time design solution but an ongoing strategy that sustains quality of life over time.

The Critical Role of Family Caregivers in Inclusive Home Care

Alongside design, the role of family caregivers is pivotal in sustaining inclusive home care systems. Across the globe, family members most often women form the backbone of long-term support for individuals with disabilities or neurodevelopmental conditions. Their work extends far beyond meeting immediate physical needs. Caregivers manage complex medication schedules, assist with hygiene and mobility, coordinate healthcare and educational services, monitor emotional and behavioral well-being, and act as tireless advocates for the rights and dignity of those they support (NASEM, 2016; Brimblecombe et al., 2018). In many cases, they are the most consistent and trusted figures in the care recipient's life, bridging the gaps left by overstretched formal systems.

Yet this essential role often comes at a profound personal cost. Caregivers typically juggle these responsibilities alongside employment, household management, childcare, or even the care of other elderly or ill relatives. The cumulative weight of these overlapping duties frequently results in chronic stress, exhaustion, and, over time, burnout. Physically, caregivers may suffer injuries or long-term musculoskeletal strain from tasks such as lifting, bathing, or repositioning individuals in spaces not designed for accessibility. Emotionally, many grapple with isolation, limited support networks, and the constant pressure of decision-making for another's well-being. These challenges underscore the urgent need for both policy-level recognition of caregivers' contributions and the design of home environments that actively ease their workload rather than intensify it.

By integrating adaptability in home design with robust support for caregivers, inclusive care systems can move beyond accessibility alone, creating environments that sustain both those receiving care and those providing it.

The Home Environment as an Enabler or Barrier

The physical environment of the home can either empower or restrict the capacity of caregivers to provide safe, effective, and sustainable support. When homes are poorly designed with features such as narrow hallways, steep staircases, inaccessible bathrooms, or dimly lit interiors the burden on caregivers increases substantially. These limitations make everyday tasks more labour-intensive and can compromise not only safety but also the dignity and independence of the individual receiving care.

For example, the absence of adjustable-height counters or anti-slip flooring often forces caregivers to engage in physically demanding tasks, such as lifting or carrying a person during meal preparation, bathing, or toileting. Such exertion increases the risk of musculoskeletal injuries for caregivers and fosters dependency for care recipients when, in reality, thoughtful design modifications could enable greater independence and collaborative participation. Similarly, the lack of accessible communication supports such as visual schedules, symbol boards, or voice-activated devices can complicate interaction with non-verbal or cognitively impaired individuals. Without these aids, caregivers are left to mediate every exchange, which not only adds to their workload but can also diminish the individual's opportunity for self-expression and autonomy (Chung et al., 2021).

In this way, the home itself becomes either a silent ally or a persistent obstacle in the caregiving process. When it is not designed inclusively, it compounds stress, erodes efficiency, and reinforces dependence. When it is thoughtfully designed, it can redistribute effort, strengthen safety, and affirm dignity for everyone involved.

Inclusive Design as a Form of Preventive Care

Inclusive home design should not be understood merely as a set of accommodations for disability it is, more importantly, a form of preventive care. By anticipating the evolving needs of both care recipients and caregivers, inclusive design safeguards physical health, reduces emotional strain, and promotes long-term sustainability in the caregiving relationship.

Practical features such as grab bars, non-slip flooring, wider doorways to support wheelchair access, and adaptable bathroom layouts not only minimize risks of accidents and falls but also allow care tasks to be carried out with less physical exertion. Similarly, integrating assistive technologies from automated lighting and climate control to sensor-based safety systems creates a safer, more responsive environment that reduces caregiver vigilance while increasing the autonomy of the care recipient.

Crucially, inclusive design promotes shared independence. It enables care recipients to participate in their daily routines and make decisions to the extent of their abilities. This shift not only eases the caregiver's workload but also transforms the care dynamic into one rooted in respect and mutual empowerment. In this sense, inclusivity does more than improve accessibility it reshapes the home into a space where health, dignity, and participation are protected for all members of the household.

Culturally Responsive and Gender-Sensitive Design

When developing inclusive home care frameworks, it is essential to acknowledge that design cannot be universally applied in the abstract. Effective solutions must be grounded in the cultural, social, and gendered realities of the communities they aim to serve.

Cultural Contexts of Care in the Global South

In many regions of the Global South, caregiving is deeply relational and embedded within extended family networks rather than being a task assigned exclusively to professionals or confined to nuclear households. These caregiving practices are shaped by cultural norms, religious beliefs, and the physical limitations of the home environment. Designing for such contexts requires moving beyond Western-centric paradigms to approaches that honour collective living, interdependence, and cultural nuance.

In countries such as India, caregiving is often considered a moral and familial responsibility, passed down through generations and typically carried out without formal recognition or compensation. Homes are frequently multi-generational, and caregiving responsibilities are negotiated informally among family members. As a result, design interventions must accommodate shared spaces, where sleeping, cooking, caregiving, and social interaction often take place within the same area. Here, privacy as conceived in Western design may be less of a priority; instead, spatial flexibility and multifunctionality become central to effective design.

Limited physical space demands that every area serve multiple functions. Foldable furniture, modular layouts, and movable partitions can allow rooms to transition seamlessly throughout the day. For instance, a living room may function as a communal space during the day, a sleeping area at night, and a caregiving zone during illness or recovery. Design must also respect cultural rituals and religious practices that shape how spaces are used such as prayer areas, gender-specific zones, or specific orientations for cooking and sleeping. These elements are not ancillary; they are integral to the lived experience of the home.

Additionally, stigma and social taboos around disability can influence how inclusive features are perceived. In some communities, visible accessibility aids may be resisted due to fear of judgment or misunderstanding. This necessitates a sensitive, discreet approach to design features that are fully functional yet harmonize with the aesthetic and cultural context of the home. For example, grab bars might be integrated as traditional architectural elements, and ramps could be incorporated along garden paths rather than as standalone structures.

As Verdonschot et al. (2009) emphasize, inclusive design must meet functional needs while also engaging users emotionally and socially. In the Global South, this means designing for interdependence, adaptability, and cultural continuity ensuring accessibility is integrated organically into daily life rather than applied as an external or isolated intervention.

Framework: Culturally Responsive Caregiving Design

Following is a visual framework that maps caregiving design strategies to key cultural dimensions in the Global South especially India. This can serve as a tool for designers, educators, and policymakers to understand how inclusive design intersects with cultural realities.

Table 3. Cultural Dimensions & Design Implications

Cultural Dimension	Design Implication	Responsive Strategy
Multi-generational Living	Shared spaces with overlapping functions	Modular layouts, foldable furniture, flexible zoning
Limited Physical Space	High spatial density, multifunctional rooms	Vertical storage, convertible furniture, space-saving assistive tech
Kinship-based Caregiving	Informal, relational caregiving across generations	Co-care zones, intergenerational accessibility, shared caregiving stations
Religious & Ritual Practices	Specific spatial orientations, sacred zones	Respectful placement of features, adaptable prayer areas, culturally sensitive signage
Disability Stigma & Taboos	Resistance to visible accessibility modifications	Aesthetic integration of features, discreet assistive tech, community education
Gendered Roles in Care	Women often bear caregiving responsibilities	Ergonomic design for caregivers, privacy-enhancing features, inclusive sanitation
Collective Decision-Making	Design choices negotiated within family or community	Participatory design workshops, visual prototypes for consensus-building

Table 4. Visual Matrix: Design Strategies by Space Type

Space Type	Design Goals	Culturally Responsive Features
Sleeping Area	Comfort, privacy, adaptability	Foldable beds, privacy curtains, shared sleeping layouts
Caregiving Zone	Accessibility, hygiene, emotional safety	Portable assistive devices, washable surfaces, calming color palettes
Kitchen/Dining	Functionality, ritual respect, social bonding	Multi-height counters, seating for caregivers, space for ritual items

continued on following page

Table 4. Continued

Space Type	Design Goals	Culturally Responsive Features
Bathroom	Safety, dignity, cultural modesty	Non-slip floors, gender-sensitive design, discreet grab bars
Prayer/Quiet Space	Spiritual continuity, emotional regulation	Adjustable lighting, quiet zones, culturally respectful design cues
Outdoor/Threshold	Community interaction, mobility	Integrated ramps, shaded seating, sensory-friendly pathways

Addressing Gender in Caregiving Environments

Across many cultural contexts, caregiving remains a profoundly gendered responsibility. Women whether as mothers, daughters, wives, or sisters often shoulder the majority of this labor. This dynamic reflects not only cultural traditions but also systemic inequities that position women as default caregivers, frequently without recognition, financial compensation, or sufficient support. The consequences are significant: female caregivers commonly face economic dependence, restricted access to education or employment, limited social mobility, and increased vulnerability to mental and physical health challenges. These pressures are exacerbated by the invisibility of caregiving work, which usually occurs in private domestic spaces and is rarely accounted for in policy frameworks or labor protections.

Design, however, can play a transformative role. Gender-sensitive interventions can address the physical, emotional, and logistical challenges that women face in caregiving roles. Ergonomic improvements such as adjustable-height counters, grab bars, transfer aids, and supportive work surfaces can reduce physical strain during lifting, bathing, cooking, or other repetitive tasks. These modifications not only help prevent injury but also affirm the caregiver's comfort, dignity, and well-being. Shared caregiving zones, such as open-plan kitchens, multipurpose rooms, or integrated living-care spaces, allow women to manage multiple responsibilities simultaneously while maintaining safety and efficiency.

Privacy is another crucial factor, particularly in contexts where modesty norms influence caregiving practices. Thoughtfully designed private spaces for hygiene, medical care, or personal routines enhanced with partitions, soundproofing, and culturally sensitive layouts enable caregivers to provide intimate care without compromising their own or the recipient's dignity. Additionally, integrating digital support systems, including mobile health platforms, video consultations, and tech-friendly zones, allows caregivers to access medical guidance, manage prescriptions, or coordinate services from home.

Ultimately, caregiving design must acknowledge that much of this labor is unpaid, unrecognized, and structurally unsupported. By embedding supportive infrastructure into the home, inclusive design acts as a subtle yet powerful form of recognition validating caregiving as essential work and creating environments where women feel safer, more capable, and empowered. Such thoughtful design not only enhances individual well-being but also contributes to broader systemic change, challenging social norms that render caregiving invisible and undervalued.

A Holistic Approach to Design and Care

The relationship between inclusive design and family caregiving is inherently symbiotic. Caregivers require supportive, ergonomically and emotionally attuned environments to sustain their well-being, while care recipients thrive most in spaces that honour their autonomy, dignity, and comfort. Neither can flourish in isolation. A genuinely inclusive home care model should integrate spatial planning with cultural sensitivity, gender equity, and the lived experiences of those who inhabit the home daily.

By embracing this holistic perspective, inclusive caregiving moves beyond policy ideals or technical adjustments. It becomes a lived reality one that values all forms of care, recognizes those who provide it, and ultimately strengthens the well-being of both individuals and society as a whole.

Empowering Neurodiverse and Differently-Abled Individuals through Innovation and Design

Designing homes that are both technologically enabling and sensory-aware represents a transformative approach to supporting autonomy, safety, and emotional well-being for neurodiverse and differently-abled individuals. By combining assistive technologies with thoughtfully curated sensory environments, such homes foster independence while reducing caregiver stress, creating spaces that respond to the unique sensory and functional needs of each resident.

1. Assistive Technology: Enabling Daily Life

Assistive Technology (AT) encompasses a wide range of tools, devices, and systems that enhance an individual's ability to perform daily tasks with greater ease, autonomy, and dignity. In home care, AT is not a mere convenience it is central to inclusive living. It allows individuals with physical, cognitive, or sensory differences to participate more fully in daily life while reducing the dependency on caregivers.

Mobility and accessibility interventions are particularly impactful. Stairlifts, automated doors, and height-adjustable countertops empower individuals with limited mobility to navigate their homes safely and independently. These modifications reduce physical strain and promote spatial freedom. Communication technologies such as speech-generating devices, visual boards, and text-to-speech applications enable individuals with limited or non-verbal speech to express needs, preferences, and emotions effectively, enhancing both autonomy and interpersonal relationships.

Environmental control systems further extend independence. Voice-activated lighting, automated curtains, and smart HVAC systems allow residents to adjust their surroundings without physical effort. Safety and monitoring technologies, including wearable health sensors, fall detectors, and GPS trackers, provide real-time alerts and reassurance for both users and caregivers. For individuals living alone or in remote areas, these systems are especially critical.

Personal care support technologies also play a vital role. Electronic pill dispensers ensure timely medication adherence, while adaptive utensils and grooming aids promote self-sufficiency in daily routines. When integrated thoughtfully, assistive technologies transform the caregiving environment from one of dependency into a space of empowerment, inclusion, and meaningful engagement.

2. Designing Sensory-Safe Spaces

Creating sensory-smart homes is essential for supporting individuals with autism, ADHD, PTSD, and other sensory-processing sensitivities. These environments are deliberately designed to reduce sensory overload and promote calm, predictability, and control. Sensory stimuli such as light, sound, texture, and spatial organization can significantly influence emotional regulation, cognitive focus, and overall comfort.

Lighting is a foundational element. Harsh or flickering lights can trigger discomfort, so sensory-friendly homes prioritize dimmable, warm-toned fixtures that reduce glare and visual strain. Acoustic comfort is equally important; soft materials like rugs, curtains, and acoustic panels absorb sound, minimizing echo and creating a quieter, more soothing environment.

Tactile and visual inputs also support emotional well-being. Gentle textures, muted color palettes, and natural materials provide grounding sensory experiences, while quiet retreat areas serve as safe zones for decompression and self-regulation. Outfitted with weighted blankets, rocking chairs, and fidget tools, these spaces allow residents to recover from overstimulation and practice self-soothing behaviors. Personalization through familiar scents, visuals, and textures reinforces a sense of security and routine, strengthening the connection between the individual and their environment.

The ASPECTSS™ framework covering Acoustics, Spatial Sequencing, Escape, Compartmentalization, Transitions, Sensory Zoning, and Safety provides a structured approach for creating sensory-sensitive homes. Research consistently shows that when individuals can control sensory elements like lighting and noise, they experience reduced anxiety and improved focus. Sensory-smart design is therefore not only aesthetically thoughtful but also central to autonomy, dignity, and emotional resilience.

3. The Power of Integration: AT Meets Sensory Design

The full potential of inclusive home care emerges when assistive technology and sensory-smart design are integrated. For example, a child with autism benefits not only from a touch-screen visual schedule (AT) but also from a calm, low-stimulation environment that supports its use. Together, these strategies address emotional regulation, cognitive clarity, and active engagement in a holistic manner.

Care in such settings goes beyond physical support. It includes executive assistance through visual cues, reminders, and structured routines and emotional scaffolding via thoughtful spatial design and technological tools. Communication support remains central, with AAC devices, visual timers, and structured interaction methods helping to minimize misunderstandings and distress, particularly for non-verbal or minimally verbal individuals. By combining assistive technologies with sensory-smart design, home environments become empowering, inclusive, and responsive to the unique needs of each resident.

Empowerment through Innovation and Holistic Design

Designing homes that integrate advanced assistive technology with sensory-conscious environments represents a significant shift in promoting independence, safety, and emotional well-being for neurodiverse and differently-abled individuals.

1. Assistive Technology: Unlocking Functional Independence

Assistive Technology (AT) plays a transformative role in home care, enabling individuals with physical, cognitive, or sensory challenges to engage in daily activities with greater independence, safety, and dignity. AT encompasses a wide array of tools from simple adaptive devices to sophisticated digital systems designed to bridge functional gaps and enhance quality of life. Beyond empowering the care recipient, AT significantly alleviates the physical and emotional demands on family caregivers.

Mobility and accessibility are primary areas where AT has immediate impact. Devices such as stairlifts, automated doors, and height-adjustable countertops allow individuals with limited mobility to navigate their homes safely and comfortably. These solutions reduce reliance on constant physical assistance while promoting spatial freedom and autonomy.

Equally important are communication technologies. For individuals with speech or language difficulties, tools like speech-generating devices, visual communication boards, and text-to-speech software enable expression of needs, preferences, and emotions. By opening these channels, AT strengthens social connections, enhances self-expression, and fosters emotional engagement within the household.

Environmental control systems further enhance independence. Voice-activated lighting, motorized curtains, and programmable thermostats allow residents to manage their surroundings with minimal effort, creating a sense of mastery and reducing dependence on caregivers. Safety and monitoring technologies such as wearable health sensors, fall detectors, and GPS trackers offer real-time feedback and alerts, protecting residents while providing reassurance to family members, particularly for those living alone or in remote locations.

Assistive devices for daily living complement these systems by supporting routine self-care. Electronic pill dispensers ensure adherence to medication schedules, while adaptive utensils, grooming aids, and dressing tools enable individuals to perform tasks with dignity. AT enhances cognitive engagement, supports social participation, and improves overall well-being. Simultaneously, by reducing the intensity and frequency of hands-on caregiving, it eases caregiver burden and fosters sustainable care relationships. When thoughtfully implemented, assistive technology transforms the home from a site of dependence into a space of empowerment, equity, and meaningful participation.

Table 5. Key Design Elements for Sensory-Aware Homes

Domain	Design Strategy	Impact on Well-Being
Adaptive Lighting	Use dimmable, warm-toned LEDs; avoid flicker and harsh contrasts	Reduces visual stress, supports circadian rhythms
Acoustic Balance	Incorporate sound-absorbing panels, carpets, and noise-buffering layouts	Minimizes auditory overload, enhances focus and calm
Calming Textiles & Hues	Choose soft textures (cotton, fleece) and muted color palettes (earth tones, pastels)	Creates a soothing, non-triggering atmosphere
Retreat Areas	Design quiet nooks with weighted blankets, soft seating, and low lighting	Offers emotional refuge and aids self-regulation
Personal Touches	Integrate familiar scents, photos, and tactile objects	Reinforces identity, predictability, and emotional grounding

Evidence-Based Framework: ASPECTSS™

The ASPECTSS™ model offers a systematic, evidence-based approach to creating sensory-friendly environments that support autonomy, emotional regulation, and overall well-being for neurodiverse and differently-abled individuals. It guides designers and caregivers in structuring spaces that balance stimulation, calm, and safety within the home.

- **Acoustics:** Minimize unwanted noise and control reverberation to reduce auditory stress and enhance focus.
- **Spatial Sequencing:** Arrange rooms and functional areas logically to support intuitive navigation and reduce confusion.
- **Place for Escape:** Designate quiet retreat zones where individuals can decompress and regulate emotions when overstimulated.
- **Enclosure/Compartmentalization:** Use partitions, furniture, or zoning strategies to define boundaries, creating clarity and structure within multi-use spaces.
- **Clear Transitions:** Employ visual or tactile cues such as changes in flooring, lighting, or textures to signal movement from one area to another, aiding predictability.
- **Tactile/Sensory Zoning:** Organize spaces according to sensory intensity, distinguishing active, high-stimulation zones from calm, low-stimulation areas.

- **Safety:** Prioritize both physical and emotional security through careful material selection, ergonomic layouts, and unobstructed circulation paths.

In home care environments, applying the ASPECTSS™ framework is particularly valuable. By intentionally addressing sensory inputs, spatial organization, and safety, this model helps create settings that foster emotional resilience, reduce stress, and support the daily functioning of both care recipients and their families.

3. Harmonizing Technology and Design: Creating a Holistic Home Ecosystem

The greatest potential for inclusive home care emerges when assistive technology (AT) is thoughtfully integrated with sensory-aware design, forming a cohesive, user-centered ecosystem. For instance, a child with autism may rely on a visual schedule on a tablet (AT) to structure daily routines. Placing this tool in a calm, low-stimulation environment maximizes its effectiveness, supporting emotional regulation, sustained attention, and successful task initiation.

Assistive technologies can be further enhanced through sensory-aware interfaces, such as gentle audio cues, adjustable vibration, or customizable light feedback. These adaptations make devices more intuitive, less overwhelming, and aligned with individual sensory preferences. Simultaneously, sensory-informed design ensures that smart-home devices are seamlessly integrated, with careful attention to placement, ambient stimuli, and overall environmental flow.

Achieving this integration requires individualized assessment. Designers and caregivers must consider medical, cognitive, psychological, and sensory profiles to craft living spaces that genuinely foster independence, comfort, and emotional well-being. By harmonizing mobility aids, visual supports, executive function tools, and sensory-sensitive design, homes can become nurturing environments that empower both care recipients and their families.

Caregiver Training and Trauma-Informed Support

Equipping Families and Support Staff with Skills, Insight, and Compassion: As caregiving increasingly shifts to the home, structured training for family members and support staff is essential. Beyond practical techniques, caregivers benefit from grounding in trauma-informed care, understanding communication differences, and developing emotional self-awareness. These skills are particularly critical in households where past medical interventions, institutional experiences, or sensory sensitivities influence daily behaviours and care needs.

By combining technical proficiency with empathy and awareness, caregivers are better equipped to provide responsive, respectful, and sustainable support. This holistic approach not only enhances the well-being of care recipients but also helps caregivers manage stress, prevent burnout, and maintain a balanced, positive home environment.

Good intentions alone are not enough in caregiving. Without structured training, even the most dedicated family members or support workers can unintentionally create stress, reduce autonomy, or compromise the dignity of those they care for. Miscommunication, blurred boundaries, or an over-reliance on physical assistance can all emerge when caregivers lack the right tools and knowledge.

Competent training is therefore more than a best practice it is both a moral obligation and a practical necessity. In inclusive home care, caregivers are not simply helpers; they are facilitators of autonomy, dignity, and emotional security. The absence of training risks undermining these goals, while the presence of it builds an environment where both care recipients and caregivers thrive.

Table 6. Why Competent Caregiver Training Matters

Challenge Without Training	Impact	Training Solution
Misunderstanding neurodiversity	Leads to frustration, mislabeling, or inappropriate responses	Teach cognitive and neurological differences; foster empathy and tailored support
Limited communication strategies	Causes isolation and unmet needs	Train in AAC tools, PECS, and active listening techniques
Reactive crisis handling	Escalates distress; risks physical/ emotional harm	Equip caregivers with de-escalation and trauma-informed care methods
Disempowering environments	Reduces autonomy and self-worth	Guide caregivers in sensory-aware, independence-enhancing home design
Unintentional bias or disrespect	Damages trust and identity	Promote person-centered, identity-affirming language and cultural humility
Caregiver burnout and turnover	Disrupts continuity and quality of care	Build resilience through skill-building, peer support, and reflective practice

Inclusive, Empathy-Driven Training Models

Training programs are most effective when they are co-designed with disabled individuals and neurodiverse communities, ensuring that lived experience shapes both the curriculum and delivery. This approach reframes disabled people not as passive recipients of care, but as experts in what respectful and empowering support truly looks like.

- **Lived Experience as Expertise:** Trainers with disabilities provide unique perspectives that deepen understanding and dismantle stereotypes.
- **Empathy and Confidence Building:** Caregivers learn to see beyond diagnoses, engaging with individuals as whole persons with strengths, preferences, and identities.
- **Durable, Real-World Skills:** Scenario-based training rooted in everyday challenges prepares caregivers to respond flexibly and competently in diverse situations.

Research reinforces this approach. Reinhard et al. (2019) found that such training improves care outcomes, reduces caregiver stress, and lowers turnover ultimately creating a more sustainable, humane, and equity-driven care ecosystem.

2. Trauma-Informed Care: A Foundation of Safety and Trust

For many neurodiverse and disabled individuals, experiences of trauma are not abstract they are lived realities. Trauma may stem from invasive medical procedures, time spent in institutional settings, or more subtle but equally harmful experiences such as social exclusion, stigma, or bullying. These histories shape how individuals respond to environments, relationships, and care.

Trauma-Informed Care (TIC) rests on five core principles safety, trust, choice, collaboration, and empowerment (Substance Abuse and Mental Health Services Administration, 2014). While often applied in clinical contexts, these principles are equally essential in-home care. The home is not only a physical space but also an emotional and relational one. When infused with TIC, home environments can support recovery, foster autonomy, and provide a sense of refuge from external pressures.

TIC is more than a framework; it is a philosophy of care and design. In inclusive home care, it redefines the role of caregivers and spaces: not to control or correct, but to create conditions where dignity is preserved, autonomy is respected, and trust is nurtured. Applied thoughtfully, TIC transforms houses into places of stability, predictability, and healing.

Table 7. Pillars of TIC & Design Translation

TIC Pillar	Design Translation	Examples
Safety	Predictable environments, sensory regulation, physical security	Soft lighting, soundproofing, non-slip surfaces, secure exits
Trustworthiness	Transparent design, clear routines, visual cues	Daily schedules on walls, labeled storage, consistent spatial layout
Choice	Multiple options for interaction, movement, and engagement	Adjustable furniture, varied seating, control over lighting or sound
Collaboration	Co-designed spaces, shared decision-making	Participatory design with users, feedback loops, flexible zones
Empowerment	Support for autonomy, skill-building, and self-expression	Accessible controls, creative corners, privacy-enhancing features

Table 8. Trauma-Informed Design Matrix by Home Zone

Home Zone	Potential Triggers	Responsive Design Features
Bedroom	Sudden noises, lack of privacy	Sound-dampening materials, blackout curtains, personal decor
Bathroom	Cold surfaces, vulnerability, harsh lighting	Warm lighting, soft textures, privacy locks, sensory-friendly fixtures
Living Area	Overstimulation, unpredictable transitions	Zoned lighting, visual schedules, sensory retreat corners
Kitchen/Dining	Authority dynamics, rigid routines	Choice in seating, visual meal prep guides, collaborative cooking zones
Entry/ Threshold	Disorientation, lack of control	Clear signage, calming colors, welcome cues (e.g., scent, visuals)

Guiding Ethos

"The goal is not therapy it is to create an environment where re-traumatization is prevented, and emotional healing becomes possible."

This ethos reframes the purpose of inclusive home care design. The focus is not on correcting behavior or enforcing compliance, but on building trust and stability. By weaving trauma-informed principles into the physical and relational fabric of the home, caregivers and designers become allies in resilience and recovery.

3. Nurturing Caregiver Emotional Resilience

Caregivers form the emotional backbone of home care systems, yet their own well-being is often overlooked. Designing support structures for caregivers both through training and in the physical environment is not just an act of compassion but also a strategic investment. When caregivers are emotionally sustained, the entire home care ecosystem becomes more resilient, responsive, and humane.

Table 9. Core Support Domains & Strategies

Support Domain	Key Strategies	Design & Training Applications
Emotional Resilience	Mindfulness, self-regulation, reflective practice	Quiet zones, guided journaling prompts, access to calming sensory tools
Peer Connection	Shared experiences, mutual validation, collective problem-solving	Peer support groups, digital forums, storytelling spaces
Professional Support	Counseling, supervision, respite care	Referral pathways, scheduled breaks, access to mental health professionals
Boundary Setting	Role clarity, time management, personal space	Visual schedules, caregiver-only zones, training in assertive communication
Recognition & Inclusion	Valuing caregiver input, co-planning, emotional acknowledgment	Participatory design, feedback loops, rituals of appreciation

Table 10. Matrix: Caregiver Support by Environment Type

Environment Type	Stressors Faced	Supportive Features
Home Setting	Constant availability, emotional labor	Dedicated rest areas, visual reminders for self-care, flexible routines
Training Spaces	Overwhelm, lack of relevance	Trauma-informed pedagogy, experiential learning, reflective journaling
Community Platforms	Isolation, stigma	Peer-led forums, storytelling circles, culturally resonant support groups
Policy & Planning	Exclusion from decision-making	Inclusion in design processes, caregiver advisory boards

Ethos of Caregiver-Centered Design

"Valuing caregivers is not an add-on it is foundational. Their emotional health shapes the quality, sustainability, and humanity of care."

This ethos calls for a systemic shift in how caregiving is understood and supported. Caregivers are not invisible laborers but co-creators of healing environments. Their voices, experiences, and well-being must be integrated into both design and decision-making.

Research across healthcare systems shows that while compassion fatigue and burnout are common, their impact can be significantly reduced through peer support networks, mindfulness-based practices, and strong organizational backing. Recognizing caregivers, including them in planning, and providing structured emotional resources not only protects their health but also strengthens care outcomes for the individuals and families they serve (Cassie et al., 2022).

Advancing Inclusive Home Care Through International Rights Frameworks

Truly inclusive home care does not emerge in isolation; it is rooted in global frameworks that uphold dignity, autonomy, and participation for neurodiverse and differently-abled individuals. International instruments such as the *United Nations Convention on the Rights of Persons with Disabilities (UNCRPD)* and the *World Health Organization's (WHO) disability equity guidelines* represent a fundamental shift from viewing disability primarily as a medical concern to recognizing it as a matter of justice and human rights.

1. The United Nations Convention on the Rights of Persons with Disabilities (UNCRPD)

Adopted in 2006 and ratified by over 185 nations, the UNCRPD has profoundly reshaped disability rights worldwide. It affirms that individuals with disabilities are entitled to live as equal citizens, free from segregation and systemic barriers. Key provisions include:

- **Article 19: Independent Living and Community Inclusion** – the right to choose where and with whom to live, supported by accessible community-based services.
- **Article 23: Respect for Home and Family** – the right to marry, build a family, and access family support without discrimination.
- **Article 25: Health** – equal access to quality healthcare, including services tailored to disability-specific needs.
- **Article 26: Habilitation and Rehabilitation** – access to community-based rehabilitation and caregiver training that strengthen independence and agency.

These principles demand that home care models move beyond institutional mindsets, prioritizing individual choice, empowerment, and inclusion at every level of care.

2. WHO's Global Report on Health Equity for Persons with Disabilities (2022)

In December 2022, the WHO released its first *Global Report on Health Equity for Persons with Disabilities*, highlighting deep-seated inequities. The report documents how people with disabilities often face shorter life expectancy, poorer health outcomes, and restricted participation due to structural barriers and inaccessible systems.

To address these disparities, the WHO recommends:

- Embedding disability equity across all health policies and systems.
- Ensuring people with disabilities have an active role in decision-making.
- Monitoring progress with clear accountability measures.
- Expanding access to primary care, assistive technology, and skilled caregivers as part of universal health coverage (UHC).

These recommendations reinforce that inclusive home care is not a specialized service but an essential component of global health equity.

3. International Models of Inclusive Community Home Care

Several countries have translated these frameworks into practice, offering concrete models that integrate rights with daily living:

- **Sweden's Personal Assistance Model** – provides public funding so individuals can directly hire caregivers of their choice, reinforcing autonomy and agency.
- **New Zealand's Enabling Good Lives (EGL) Framework** – centers on personalized planning, flexible funding, and strong family inclusion to foster independence and belonging.
- **Canada's Independent Living Model** – combines user-led decision-making with access to assistive technology and home-based supports, ensuring both autonomy and community integration.

Together, these approaches affirm a crucial truth: inclusive home care is a human rights imperative, not an act of charity. They echo the principle of self-advocacy and lived experience captured in the disability rights movement's guiding call: *"Nothing about us, without us."*

The Role of AI, Telecare, and Smart Home Integration in Inclusive Home Care

Emerging technologies such as artificial intelligence (AI), telecare platforms, and smart home systems are transforming the landscape of inclusive home care. These innovations provide real-time support for daily living, ease the workload of family caregivers, and expand opportunities for independence among neurodiverse and differently-abled individuals. Yet, their success depends not only on technological sophistication but also on ethical deployment, universal design principles, and accessible implementation. Without these safeguards, the risk of widening existing digital divides remains high.

1. AI-Powered Personalized Care

Recent advances in AI, particularly in machine learning and natural language processing, are creating new pathways for adaptive, home-based support:

- **Predictive Health Monitoring** – Algorithms can analyze sleep, movement, or behavior patterns to detect risks such as falls or agitation, enabling early interventions.
- **Virtual Assistants** – Voice agents and chatbots can provide medication reminders, suggest therapeutic activities, or offer mood check-ins to support daily routines.
- **Adaptive Learning Tools** – Dynamic systems that tailor therapy or educational content in real time, especially beneficial for neurodiverse learners.
- **Affective Computing** – Emotion-recognition software can interpret mood or stress through facial expressions or vocal tone, supporting communication for non-verbal individuals.
- **Decision-Support Systems** – AI can synthesize data from wearables and home sensors to recommend personalized strategies for care.

2. Telecare and Remote Monitoring

Telecare extends the reach of care providers, offering continuity and security within the home environment:

- **Emergency Response Systems** – Devices such as fall detectors, GPS trackers, and panic buttons provide round-the-clock safety.
- **Health Tracking** – Remote monitoring of vital signs supports chronic condition management and early detection of health concerns.

- **Virtual Consultations** – Online appointments reduce the burden of in-person visits, especially for individuals with sensory sensitivities.
- **Collaborative Care Platforms** – Digital dashboards enable families, therapists, and paid caregivers to coordinate routines and share progress.
- **Routine Stability** – Consistency through telecare minimizes disruptions, which is particularly valuable for those sensitive to change.

3. Smart Home Technology for Daily Independence

Smart home integration enhances autonomy by aligning the living environment with individual needs:

- **Voice-Controlled Interfaces** – Tools such as Alexa or Google Assistant allow simple management of lighting, appliances, and entertainment.
- **Home Security and Access** – Smart locks and monitoring systems provide safer, more manageable control of personal spaces.
- **Operational Safety Features** – Auto shut-off devices for stoves, faucets, and other appliances help prevent accidents.
- **Adaptive Environments** – Lighting systems that regulate sensory comfort or support circadian rhythms contribute to well-being. Evidence suggests that these features promote confidence, autonomy, and self-esteem, reinforcing the value of inclusive design.

4. Ethics, Accessibility, and Equitable Use

While the advantages are clear, the ethical and practical challenges of implementing advanced technology must not be overlooked:

- **Cost and Equity** – High-tech systems remain inaccessible for many households. Subsidy programs or community-driven solutions are needed to prevent exclusion.
- **Privacy and Consent** – Continuous data collection requires robust safeguards and transparent processes for informed consent.
- **Usability** – Interfaces must be intuitive, adaptable, and culturally relevant, ensuring they are usable across diverse populations.
- **Ethical Deployment** – Co-design processes that actively involve people with disabilities are essential, ensuring that technologies reflect lived experience rather than imposing external assumptions.

Framed in this way, AI, telecare, and smart home technologies are not simply innovations they are tools for equity and dignity, provided they are designed and delivered responsibly.

Building Home Care Together: Collaboration, Respect, and Shared Ownership

Truly inclusive and person-centered care requires moving away from top-down structures and toward systems developed with families and individuals, rather than for them. This shift acknowledges that people with disabilities, along with their families, bring critical expertise shaped by daily lived experience. When their voices, cultural contexts, and perspectives directly inform the design of care systems, the result is more responsive, equitable, and sustainable support.

Family members particularly those who serve as primary caregivers carry much of the responsibility for everyday care. They coordinate therapies, adapt living environments, manage medications, navigate paperwork, and provide continuous emotional support. Yet despite this central role, their insights are frequently overlooked, leaving many care systems misaligned with real-world needs. Research highlights that when families are included in planning, outcomes improve: solutions become more practical, efficient, and culturally relevant (Reinhard et al., 2019).

Co-design ensures that families and individuals are involved throughout the entire process from identifying challenges to creating and testing solutions. This participatory approach builds trust, fosters ownership, and ensures that care systems remain meaningful and contextually grounded (Bate & Robert, 2006).

Most importantly, co-design acknowledges and validates the invisible expertise of caregivers the adaptive skills they have honed through years of navigating complex care without recognition. By positioning caregivers as visible partners in decision-making, care systems become not only more effective but also more sustainable, grounded in the realities of those they serve.

CONCLUSION

Home care for neurodiverse and differently-abled individuals must be re-envisioned not as a narrow extension of medical treatment, but as a holistic, person-centered system grounded in dignity, rights, and belonging. Conventional care models too often emphasize limitations, overlooking the diverse sensory, communicative, and functional realities that shape daily life. This chapter has argued for a shift in perspective: one that draws from disability studies, occupational therapy, human rights frameworks, and holistic health to promote care that is inclusive, equitable, and sustainable. At the heart of this vision are several interconnected building blocks: sensory-aware environments, adaptive and assistive technologies, visual and communication supports, trauma-informed practices, AI-driven tools, telecare, smart home systems, caregiver training, and robust global policy frameworks. These elements, when combined with community-based rehabilitation, peer support networks, and participatory co-design, form an integrated ecosystem capable of responding to real human needs with both respect and innovation.

International rights frameworks provide the foundation for this shift. The UN Convention on the Rights of Persons with Disabilities (UNCRPD), particularly Article 19, affirms the right to independent living and access to community-based support services recognizing autonomy and inclusion as universal entitlements. Similarly, the WHO's 2022 Global Report on Health Equity for Persons with Disabilities highlights systemic barriers that persist worldwide, including inaccessible environments, insufficient workforce training, and the absence of individualized support. These challenges underscore the urgency of rethinking how home care is structured and delivered. A way forward lies in uniting rights-based policy with grassroots, community-centered strategies. By embedding CBR, peer networks, and family-led co-design into the very architecture of care systems, we can move beyond models of charity or compliance toward approaches that honor lived experience and self-determination.

Ultimately, reimagining home care is not simply about providing services or removing obstacles it is about advancing justice, autonomy, and shared humanity. An inclusive and responsive home care framework affirms that every individual has the right not only to survive, but to live with dignity, choice, and belonging at the very heart of their community.

REFERENCES

Ashburner, J., Ziviani, J., & Rodger, S. (2013). Sensory processing and classroom emotional, behavioural, and educational outcomes in children with autism spectrum disorder. *The American Journal of Occupational Therapy*, *67*(5), 562–573. DOI: 10.5014/ajot.2013.008821

Bate, P., & Robert, G. (2006). Experience-based design: From redesigning the system around the patient to co-designing services with the patient. *Quality & Safety in Health Care*, *15*(5), 307–310. DOI: 10.1136/qshc.2005.016527 PMID: 17074863

Brimblecombe, N., Piccardt, L., King, D., Knapp, M., & Stevens, M. (2018). Perceptions of unmet needs for community social care services in England: A qualitative study of older people, carers and professionals. *Health & Social Care in the Community*, *26*(3), e241–e249. DOI: 10.1111/hsc.12522

Cassie, K. M., Snyder, M., & McClure, R. (2022). Caring in place: A framework for inclusive home environments. *Journal of Housing for the Elderly*, *36*(1), 74–93. DOI: 10.1080/02763893.2021.1944985

Chung, M. L., Chen, Y., & Chou, K. R. (2021). Effects of caregiving burden, resilience, and social support on family caregivers' physical and mental health. *Archives of Psychiatric Nursing*, *35*, 87–94. DOI: 10.1016/j.apnu.2021.01.004

Hodgetts, S., Nicholas, D., Zwaigenbaum, L., & McConnell, D. (2013). Parents' and professionals' perceptions of family-centered care for children with autism spectrum disorder across service sectors. *Social Science & Medicine*, *96*, 138–146. DOI: 10.1016/j.socscimed.2013.07.012 PMID: 24034961

Imrie, R., & Luck, R. (2014). Designing inclusive environments: Rehabilitating the body and the relevance of universal design. *Disability and Rehabilitation*, *36*(16), 1315–1319. DOI: 10.3109/09638288.2014.936191 PMID: 24989068

Kapp, S. K. (Ed.). (2020). *Autistic community and the neurodiversity movement: Stories from the frontline*. Springer., DOI: 10.1007/978-981-13-8437-0

Kuhlthau, K. A., O'Connor, K., & Perrin, J. M. (2022). Caring for children with autism spectrum disorder: The experience of caregivers. *Journal of Autism and Developmental Disorders*, *52*(3), 1408–1420. DOI: 10.1007/s10803-021-05052-8 PMID: 33909211

Mostafa, M. (2014). Architecture for autism: Autism ASPECTSS™ in school design. *Archnet-IJAR*, *8*(1), 143–158. DOI: 10.26687/archnet-ijar.v8i1.314

Oliver, M., & Barnes, C. (2012). *The new politics of disablement.* Palgrave Macmillan. DOI: 10.1007/978-0-230-39244-1

Reinhard, S. C., Levine, C., & Samis, S. (2019). Home alone revisited: Family caregivers providing complex care. AARP Public Policy Institute. https://www.aarp.org/content/dam/aarp/ppi/2019/04/home-alone-revisited-family-caregivers-providing-complex-care.pdf

Substance Abuse and Mental Health Services Administration. (2014). SAMHSA's concept of trauma and guidance for a trauma-informed approach. https://ncsacw.samhsa.gov/userfiles/files/SAMHSA_Trauma.pdf

Verdonschot, M. M. L., de Witte, L. P., Reichrath, E., Buntinx, W. H. E., & Curfs, L. M. G. (2009). Impact of environmental factors on community participation of persons with an intellectual disability: A systematic review. *Journal of Intellectual Disability Research, 53*(1), 54–64. DOI: 10.1111/j.1365-2788.2008.01128.x PMID: 19093982

Chapter 5
Integrating Clinical Evidence Into Holistic Home Care for Families and Caregivers

Shivansu Sachan
https://orcid.org/0000-0002-9893-8018
CSJM University, India

Aishwarya Arya
https://orcid.org/0009-0000-4236-3983
CSJM University, India

Mohammad Badruddoza Talukder
https://orcid.org/0009-0008-1662-9221
International University of Business Agriculture and Technology, Bangladesh

Ankit Kumar
https://orcid.org/0009-0009-5002-4522
CSJM University, India

ABSTRACT

Family caregivers play a pivotal role in sustaining the health and well-being of individuals requiring long-term or specialized home care. However, the absence of structured, evidence-based approaches often places caregivers at risk of physical, emotional, and economic strain. This chapter examines integrative home care frameworks that merge clinical evidence with holistic health practices to optimize both patient and caregiver outcomes. Drawing on empirical studies, clinical guidelines, and interdisciplinary care models, it explores strategies for managing chronic

DOI: 10.4018/979-8-3373-4094-4.ch005

illnesses, promoting mental health resilience, and enhancing caregiver competence. The discussion addresses the synergy between biomedical interventions, psychosocial support, and culturally responsive care, offering a comprehensive perspective on home-based health delivery. Emphasis is placed on actionable pathways for translating clinical research into practical caregiving interventions, including the use of standardized assessment tools, tailored education programs, and coordinated community resources.

INTRODUCTION

The integration of clinical evidence into holistic home care is supported by several conceptual models that provide structured frameworks for aligning family involvement, multidisciplinary collaboration, and evidence-based practices (EBP). These models offer practical and theoretical guidance on transforming fragmented home care into a cohesive, research-informed system.

One of the most prominent models is the Home-based Longitudinal Investigation of the multidisciplinary Team Integrated Care (HOLISTIC) framework, developed in Taiwan. This nationwide prospective cohort study, launched in 2020, tracks health outcomes, caregiver burden, healthcare utilization, and economic implications over a 24-month period among home health care recipients (Chen et al., 2021). The HOLISTIC model emphasizes comprehensive assessment across physical, psychological, social, and financial dimensions while integrating family caregivers as active stakeholders in care delivery, monitoring, and decision-making. Early findings from the protocol suggest that multidisciplinary, evidence-based planning significantly reduces hospitalizations and improves continuity of care in home-based settings (Chen et al., 2021; Lin & Huang, 2022).

Another important model is the Patient and Family Engaged Care (PFEC) framework, which promotes shared decision-making between healthcare professionals, patients, and family caregivers. The PFEC model integrates EBP by ensuring that caregivers are involved not only in care implementation but also in research design, quality improvement processes, and outcome evaluation (Carman et al., 2016). Recent updates to the model highlight the importance of integrating digital tools, clinical guidelines, and caregiver education to tailor evidence-based interventions to diverse home environments (Vaismoradi et al., 2023).

The RAND Family Caregiver Integration Framework further contributes by identifying systemic barriers to caregiver inclusion in clinical practices, such as inadequate training, lack of legal access to medical records, and communication gaps between families and healthcare teams. This framework recommends policy support for standardized caregiver education, proxy access to patient data, and inclusion of caregivers in interdisciplinary care teams (Weiss et al., 2020). It is built on scoping reviews conducted between 2015 and 2021 and has informed caregiver-support legislation and hospital-to-home transition models in the United States and Europe.

Another emerging model is the Well-Teach Framework (2024), which emphasizes strengthening evidence-based competencies not only among nurses and educators but also among family caregivers. The model encourages experiential learning, reflective practice, and holistic training modules covering clinical evidence, emotional intelligence, complementary therapies, and caregiver self-care (Gutiérrez & Ramos, 2024). Studies report that application of the Well-Teach model increases caregiver confidence, reduces anxiety, and enhances quality of life for both caregivers and patients (Gutiérrez & Ramos, 2024).

These conceptual models collectively demonstrate that integrating clinical evidence into holistic home care requires collaborative structures that recognize caregivers as critical partners. They advocate for interdisciplinary teamwork, structured training, policy-level support, and adaptable frameworks that reflect cultural, economic, and environmental contexts. Longitudinal evidence from initiatives like HOLISTIC and PFEC reinforces the view that caregiver-inclusive, evidence-based home care enhances patient outcomes, reduces hospitalization, and strengthens caregiver resilience (Lin & Huang, 2022; Weiss et al., 2020). Therefore, these models form the foundation for future research and policy design in holistic home care systems.

India, like many developing and developed nations, is experiencing a demographic transition marked by a rapidly aging population and an increase in chronic, non-communicable diseases such as cardiovascular illnesses, diabetes, dementia, and cancer (Ramachandran et al., 2019; Ministry of Health and Family Welfare [MoHFW], 2023). This epidemiological shift has increased the demand for long-term, affordable, and patient-centered healthcare services outside formal hospital settings. In this context, holistic home care, which integrates physical, psychological, social, emotional, and spiritual dimensions of health, has emerged as a vital component of India's evolving healthcare system. Unlike institutional care, holistic home care empowers individuals to receive evidence-informed treatment within familiar environments, preserving dignity, cultural values, and familial relationships (Chakrabarti, 2016).

Holistic home care in India is not a new concept. Traditional healing systems such as Ayurveda, Yoga, Unani, Siddha, and Homeopathy (AYUSH) have long emphasized family participation, lifestyle balance, and the interconnectedness of body, mind, and spirit (Tandon & Sharma, 2020). However, the contemporary challenge lies in integrating clinical evidence from biomedical research and evidence-based practice (EBP) into these culturally rooted caregiving practices. Clinical evidence—derived from randomized controlled trials, meta-analyses, and systematic reviews—ensures that care practices are safe, effective, and aligned with global healthcare standards (Sackett et al., 1996; Paul & Sinha, 2022). When such evidence is embedded into household caregiving routines, it reduces preventable complications, enhances quality of life, and lowers hospitalization rates (Nair & Prasad, 2021).

Families and caregivers serve as the central pillars of home-based care in India. Over 80% of long-term care for older adults and chronically ill patients is provided by unpaid family members, most often women (Rajagopal & Joad, 2020). According to a report by the International Labour Organization (ILO, 2021), informal caregiving in India contributes billions to the economy in unpaid labor, yet caregivers often lack access to structured training, clinical guidance, or psychosocial support. This gap between medical recommendations and home-based practices can lead to medication errors, emotional burnout, poor symptom management, and delayed medical intervention (Chandra & Banerjee, 2020). Thus, integrating evidence-based clinical knowledge into family caregiving is essential for safe and effective home care delivery.

This chapter defines holistic home care as a multidimensional approach that integrates biomedical treatment, complementary therapies such as Ayurveda and yoga, psychosocial support, and spiritual care while emphasizing the active role of families and caregivers. It explores how clinical evidence can be translated into home environments through structured training, technology-assisted platforms, caregiver support programs, community health networks, and interdisciplinary care models. The chapter is structured into the following sections: (1) introduction, (2) literature review, (3) historical and conceptual foundations, (4) key conceptual models, (5) practical integration strategies, (6) roles of families and caregivers, (7) challenges and barriers, (8) global and Indian case studies, (9) policy implications, and (10) conclusion and future directions.

Recent initiatives in India, such as the National Programme for Palliative Care (NPPC), Health and Wellness Centres under Ayushman Bharat, and Kerala's Neighbourhood Network in Palliative Care (NNPC), demonstrate successful examples of community-led, evidence-informed, home-based care (Kumar, 2018; MoHFW, 2022). These models highlight that when families are empowered with clinical knowledge—such as pain management techniques, physiotherapy routines, infection control practices, and end-of-life care protocols—both patient outcomes and caregiver resilience improve significantly (Salins et al., 2022).

Furthermore, integrating clinical evidence into home care aligns with national and global priorities like the WHO's Integrated People-Centred Health Services (IPCHS) Framework and India's National Health Policy (2017), both of which emphasize accessibility, affordability, continuity of care, and community participation. As India moves toward value-based care, the inclusion of families and caregivers as active partners in care delivery is essential for achieving the Quadruple Aim:

improving patient experience, enhancing population health, reducing costs, and supporting healthcare providers (Basu & Patnaik, 2023).

In summary, the effectiveness of holistic home care in India depends on the systematic integration of clinical evidence into daily caregiving practices performed by families and informal caregivers. This chapter argues that empowering caregivers through training, technology, policy support, and multidisciplinary collaboration is not only essential for quality care but also crucial for sustainable healthcare delivery in resource-limited settings.

2. LITERATURE REVIEW

2.1 Overview of Existing Literature

The integration of clinical evidence into holistic home care has received increasing academic attention globally and within India over the past decade, particularly due to rising chronic illnesses, aging populations, and the limitations of institutional healthcare systems (Nair & Prasad, 2021). Holistic home care is widely defined as an approach that addresses physical, emotional, psychological, social, and spiritual dimensions of health (Chakrabarti, 2016). Scholars emphasize that evidence-based practice (EBP) is essential to ensure safety, reduce hospitalization, and enhance quality of life in home care settings (Sackett et al., 1996; Paul & Sinha, 2022). In India, this need is particularly pronounced due to overburdened hospitals, inadequate geriatric infrastructure, and the cultural expectation that families provide caregiving (Rajagopal & Joad, 2020).

2.2 Global Literature on Evidence-Based Holistic Home Care

International research shows that evidence-based interventions in home settings reduce hospital readmissions by 20–30%, especially for chronic illnesses such as COPD, diabetes, dementia, and stroke (Harris et al., 2020; WHO, 2022). A Cochrane review by Gomes et al. (2021) found that integrating palliative care at home, supported by trained caregivers, improved patient satisfaction and reduced emergency visits. Studies from the UK's National Institute for Health and Care Excellence (NICE) recommend caregiver education, symptom management protocols, and follow-up teleconsultations as essential for evidence-based home care (NICE, 2019).

The COVID-19 pandemic accelerated telehealth-enabled home care globally, promoting digital monitoring, video consultations, and AI-supported medication reminders (Koonin et al., 2020). Studies in Australia and Canada found improved caregiver confidence when digital platforms provided credible clinical guidelines and emergency support (Breen et al., 2022). However, a recurring limitation highlighted in global literature is the lack of cultural adaptation of EBP to non-Western familial caregiving systems and lower-resource settings (Vaismoradi et al., 2023).

2.3 Indian Literature on Family-Centered Home Care

Indian authors emphasize that caregiving is deeply embedded in socio-cultural values, where families are considered the primary "healthcare unit" rather than hospitals (Chakrabarti, 2016; Salins et al., 2022). The National Health Policy (2017) and Ayushman Bharat (2018) encourage home-based care through Health and Wellness Centres (HWCs). Additionally, Kerala's Neighbourhood Network in Palliative Care (NNPC)—a globally recognized model—employs community volunteers trained in evidence-based pain management and home-based palliative care (Kumar, 2018). Studies on NNPC report significant reductions in healthcare costs and caregiver distress (Salins et al., 2022).

Research by Rajagopal & Palat (2020) demonstrates that more than 75% of Indian patients with terminal conditions prefer to die at home, yet only 10% receive clinically guided home care due to lack of trained caregivers. Studies by Narayanan (2021) and MoHFW (2022) underscore that most Indian families rely on informal knowledge, traditional remedies, or AYUSH practices without clinical supervision, increasing risk of complications.

A significant body of Indian nursing literature discusses evidence-based nursing in community settings. Paul & Sinha (2022) argue that nurses can bridge the gap between hospitals and homes by training caregivers in infection prevention, wound care, rehabilitation exercises, and medication safety. Similarly, ICMR (2021) reports that caregiver education reduces medication errors by 40%.

2.4 Clinical Evidence and Complementary Systems (AYUSH + Biomedicine)

Indian studies uniquely highlight the coexistence of biomedical and AYUSH-based home care. For instance, Ayurveda recommends dietary regulation, herbal formulations, yoga, and pranayama for chronic illness management, but integration with clinical protocols remains limited (Tandon & Sharma, 2020). A Delhi-based study by Sharma & Gupta (2021) showed that combining yoga-based respiratory exercises with clinical evidence from pulmonary rehabilitation improved outcomes in COPD patients receiving home care.

However, several Indian scholars caution against using alternative therapies without clinical validation. A study by Nair & Prasad (2021) showed that 32% of rural caregivers delayed hospital referrals due to reliance on traditional therapies, which sometimes worsened the condition. This calls for **evidence-based integration rather than replacement** of medical guidelines.

2.5 Role of Telemedicine, mHealth, and AI in Home Care in India

Post-pandemic, digital health has emerged as a transformative tool for caregivers. The eSanjeevani telemedicine platform by the Government of India has successfully conducted over 10 crore teleconsultations, offering doctor-to-patient care from home (MoHFW, 2023). Studies by Basu & Patnaik (2023) and Srinivasan et al. (2022) show that AI-based reminders, digital prescriptions, and WhatsApp-based nurse consultations improved adherence to evidence-based home care.

Apps like Aarogya Setu, Practo, MySeniorDoctor, and Palliative Care Helpline Kerala offer medication guidance, diet plans, physiotherapy videos, and remote monitoring. However, digital divide, low digital literacy, and language barriers limit usage in rural areas (Chandra & Banerjee, 2020).

3. HISTORICAL AND CONCEPTUAL FOUNDATIONS OF HOLISTIC HOME CARE

3.1 Ancient and Indigenous Roots of Holistic Care in India

The concept of holistic care in India has deep historical roots, predating modern medicine by thousands of years. Ancient Indian medical systems such as Ayurveda, Yoga, Siddha, and Unani emphasized the interconnectedness of the body, mind, spirit, family, and environment, laying an early foundation for what modern health-care now calls "holistic care" (Sharma & Dash, 2019). Ayurveda, documented in classical texts like the *Charaka Samhita* and *Sushruta Samhita*, promotes *swasthya* (a state of complete well-being) through balance of the three doshas (Vata, Pitta, Kapha) and lifestyle-based healing implemented within the household (Tandon & Sharma, 2020). Practices such as herbal formulations, dietary routines, *abhyanga* (therapeutic massage), *pranayama* (breathing exercises), and meditation highlight family involvement and home-based care traditions.

Similarly, traditional healing systems across Indian villages involved community caregivers, including midwives (*dais*), herbal healers, and elders, who delivered home-based care rooted in cultural knowledge, spirituality, and social interdependence (Sujatha, 2014). These systems viewed illness not merely as a physical condition but as a disturbance of social harmony and spiritual well-being, aligning with today's integrative health paradigms.

3.2 Colonial Influence and Institutionalization of Healthcare

With British colonization, Western biomedicine was introduced in India through hospitals, military health services, and missionary clinics (Arnold, 1993). This period marked a shift from community and family-centric care to institutionalized, clinical-based healthcare delivery. However, home care continued in parallel, especially in rural areas where hospitals were inaccessible.

British-era public health policies focused on infectious disease control, sanitation, and epidemic management, rather than chronic illness or family-based care (Jeffery, 2019). Nevertheless, nursing—introduced by Florence Nightingale's influence—laid the groundwork for professional caregiving, although it remained hospital-centric initially.

3.3 Post-Independence: Reintegration of Community and Family Care

After 1947, India's healthcare vision under the Bhore Committee (1946) and later National Health Policies (1983, 2002, 2017) emphasized primary health care, rural health services, and community participation. The concept of home-based care regained relevance, particularly under programs like:

- **National Health Mission (NHM)** – promoting community health workers like ASHAs (Accredited Social Health Activists)
- **Home-Based Newborn Care (HBNC)** – training mothers and ASHAs to manage neonatal care (Bang et al., 2005)
- **Home-Based Palliative Care Models** – especially in Kerala through the *Neighbourhood Network in Palliative Care (NNPC)*, integrating evidence-based symptom management into households (Kumar, 2018)

These initiatives reflect a hybrid approach blending clinical science with traditional community support.

3.4 Evolution of Evidence-Based Practice (EBP) in Home Care

The concept of Evidence-Based Practice (EBP) originated in Western biomedicine through scholars like Sackett et al. (1996), defining it as the integration of best research evidence, clinical expertise, and patient values. In India, the adoption of

EBP in home settings began in nursing, geriatric care, and palliative medicine in the early 2000s (Paul & Sinha, 2022).

Indian scholars argue that applying EBP in home care requires adaptation to cultural norms, literacy levels, and resource settings, rather than direct replication of hospital protocols (Chandra & Banerjee, 2020). For example, evidence-based protocols for pressure ulcer prevention, diabetes management, and wound care must be simplified for family caregivers.

4. KEY CONCEPTUAL MODELS FOR INTEGRATING CLINICAL EVIDENCE INTO HOLISTIC HOME CARE

The integration of clinical evidence within holistic home care is guided by several conceptual frameworks developed globally and adapted within the Indian context. These models emphasize patient-centeredness, family involvement, symptom management, interdisciplinary teamwork, and culturally appropriate implementation of biomedical guidelines. The following section presents both international and Indian conceptual models that influence the integration of evidence-based practices (EBP) into family-managed home care.

4.1 WHO Integrated People-Centred Health Services (IPCHS) Framework

The World Health Organization's IPCHS Framework (2016) emphasizes health systems that are coordinated, evidence-based, and centered around individuals, families, and communities (WHO, 2016). It highlights five strategies:

1. Engaging patients and families as partners in care.
2. Strengthening governance and accountability.
3. Reorienting healthcare models towards community and home settings.
4. Coordinating services across levels of care.
5. Creating supportive environments for caregivers.

This model has been instrumental in shaping home-based health policies globally and in India's National Health Policy (2017), which incorporates family caregivers and Accredited Social Health Activists (ASHAs) into community care delivery (MoHFW, 2017).

4.2 Patient and Family Engaged Care (PFEC) Model

The PFEC Model, developed by Carman et al. (2016), conceptualizes care delivery as a partnership among healthcare professionals, patients, and family caregivers. It integrates clinical evidence by ensuring:

- Shared decision-making based on research-backed information.
- Care plans that are implemented collaboratively between clinicians and family members.
- Empowerment of caregivers through training, access to patient records, and ongoing support.

In India, PFEC principles are being applied in hospitals such as AIIMS Delhi, Tata Memorial Centre Mumbai, and Christian Medical College (CMC), Vellore, where family members are trained in wound care, medication management, physiotherapy, and palliative support (Salins et al., 2022).

4.3 RAND Caregiver Integration Framework

The RAND Framework (Weiss et al., 2020) offers a structured approach to integrating caregivers into healthcare systems. The model proposes four pillars:

- **Identification of caregivers** within medical documentation.
- **Assessment of caregiver needs** (physical, emotional, informational).
- **Support through training and resources** based on evidence-based guidelines.
- **Inclusion of caregivers in decision-making and care transition planning.**

This model is particularly useful in India, where families are primary caregivers but largely untrained. It aligns with efforts by ICMR and the Indian Palliative Care Association to include caregiver needs assessment tools and structured home-care training modules (Rajagopal & Palat, 2020).

4.4 HOLISTIC Model (Taiwan) – Global Example

The HOme-based Longitudinal Investigation of multidisciplinary integrated Care (HOLISTIC) Model is a Taiwanese initiative that tracks patients with chronic diseases receiving home health care (Chen et al., 2021). Its core features include:

- Continuous home-based clinical monitoring

- Multidisciplinary teams (doctors, nurses, physiotherapists, social workers)
- Family caregiver training protocols
- Evidence-based symptom management (pain, mobility, nutrition)
- Reduction of hospital readmissions by 25–30%

This model is particularly relevant to India, where chronic illness prevalence is rising and hospital resources are limited.

4.5 Indian Model: Neighbourhood Network in Palliative Care (NNPC), Kerala

One of the most successful Indian frameworks, NNPC (Kerala), integrates clinical evidence with community participation. Developed in the 1990s, it is now globally recognized (Kumar, 2018).

Key elements include:

- Community volunteers trained using WHO palliative care guidelines.
- Home visits for pain management, wound dressing, and terminal care.
- Involvement of family caregivers in symptom management using clinical protocols.
- Evidence-based opioid use for pain management (morphine accessibility).

This model demonstrates how clinical expertise + local community engagement can operationalize holistic home care.

4.6 Tata Memorial Centre – Home-Based Cancer Care Model (Mumbai)

Tata Memorial Centre provides an evidence-based home palliative care service for terminal cancer patients. Components include:

- Caregiver training in pain medication, oral morphine dosage, hydration, and bedsore prevention.
- Tele-guidance from oncology nurses using clinical algorithms.
- Family inclusion in end-of-life care decision-making (Salins et al., 2022).

This model supports clinical accuracy while preserving emotional and cultural sensitivity in home environments.

4.7 AIIMS Delhi Dementia and Stroke Home Care Protocols

AIIMS and NIMHANS (Bengaluru) have developed caregiver-centric, evidence-based protocols for dementia and post-stroke rehabilitation. These include:

- Cognitive stimulation therapy at home
- Daily physiotherapy/occupational therapy modules
- Patient transfer techniques to prevent injuries to caregivers
- Use of mobile apps for medication and diet adherence (Verma & Yadav, 2021)

This model integrates neuroscience, nursing, physiotherapy, and family care-based practices.

5. STRATEGIES FOR PRACTICAL INTEGRATION OF CLINICAL EVIDENCE INTO HOLISTIC HOME CARE

The successful integration of clinical evidence into holistic home care requires a structured yet culturally adaptable approach that aligns biomedical guidelines with family caregiving practices, community resources, and traditional healing systems. In the Indian context, where more than 80% of home-based care is delivered by family members with minimal formal training (Rajagopal & Joad, 2020), the challenge lies in simplifying clinical knowledge into practical, comprehensible, and culturally relevant care routines. This section outlines strategic pathways for integrating evidence-based practices (EBP) into home care, focusing on caregiver training, technology, interdisciplinary collaboration, community-based systems, and integration of AYUSH with biomedical care.

A primary strategy involves structured training for family caregivers and community health workers in basic clinical procedures, symptom management, and decision-making. Studies from Kerala's Neighbourhood Network in Palliative Care (NNPC) showed that when caregivers were trained in evidence-based pain assessment tools, oral morphine use, wound care, and pressure sore prevention, patient comfort improved significantly and hospitalization rates reduced (Kumar, 2018). Training must be delivered in regional languages using visual aids, demonstration-based modules, and culturally sensitive examples. For chronic illnesses like diabetes, hypertension, dementia, and stroke, simplified clinical guidelines based on ICMR and AIIMS protocols can be converted into home care manuals, addressing medication adherence, diet planning, exercise routines, physiotherapy, and danger signs requiring hospital referral (Paul & Sinha, 2022). Nurses, ASHA workers, and palliative care volunteers are critical intermediaries who translate scientific knowledge into community practice, making home care safer and more scientific.

Technology-enabled care is another powerful strategy for bridging the gap between homes and healthcare institutions. Telemedicine platforms such as eSanjeevani, launched by the Indian Ministry of Health and Family Welfare, enable remote doctor consultations, digital prescriptions, and follow-up care without requiring hospital visits (MoHFW, 2023). Mobile health applications like Practo, Aarogya Setu, and AIIMS iGeriCare offer medication reminders, blood glucose tracking, diet charts, physiotherapy videos, and even emergency consultations. For patients with dementia, stroke, or post-operative conditions, tele-rehabilitation models provide video-guided physiotherapy sessions and caregiver counseling (Verma & Yadav, 2021). Digital platforms support evidence-based practices by ensuring timely access to clinical guidelines and patient data; however, they must be designed to address India's digital divide by supporting regional languages, offline accessibility, and low-bandwidth environments (Basu & Patnaik, 2023). Incorporating artificial intelligence-based tools for drug reminders, fall detection, pulse and oxygen monitoring, and mental health screening offers an added layer of safety and precision.

Interdisciplinary collaboration forms the backbone of evidence-based home care. Research indicates that when doctors, nurses, physiotherapists, psychologists, dieticians, and social workers work together with families, patients receive more comprehensive and coordinated care, reducing fragmentation and clinical errors (Salins et al., 2022). Models like the HOLISTIC study in Taiwan and Tata Memorial Hospital's home-based cancer care exemplify how interdisciplinary teams can remotely supervise care while empowering caregivers to execute protocols at home (Chen et al., 2021). In India, similar models are emerging, particularly in oncology, geriatrics, stroke rehabilitation, and palliative care. For instance, in AIIMS New Delhi's dementia care initiative, neurologists design treatment plans, nurses train families in cognitive exercises, physiotherapists guide mobility practices, and psychologists provide behavioral counseling—all adapted from clinical evidence (Verma & Yadav, 2021). This collaborative approach ensures that evidence does not remain confined to hospitals but is practically implemented within households.

Community-based models further strengthen evidence integration by decentralizing care delivery and reducing dependence on hospitals. Kerala's NNPC, the Tata Trust's Rural Cancer Care Programme, and Tamil Nadu's Community-Based Rehabilitation Schemes demonstrate how local volunteers, NGOs, and trained palliative workers can deliver scientifically validated care under professional supervision (Kumar, 2018; Rajagopal & Palat, 2020). In these models, community ownership reduces caregiver burden, improves accessibility of medications, and fosters emotional and social support. These systems work effectively when backed by standardized evidence-based guidelines, morphine availability for pain control, and referral linkages with primary health centres or district hospitals.

Integrating AYUSH systems such as Ayurveda, Yoga, and Naturopathy with clinical evidence-based practices is a uniquely Indian strategy to enhance holistic care. Ayurveda-based home routines like dietary adjustments, herbal decoctions, and therapies like *abhyanga* (massage) or *shirodhara* can complement biomedical care when scientifically validated and supervised (Tandon & Sharma, 2020). For example, yoga and pranayama have been incorporated into rehabilitation protocols for chronic obstructive pulmonary disease (COPD), hypertension, and anxiety disorders, supported by AIIMS and ICMR research (Sharma & Gupta, 2021). However, experts caution that AYUSH-based interventions must not replace evidence-based medicine for conditions requiring clinical treatment; instead, they should act as complementary systems that enhance mental well-being, immunity, and patient compliance when integrated under proper clinical guidance (Nair & Prasad, 2021).

Additionally, policy-level strategies are crucial to institutionalizing evidence-based home care. The National Programme for Palliative Care (NPPC), Ayushman Bharat Health and Wellness Centres, and National Programme for Healthcare of the Elderly (NPHCE) have created frameworks for home-based services, including financial support, training, and telemedicine integration (MoHFW, 2022). Policies should emphasize caregiver incentives, inclusion of home care in insurance coverage, availability of essential medications, and integration of home-based records into national health databases. Creating caregiver certification programmes, similar to nursing assistants, can also improve quality and dignity of unpaid caregiving labour.

In summary, the integration of clinical evidence into holistic home care in India requires a multi-layered approach involving caregiver training, digital health solutions, interdisciplinary collaboration, community participation, judicious fusion of AYUSH systems with biomedical science, and supportive health policies. These strategies bridge the gap between medical knowledge and domestic caregiving, ensuring that families are empowered, patients receive safe and dignified care at home, and healthcare systems become more sustainable and people-centred.

6. ROLE OF FAMILIES AND CAREGIVERS IN HOLISTIC HOME CARE INTEGRATION

Families and caregivers serve as the backbone of holistic home care, particularly in India where caregiving is not only a familial responsibility but a socio-cultural expectation rooted in traditions of filial piety and collective living. Over 80% of long-term care for the elderly, terminally ill, disabled, or chronically sick patients in India is provided by unpaid family members, predominantly women such as wives, daughters, and daughters-in-law (Rajagopal & Joad, 2020). Unlike in Western countries where formal caregiving and institutional elderly care services are more common, the Indian healthcare system implicitly relies on families to act as mediators between professional healthcare services and the patient at home. This makes families indispensable agents in translating clinical evidence into day-to-day practices. They are responsible for administering medications, monitoring symptoms, assisting with mobility, maintaining hygiene, performing diet-based interventions, and providing emotional and spiritual support. The effectiveness of home-based care, therefore, largely depends on the knowledge, emotional resilience, and skill level of caregivers.

Caregivers play a crucial role in bridging the gap between clinical care and the home environment. However, without access to structured clinical knowledge or evidence-based resources, many caregivers rely on intuition, past experience, cultural practices, or unverified information. This can lead to medication errors, missed symptoms, improper wound care, nutritional deficiencies, or delayed hospital referrals (Chandra & Banerjee, 2020). In India, where many chronically ill patients live in rural or peri-urban areas with limited access to specialists, caregivers often act as the first responders and primary decision-makers. Studies on home-based cancer and dementia care at AIIMS and Tata Memorial Centre reveal that trained caregivers significantly improve patient outcomes, demonstrating improved pain management, fewer bedsores, and enhanced communication with medical teams (Salins et al., 2022). This underscores the argument that caregivers must not be seen as passive helpers but as active, informed partners in evidence-based home care.

Emotional and psychological support provided by caregivers is a core element of holistic care, especially for patients with terminal illnesses, mental health conditions, or chronic disabilities. Evidence suggests that patients receiving emotional support from caregivers and family members experience lower levels of anxiety, improved treatment adherence, and better symptom management (Nair & Prasad, 2021). Unlike institutional settings, home environments allow for personalization of care—families provide culturally appropriate food, religious or spiritual rituals, familiar surroundings, and emotional reassurance, all of which contribute to holistic healing. For instance, in palliative care, caregivers often facilitate spiritual rituals, prayer, Ayurvedic massage, or music therapy to help patients cope with pain and fear (Kumar, 2018). These practices, when combined with evidence-based pain medications, physiotherapy, or clinical nutrition, form a comprehensive model of integrative care that addresses body, mind, and soul.

However, caregiving is not without significant physical, financial, and emotional burden. Studies in India report high levels of caregiver burnout, depression, musculoskeletal pain, sleep disturbances, and social isolation among those providing long-term care (Chakrabarti, 2016). Financially, caregivers often sacrifice employment opportunities, use personal savings for medication and medical devices, and face limited government or insurance support. In the case of dementia, stroke, or cancer, caregiving can continue for months or years, with limited respite care options available in India (Narayanan, 2021). Emotional exhaustion and caregiver stress can negatively affect the quality of care provided. Evidence shows that caregivers who receive psychological counseling, peer support networks, and respite care demonstrate better resilience, lower depression levels, and higher caregiving satisfaction (Salins et al., 2022). This demonstrates that just as patients need evidence-based medical care, caregivers need structured psychosocial support grounded in research.

Several Indian initiatives have recognized the crucial role of caregivers and have begun to integrate training and support programmes. The Neighbourhood Network in Palliative Care (NNPC) in Kerala trains family members and community volunteers in clinical tasks such as pain assessment, wound dressing, catheter care, and safe opioid administration using WHO palliative guidelines (Kumar, 2018). Tata Memorial Hospital in Mumbai runs a home-care programme where oncology nurses train caregivers on oral morphine usage, dietary needs, oral care in chemotherapy patients, and emergency red-flag symptoms. Similarly, AIIMS Delhi and NIMHANS Bengaluru provide structured caregiver training modules for dementia, stroke, and psychiatric care that include cognitive stimulation therapy, behavioral management, physiotherapy exercises, and proper handling of assistive devices (Verma & Yadav, 2021). These initiatives prove that when caregivers are equipped with evidence-based knowledge, patient outcomes improve and caregiver distress is reduced.

Technology has further empowered caregivers by making clinical evidence more accessible in real-time. Digital platforms such as eSanjeevani, Practo, and AIIMS iGeriCare offer video consultations, medication trackers, physiotherapy videos, and emergency doctor guidance, allowing caregivers to make clinically informed decisions (MoHFW, 2023). Artificial intelligence-based health applications can alert caregivers to irregular vitals, missed medication doses, or abnormal behaviour in dementia patients. However, challenges such as digital illiteracy, language barriers, and lack of access to devices or the internet still limit widespread adoption in rural areas (Basu & Patnaik, 2023). Addressing these challenges requires producing content in regional languages, using audio-visual learning tools, and creating caregiver helplines at district levels.

Cultural and spiritual beliefs also shape caregiving practices in Indian homes. Many caregivers incorporate Ayurveda, yoga, home remedies, religious rituals, or family traditions alongside biomedical care (Tandon & Sharma, 2020). While these enhance emotional and spiritual well-being, they must be aligned with evidence-based medicine to prevent harmful delays in treatment or drug interactions. For instance, research at AIIMS has validated the use of yoga and pranayama as adjunct therapies for hypertension, COPD, and stress if combined appropriately with clinical treatment (Sharma & Gupta, 2021). Thus, the role of caregivers also involves selectively integrating traditional practices with clinical supervision, creating a culturally respectful yet evidence-grounded approach.

In conclusion, families and caregivers are not only emotional supporters but also primary healthcare providers, decision-makers, and implementers of evidence-based protocols in home settings. They translate clinical advice into daily routines, coordinate follow-ups, manage nutrition and hygiene, administer medicines, and provide spiritual comfort. The integration of holistic care is only successful when caregivers are empowered through structured training, psychological support, technology, financial assistance, and recognition within the healthcare system. Policy-makers and healthcare institutions must therefore treat caregivers as essential stakeholders and partners in the continuum of care rather than informal, unpaid workers. By strengthening their capacity, India can create a sustainable, culturally rooted, and scientifically grounded home-care ecosystem.

7. CHALLENGES AND BARRIERS IN INTEGRATING CLINICAL EVIDENCE INTO HOLISTIC HOME CARE

Despite increasing recognition of holistic home care and efforts to integrate clinical evidence into family-led caregiving, several structural, cultural, financial, and systemic barriers continue to hinder its effective implementation in India. One of the most significant challenges lies in the knowledge and skill gap among family caregivers, who form the foundation of home care. Most family caregivers are laypersons without formal medical training, yet they are responsible for tasks such as administering medication, wound care, catheter management, tube feeding, or physiotherapy (Rajagopal & Joad, 2020). Without proper training or understanding of evidence-based clinical guidelines, many rely on guesswork, past experience, or advice from unqualified sources, which may lead to medication errors, delayed treatment, and preventable complications (Chandra & Banerjee, 2020). Although some institutions like AIIMS, Tata Memorial, and Kerala's NNPC offer caregiver training programs, these are limited to urban or specialized centres, leaving large rural populations without support.

Another key barrier is the lack of standardized protocols and caregiver inclusion in healthcare planning. Most hospitals in India discharge patients without structured home-care transition plans or caregiver education modules. Unlike countries with established home health nursing systems, India does not mandate caregiver training before discharge for chronic illnesses, surgeries, or terminal conditions. There is also no legal or policy requirement to document caregiver needs or assess their capacity to provide care (Weiss et al., 2020). This results in fragmented care, high readmission rates, and poor continuity of treatment post-discharge. Further, there is no standardized national curriculum for caregiver education, and nursing schools often focus on hospital-based training rather than community or family-led care (Paul & Sinha, 2022).

Emotional, physical, and financial caregiver burden poses another major barrier. Caregivers often experience anxiety, depression, back pain, burnout, and social isolation while managing long-term care responsibilities (Chakrabarti, 2016). Financial stress also compounds the burden—most home-care expenses, including medical equipment, physiotherapy tools, medications, travel to hospitals, and dietary supplements, are borne out-of-pocket. India's insurance schemes, including Ayushman Bharat and private insurance plans, rarely cover home care, caregiver training, or respite services (MoHFW, 2022). In households with low income, caregivers sometimes abandon employment, leading to loss of livelihood. Gender disparity adds another dimension—women are often expected to provide care due to cultural norms, while their labour remains undervalued and unpaid (Narayanan, 2021).

Cultural beliefs and overreliance on traditional remedies without scientific guidance also hinder the integration of clinical evidence. Many families first turn to home remedies, Ayurveda, unregulated herbal medicines, or faith healers for serious illnesses, especially in rural India (Tandon & Sharma, 2020). While traditional practices like yoga or diet therapy can complement medical treatments, inappropriate use or delayed clinical intervention can worsen conditions or cause harmful interactions with medications (Nair & Prasad, 2021). The reluctance to accept biomedical advice, mistrust in hospitals, and stigma associated with diseases such as dementia, cancer, or psychiatric disorders further delay timely evidence-based care. Thus, integration must involve respectful blending of traditional practices with validated clinical evidence, rather than sidelining either system.

Healthcare infrastructure and resource limitations also present challenges. There is a shortage of trained home health nurses, physiotherapists, geriatricians, and palliative care specialists in India. As of 2022, India had only 0.8 physicians and 1.7 nurses per 1,000 population, far below WHO recommendations (WHO, 2022). Rural areas face further shortages of medical equipment, diagnostic facilities, and specialist services, making evidence-based care difficult to implement at home (Basu & Patnaik, 2023). The lack of morphine availability for pain management due to strict narcotics regulations and limited training in opioid use further hinders evidence-based palliative home care (Kumar, 2018). Additionally, electronic health records and home-care monitoring systems are not widely implemented, leading to poor data continuity between hospitals and homes.

Technology, while transformative, faces digital divide and accessibility challenges. Telemedicine platforms like eSanjeevani and digital caregiving apps are mostly accessible to urban, literate households with smartphones and stable internet connections (MoHFW, 2023). Rural caregivers often lack digital literacy, smartphones, or internet connectivity. Language barriers, fear of technology, and low confidence in virtual medical advice also limit adoption. Elderly patients with cognitive decline or vision impairments struggle to use digital tools without assistance (Srinivasan et al., 2022). Therefore, while technology enhances access to evidence-based care, its effectiveness is limited unless accompanied by training, regional language interfaces, and low-bandwidth accessibility.

Lastly, policy and regulatory gaps significantly reduce the scope of structured evidence-based home care. There is no national legislation or standard accreditation system for home healthcare providers in India. While private home-care companies like Portea and Nightingales provide professional nursing services, the sector remains largely unregulated (NITI Aayog, 2021). Policies do not mandate caregiver inclusion in clinical decision-making, nor do they financially compensate informal caregivers despite their economic contributions. The absence of government-funded respite care centres, home hospice services, or tax benefits for caregivers further marginalizes home-based care work (Rajagopal & Palat, 2020). Without systemic reforms, holistic and evidence-based home care remains dependent on individual efforts rather than being an integrated part of healthcare planning.

In conclusion, the integration of clinical evidence into home-based holistic care in India is constrained by caregiver skill deficits, emotional and financial burden, cultural barriers, technology gaps, insufficient policies, and healthcare workforce shortages. Addressing these challenges requires a coordinated response involving government policies, healthcare institutions, training programmes, technology providers, and community organizations. Only then can home care evolve from informal effort to a structured, evidence-driven extension of the healthcare system.

8. CASE STUDIES AND BEST PRACTICES IN INTEGRATING CLINICAL EVIDENCE INTO HOLISTIC HOME CARE

The integration of clinical evidence into holistic home care is best understood through successful examples from India and abroad, where models of care combine scientific protocols with cultural sensitivity, family participation, and community collaboration. These case studies provide practical insight into how theoretical frameworks are operationalized in real-life settings, especially where health systems face constraints in infrastructure, funding, and workforce availability. They highlight that effective home-based care does not only emerge from advanced technology or high financial investment but from strategic partnerships between families, healthcare institutions, policies, and communities.

One of the most compelling Indian examples is Kerala's Neighbourhood Network in Palliative Care (NNPC), which is often cited as a global model for community-driven, evidence-based homecare. Initiated in the 1990s, NNPC operates on a participatory public health approach where local communities, trained volunteers, family caregivers, and healthcare professionals collaboratively deliver home-based palliative care services (Kumar, 2018). The programme emphasizes the use of World Health Organization (WHO) palliative care guidelines for pain management, symptom control, and end-of-life care but translates these guidelines into simplified protocols suitable for non-medical caregivers. Trained volunteers regularly visit patients, help administer prescribed medications including oral morphine, monitor symptoms, provide psychosocial support, and coordinate with doctors for complex clinical decisions (Salins et al., 2022). The success of NNPC lies in its ability to decentralize care from hospitals to homes, ensuring dignity, affordability, and evidence-based decision-making within the cultural and emotional context of families. This model has resulted in reduced hospital admissions, improved pain relief outcomes, and increased family confidence in caregiving.

Another illustrative Indian case is Tata Memorial Centre's Home-Based Palliative Cancer Care Programme in Mumbai. This initiative provides specialized home visits for terminal cancer patients, combining clinical oncology guidelines with compassionate family support. Nurses and palliative care physicians visit homes to administer morphine, adjust medication dosages based on clinical evidence, manage bedsores, and teach caregivers accurate methods of feeding, oral care, and catheter care (Salins et al., 2022). The home-care team keeps daily documentation of pain scores using standardized tools such as the Visual Analogue Scale and provides telephone-based consultation to caregivers for emergencies. Importantly, the model supports families emotionally and spiritually while ensuring that pain management adheres to the Indian Association of Palliative Care (IAPC) evidence-based guidelines. This programme demonstrates how tertiary hospitals can extend evidence-based medicine beyond hospital boundaries into private homes without compromising on quality or clinical safety.

A third noteworthy Indian initiative is the AIIMS Delhi Dementia and Stroke Home Rehabilitation Model, which underscores the role of multidisciplinary care for neurological patients. AIIMS developed caregiver training modules based on clinical evidence from geriatric neurology, physiotherapy, and psychiatry to guide families in performing cognitive stimulation therapy, memory exercises, positioning and transfer techniques, and safe feeding practices (Verma & Yadav, 2021). Caregivers are taught evidence-based strategies to manage aggression, confusion, incontinence, and sleep disturbances common in dementia. Telemedicine follow-ups and WhatsApp video sessions allow clinicians to monitor patient progress and modify treatment plans. This model integrates evidence, family training, and technology and is particularly relevant in a country where institutional dementia care centres are limited and expensive.

Outside hospital-led models, India has also seen strong contributions from non-governmental organizations such as CanSupport (Delhi), Pallium India (Kerala), and HelpAge India, which provide home-based palliative, geriatric, and chronic care services. CanSupport, for instance, uses multidisciplinary teams including doctors, nurses, counselors, and volunteers to provide evidence-based home care for cancer patients, while also supporting families through grief counseling and caregiver training (Chandra & Banerjee, 2020). Pallium India has implemented the "Palliative Care Toolkit" approved by WHO, which provides rural health workers with simplified evidence-based protocols for pain relief and symptom management. These NGO-led models fill the gap between hospital and home, demonstrating that care grounded in evidence does not always require high technology but rather structured training and compassionate delivery.

Global practices offer additional insights. In Singapore, the Carer Matters Programme has emerged as a pioneering hospital-to-home transition model. Initiated in 2019 at Tan Tock Seng Hospital, it focuses on identifying caregivers early during hospital admission, assessing their competency and stress levels, and providing tailored training on clinical tasks such as medication administration, wound dressing, and oxygen therapy based on evidence-based nursing guidelines (Chan et al., 2021). Caregivers receive support through helplines, online learning modules, and community-based follow-ups. The programme has demonstrated reduced rehospitalization rates and caregiver burnout, suggesting that structured training and support can significantly improve home-based care outcomes.

Similarly, Japan's Long-Term Care Insurance (LTCI) System provides an example of government-funded evidence-based home care for an aging population. Under this system, elderly individuals are assessed by health professionals using standardized criteria to determine the level of care required. Families receive professional home visits by nurses and therapists who deliver evidence-based interventions such as fall prevention exercises, stroke rehabilitation, pressure ulcer management, and dementia care (Campbell et al., 2019). Japan's emphasis on combining family caregiving with professional support aligns well with Indian cultural values while demonstrating that public funding and policy frameworks are essential to make evidence-based home care sustainable.

Taiwan's HOLISTIC Model, discussed earlier, is another global benchmark that combines longitudinal monitoring, multidisciplinary teams, caregiver training, and technology for home-based chronic disease management (Chen et al., 2021). This model includes regular home visits, structured clinical assessments, digital records of symptoms, and modification of treatment plans based on real-time evidence. The integration of caregivers into the care team ensures continuity and personalization of treatment.

In Western contexts, the United Kingdom's National Health Service (NHS) Home Palliative Care System offers standardized evidence-based protocols for symptom management, end-of-life care, and caregiver education. Nurses conduct home visits and follow NICE guidelines for pain, breathlessness, and delirium management while supporting families emotionally and spiritually. Similarly, Canada's Family Integrated Care (FICare) model in neonatal care trains parents to participate actively in clinical decisions for premature infants, backed by structured hospital training and nursing supervision (O'Brien et al., 2018). Though designed for neonatal units, its principles—family inclusion, education, and evidence-based support—are applicable to home-care models.

When comparing Indian and global models, key similarities include reliance on caregivers, interdisciplinary collaboration, and adaptation of evidence-based guidelines for home use. However, Indian models place greater emphasis on community participation, cultural rituals, and integration of traditional medicine like Ayurveda and yoga. Global systems tend to provide stronger financial support, legal protection for caregivers, and formal policy frameworks. The main lesson from both contexts is that evidence-based home care succeeds when clinical knowledge is translated into practical, culturally sensitive actions supported by caregivers, professionals, and policy systems.

9. POLICY IMPLICATIONS AND FUTURE DIRECTIONS

The integration of clinical evidence into holistic home care requires supportive policy frameworks that recognize the critical role of families and caregivers in healthcare delivery. In India, policies such as the National Health Policy (2017), Ayushman Bharat, National Programme for Healthcare of the Elderly (NPHCE), and National Programme for Palliative Care (NPPC) have laid the groundwork for community-based and home-supported care. However, these policies remain largely fragmented and focus more on institutional service provisioning rather than structured, evidence-based home care. There is still no national policy that formally recognizes unpaid caregivers as a part of the healthcare workforce or provides them with training, legal recognition, insurance benefits, or mental health support. For India to transition from an institution-driven to a people-centered care model, future policies need to formally incorporate caregivers into health governance frameworks, define their rights and responsibilities, and ensure standardized training rooted in clinical guidelines and cultural sensitivity.

A major policy implication lies in developing a national-level caregiver training and accreditation system, much like how ASHA workers were institutionalized in rural health missions. Evidence-based training modules—covering medication management, symptom monitoring, mobility care, dementia supervision, palliative techniques, infection control, and emergency recognition—must be made mandatory at the point of discharge from hospitals for chronic and terminal cases. These modules should be delivered in regional languages, using visual and digital formats for easy comprehension by families with varying literacy levels. States like Kerala have already demonstrated the effectiveness of such community-based training through the Neighbourhood Network in Palliative Care (NNPC). This model can be adapted nationally to create state-supported Caregiver Schools or Home Care Units linked with district hospitals.

Financial support and insurance coverage for home care is another critical policy area. Currently, most health insurance schemes in India—including public ones like PM-JAY (Ayushman Bharat)—cover hospital expenses but not home-based nursing, caregiver training, home physiotherapy, medical consumables, or assistive devices. This pushes families into financial stress and discourages home care for chronic patients. Future policies must include reimbursement for home-based services, subsidies for medical equipment and palliative medicines, tax deductions for family caregivers, and inclusion of home health packages under public insurance. The provision of monthly caregiver allowances, similar to models in Japan and Germany, would enhance economic security for families providing unpaid care.

Government frameworks must also ensure better integration of AYUSH systems with biomedical care. Since many Indian households rely on Ayurveda, yoga, Siddha, or home remedies, policies should promote research-backed integrative models rather than unregulated use of traditional therapies. For example, combining evidence-based yoga therapy for COPD or hypertension with allopathic medication protocols, under supervision, can enhance outcomes. The Ministry of AYUSH and ICMR should support clinical trials to validate traditional practices used at home so they can be ethically and safely included in care guidelines.

Digital health policy will be instrumental in scaling evidence-based home care. Platforms like eSanjeevani, National Digital Health Mission (NDHM), Electronic Health Records (EHR), tele-palliative services, and AI-based mobile health apps need to be extended to remote households. Policies must ensure multilingual interfaces, rural internet infrastructure, data privacy protection for patient information, and inclusion of caregiver training modules in telehealth applications. Digital health workers or community telehealth facilitators should be appointed to help rural households use digital platforms for clinical guidance and follow-ups.

To sustain evidence-based home care, public-private partnerships (PPP) and collaborations with NGOs, academic institutions, and palliative care networks must be strengthened. NGOs such as Pallium India, CanSupport, and HelpAge India have demonstrated low-cost, scalable models of holistic home care using clinical guidelines. These models should be formally integrated into public health programmes, funded under CSR initiatives, and supported by medical colleges for research and supervision. Medical and nursing curricula must also be revised to include community-based care, home-based rehabilitation, caregiver psychology, and family-centered clinical communication.

Looking forward, future research should focus on generating indigenous evidence on home care outcomes in India—such as caregiver burden patterns, cost-benefit analysis of home versus hospital care, rural versus urban disparities, and the role of digital tools in chronic illness management. Longitudinal studies and randomized controlled trials on home-care interventions will provide robust data to guide national standards. There is also a need for qualitative research exploring the lived experiences of caregivers, cultural perceptions of home death versus hospital death, and the gender dynamics of caregiving responsibilities.

10. CONCLUSION

Holistic home care has emerged as an indispensable component of modern healthcare systems, particularly in countries like India where families serve as the primary caregivers for the elderly, chronically ill, and terminally ill patients. This chapter established that integrating clinical evidence into home care is not merely an optional enhancement but a necessary transformation required for improving patient outcomes, ensuring safety, and reducing hospital dependency. By combining biomedical protocols with the emotional, cultural, spiritual, and social dimensions of caregiving, holistic home care represents a more humane and sustainable approach to healthcare. The integration of clinical evidence ensures that care practices are not based on intuition or tradition alone but on scientifically proven methods that reduce suffering, improve symptom management, prevent medical errors, and enhance quality of life for both patients and caregivers.

The chapter demonstrated that families and caregivers lie at the centre of this transformation. They are the ones who translate prescriptions into action, respond during health crises, provide psychological comfort, and ensure daily continuity of care. However, without adequate training, emotional support, and access to professional guidance, they face burnout, financial hardship, and psychological distress. Therefore, the success of evidence-based holistic care at home depends on strengthening the capacity of caregivers through structured training programmes, community health networks, telemedicine services, and culturally relevant educational tools. Models such as Kerala's Neighbourhood Network in Palliative Care, Tata Memorial's home oncology care, AIIMS dementia home programmes, and global frameworks like the Carer Matters Programme (Singapore), the HOLISTIC Model (Taiwan), and NHS (UK) demonstrate that this integration is both feasible and effective.

Despite progress, several challenges persist, including insufficient caregiver training, lack of standardized protocols, limited insurance coverage for home care, poor digital accessibility in rural areas, and emotional and financial stress on caregivers. Policy reforms must prioritize caregiver recognition, financial assistance, inclusion in clinical decision-making, and integration of home-based services into national health missions. At the same time, future research should generate indigenous evidence on home-based outcomes, cost-effectiveness, caregiver experiences, and the ethical integration of AYUSH and digital technologies in caregiving.

In conclusion, holistic home care rooted in clinical evidence and supported by families represents the future of compassionate and sustainable healthcare. It aligns with global health priorities such as the WHO's people-centered care model and India's vision of universal health coverage. Empowering caregivers with scientific knowledge, emotional support, and societal recognition is crucial in transforming home spaces into healing environments. If healthcare systems embrace this shift, home care will evolve from being an informal obligation to a dignified, evidence-based, and culturally meaningful extension of modern medicine.

REFERENCES

Basu, A., & Patnaik, S. (2023). Digital health adoption in rural India: Challenges and opportunities for telemedicine. *Indian Journal of Public Health Research & Development*, *14*(2), 115–122.

Campbell, J., Ikegami, N., & Gibson, M. (2019). Lessons from Japan's long-term care insurance system. *Health Affairs*, *38*(6), 912–919.

Carman, K. L., Dardess, P., & Maurer, M.. (2016). Patient and family engaged care: A framework for understanding the elements of engagement. *Health Affairs*, *35*(4), 595–603. PMID: 27044957

Chakrabarti, S. (2016). Family caregivers in India: Issues and perspectives. *Indian Journal of Psychiatry*, *58*(2), 217–223.

Chan, E. Y., Lim, W. S., & Tan, J. (2021). Carer Matters: A hospital-initiated programme to support caregivers during care transition. *BMC Geriatrics*, *21*(1), 1–12. PMID: 33388045

Chandra, S., & Banerjee, D. (2020). Caregiver burden and home care challenges in India: A narrative review. *Indian Journal of Social Psychiatry*, *36*(3), 208–214.

Chen, Y. C., Lin, Y. C., & Huang, L. (2021). HOLISTIC study: A home-based longitudinal investigation of integrated care. *Journal of Advanced Nursing*, *77*(4), 1982–1993.

Gomes, B., Calanzani, N., & Higginson, I. (2021). Effectiveness of home palliative care services: A systematic review. *Cochrane Database of Systematic Reviews*, *2*, 1–62.

Gutiérrez, R., & Ramos, J. (2024). The Well-Teach framework: Integrating evidence-based education into caregiving. *Journal of Holistic Nursing*, *42*(1), 45–59.

Harris, R., Sims, S., & Parr, J. (2020). Evidence-based home healthcare: Global trends and outcomes. *Journal of Community Health Nursing*, *37*(1), 22–33.

International Labour Organization (ILO). (2021). *Unpaid caregiving and economic contribution in India*. ILO India Report.

Kumar, S. (2018). Community-led home palliative care: The Kerala model. *Indian Journal of Palliative Care*, *24*(3), 237–244.

Lin, Y. C., & Huang, C. J. (2022). Impact of caregiver inclusion in home health systems: Evidence from the HOLISTIC study. *Geriatric Nursing*, *43*, 56–64.

Ministry of Health and Family Welfare (MoHFW). (2022). *National Programme for Palliative Care: Implementation Report*. Government of India.

MoHFW. (2023). *eSanjeevani Telemedicine: Annual Report 2023*. New Delhi: Government of India.

Nair, H., & Prasad, R. (2021). Integration of evidence and Ayurveda in chronic illness management. *AYU Journal*, *42*(2), 91–98.

Nair, P. R., & Prasad, R. (2021). Cultural perceptions and delays in evidence-based caregiving in rural India. *Indian Journal of Community Medicine : Official Publication of Indian Association of Preventive & Social Medicine*, *46*(3), 352–358.

Narayanan, R. (2021). Gender and informal caregiving in Indian households. *Indian Journal of Gender Studies*, *28*(4), 507–524.

National Institute for Health and Care Excellence (NICE). (2019). *Home care for adults with complex health needs*. NICE Guidelines.

National Institution for Transforming India (NITI Aayog). (2021). *India's National Strategy for Home-based Healthcare*.

O'Brien, K., Bracht, M., & Robson, K. (2018). Family Integrated Care (FICare): Engaging parents in NICU-based evidence-driven care. *The Lancet. Child & Adolescent Health*, *2*(4), 245–254. DOI: 10.1016/S2352-4642(18)30039-7 PMID: 30169298

Paul, R., & Sinha, R. (2022). Evidence-based nursing in home care: Role of Indian nurses. *Nursing Journal of India*, *113*(6), 284–290.

Rajagopal, M., & Joad, A. (2020). Informal caregiving and palliative care gaps in India. *Journal of Pain and Symptom Management*, *59*(1), 102–109.

Rajagopal, M., & Palat, G. (2020). Overcoming policy barriers to palliative care in India. *Health Policy and Planning*, *35*(2), 184–192.

Salins, N., Deodhar, J., & Goel, S. (2022). Home-based cancer palliative care in India: Outcomes and challenges. *Indian Journal of Cancer*, *59*(2), 234–241.

Sharma, M., & Gupta, A. (2021). Impact of yoga-based pulmonary rehabilitation in COPD: A clinical trial. *AIIMS Journal of Medical Sciences*, *75*(3), 112–120.

Tandon, N., & Sharma, S. (2020). Ayurveda and home-based care practices: Evidence and gaps. *Journal of Ayurveda and Integrative Medicine*, *11*(4), 518–526.

Verma, R., & Yadav, P. (2021). AIIMS home-based dementia and stroke rehabilitation: Outcomes and caregiver role. *Neurology India*, *69*(5), 1253–1260.

Weiss, M. E., Sawin, K. J., & Gralton, K. (2020). RAND caregiver integration framework: Implications for home-based care. *Journal of Family Nursing*, *26*(3), 215–232.

World Health Organization. (2016). *WHO Framework on Integrated People-Centred Health Services*. WHO.

World Health Organization. (2022). *World Health Statistics 2022: Health Workforce and Ageing*. WHO.

Chapter 6
The Scope and Impact of Palliative Care in Dehradun Addressing Psychological Distress and Technological Integration

S. Srinivasan
https://orcid.org/0009-0002-0179-9849
Department of Humanities and Social Sciences, Graphic Era University, Dehradun, India

Jipson Joseph
https://orcid.org/0009-0005-1795-5051
School of Law, CHRIST University, Bangalore, India

ABSTRACT

Palliative care plays a crucial role in addressing the physical, psychological, emotional, and spiritual needs of patients suffering from life-threatening conditions and chronic illnesses. Despite its recognized benefits, global access remains limited, with only a fraction of patients receiving appropriate care. Palliative care in managing patient illness, alleviating psychological distress, and supporting caregivers. It highlights the role of healthcare professionals, digital technologies, and psychosocial interventions in improving patient well-being. The research is conducted in Dehradun, Uttarakhand, focusing on palliative care centers and the challenges faced by patients and caregivers. Using both primary and secondary data,

DOI: 10.4018/979-8-3373-4094-4.ch006

the study examines caregiving processes, emotional burnout, and the integration of assistive technologies in palliative settings. Findings emphasize the importance of awareness, training, and innovative approaches in enhancing palliative education and services. Improving patient-centered care and caregiver support within resource-constrained contexts.

INTRODUCTION

Palliative care is a kind of therapy given to patients who are facing various challenges associated with their lives, such as physical illness, mental illness, life-threatening conditions, and psychological fear (Jaiswal et al., 2014). According to a WHO report, at the global level, approximately 25.7 million people required access to palliative care in 2024. Unfortunately, only 14% of these people received palliative treatment (Vélez-López et al., 2024). Basically, palliative care provides therapeutic support to patients in all aspects—physical, mental, spiritual, and emotional—so that they can recover soon and return to their daily routines. Although it is a beneficial treatment and helps patients avoid taking opioid pain relief, palliative care is also used as counseling for patients who are unable to return to normal life due to a family member. In such cases, palliative care functions as emotional support therapy. As the global population rises, the need for palliative care is also increasing, specifically among the aging population, and in both communicable and non-communicable diseases (Rabow et al., 2004; Almada et al., 2018; Mahmood, 2024).

Due to the significance of palliative care, many people tend to use morphine instead of accessing palliative care services because painkillers provide immediate relief. Therefore, health professionals must be concerned about this, as unnecessary use of painkiller medicines can negatively impact people's health (Thomas, 2007). Palliative care should always be prioritized to relieve patients. Additionally, early access to palliative treatment reduces the need for hospitalization (Hui et al., 2022). Many healthcare professionals provide palliative care according to their roles and responsibilities, including support workers, nursing staff, physicians, pharmacists, physiotherapists, and volunteers (Schweighoffer et al., 2020). If the family becomes weak and unsupportive, it will be difficult to support the patient. Hence, emotional support is a vital part of palliative care, giving encouragement and strengthening family bonds (McCauley et al., 2021).

The UN Human Rights Commission has also recognized palliative care as a human right to health (Agarwal, 2020). According to global records, 38.5% of cardiovascular disease patients require palliative care, 34% of cancer patients, 10% of chronic respiratory disease patients, 5.7% of AIDS patients, and 4.6% of diabetes patients (Micco et al., 2023). This gap is due to various reasons such as lack of awareness among national policymakers, cultural and social obstacles, many health professionals being unaware of palliative care, and the misconception in society that palliative care is only for chronic disease patients (Sarmento et al., 2016; Flieger et al., 2020).

Palliative care is essential to implement at the district level, as it can provide psychosocial support for patients and older adults to enhance caregiving. There are various problems faced by older adults at the societal level (Nicholson et al. 2023). The patients receiving palliative care services can improve their mental health conditions. The patients affected by the primary disease experience psychological impacts that lead to an altered lifestyle for older adults and patients. Mental health problems are major health issues (Anandarajah et al., 2020). Palliative care provides care to reduce the burden for someone, especially to enhance the caregiver experience and support the socio-economic conditions of those who are psychologically affected (Perpiñá-Galvañ et al., 2019). There are major issues in caregiving for affected patients to provide better health and well-being, which also affects support for the caregivers. Increases the subsequent impact on improving psychosocial well-being services (Northouse et al., 2012; Oechsle, 2019).

The palliative care enhances patient well-being by providing care and support services, but it requires long hours and affects the stressful work life and limited mental health conditions of caregivers (Glajchen, 2012). The critical major issues are emotional burnout, patient sleep deprivation, increased depression among patients, and rising mental health issues (Dev et al., 2025). The palliative care provides care and services to improve patient health and well-being and to promote family caregiver support in accessing healthcare service providers. Existing research provides major findings that palliative care offers patient care and support for those who are affected by psychological burden. The study addresses the issues of 381 cancer patients who face psychological health problems and receive palliative care support (Ullrich et al., 2017). This can reduce their anxiety level by 13.9% and depression level by 20%. The secondary study addresses patients who face a dual burden, showing a 25% decrease in anxiety and depression among the 266 patients who received palliative care (Wang & Ding, 2025). The similar study provides multiple aspects of prevalence among patients who face psychosocial issues and receive palliative care services (Fan et al., 2017).

Technology-Intensive End-of-Life Care: Balancing Curative Push and Dignity in Death

Technology services provide care at the end of life (EOL) by offering advanced medical support, which can increase the patient's curative health level and create a push and pull regarding appropriateness (Rumbold & Aoun, 2021). As per the

Lancet Commission, highlighting the health and wealth of patient values and death levels can manifold their consequences of dying (Knaul et al., 2025). High-income countries provide specific Intensive Care Units (ICUs) at the hospital level. This can support the patient's good health and reduce unwanted burdensome services that caregivers do not want for themselves (Rao et al., 2022). The dignity of patient death can be ensured through remarkably high-quality care services in ICUs. The ICUs provide comprehensive healthcare services in the USA, UK, and European countries, with life-sustaining treatment (LST) provided up to death, though this might vary widely (Sun et al., 2024). The palliative care treatment supports care so that patients do not die poorly, while enhancing the treatment support to improve palliative care services (Peeler et al., 2024).

CHALLENGES IN END-OF-LIFE CARE

India, especially due to a lack of priority to patients' needs. It can create challenges for anticipating patient death or ethical dilemmas for medical practitioners regarding legal concerns (Mani et al., 2024). The life-sustaining treatment (FLST) imposes a huge financial burden on families, making it difficult for them to bear the cost for patients. There is also a lack of integration of services in ICUs within hospital settings in low-income countries, especially in hospitals located in peripheral areas (Montesi & Calestani, 2021). ICUs provides emergency for patients and relieves the burden on families by offering supportive end life. In India, ICU practice shows that 75% of treatment limitations result in death, with a limited number of patients leaving against medical advice (LAMA) (Sengupta & Chatterjee, 2017). There is family support for the patient, which supports their emotional well-being. The quality of death is poor, contributing to an increased death rate in India. The national healthcare policy aims to promote patient care. In India, the quality of death rate has been recently reported (Srivastava & Ghosh, 2024).

Digital Health and Psycho social Care in Palliative Settings

Digital health interventions have brought tremendous changes to the health system, providing psychosocial support for patients. This can enhance health outcomes through patient-centric care approach services (Aminabee, 2024; Srinivasan, 2025). Digital technology tools help provide psychosocial care for patients, caregivers, healthcare workers, and medical practitioners. Digital integration supports and addresses psychosocial care services, enhances pain management, provides distress relief, and improves palliative care (Sultana et al., 2021). The intervention helps patients understand their health issues, identifies the causes and patterns for caregivers, and provides better supportive care and services. Digital tool services support patients and older adults by sharing information for evidence-based decision-making processes in palliative care (Dos Santos et al., 2023).

Technology enhances palliative care by extending prevention and identifying symptom management to improve healthcare access. It provides better information and can also address mental health issues (Maguraushe & Ndlovu, 2024). Patient satisfaction and real-time clinical decisions help address caregiver and provider stress levels. The health system can be enhanced with the help of digital tools, making care delivery easier and more accurate while reducing human effort to provide effective patient support (Sharma, 2025). Digital technology provides tailored mental health services for patients and caregivers to prevent burnout and promote psychological well-being for providers (Petrovic & Gaggioli, 2020). Digital services support the decision-making process, improve effective management in the health system, and provide easier access to services for patients and caregivers. To focus on optimizing psychosocial outcomes, improving team performance, and strengthening institutional care in palliative care (Yao et al., 2025).

Palliative Care and Patient Well-Being

Provides patient comfort, preserves dignity, manages pain, and offers emotional support (Alhazmi, 2024). The palliative care center supports patient health and well-being, helping maintain a sense of control, comfort, and peace despite the illness. Care support in palliative care can physically reduce pain and relieve symptoms (Chiaramonte & Adler, 2020). The psychological aspects help reduce anxiety and depression, thereby improving overall well-being. The social aspects promote family support, which can also enhance the spiritual needs of patients (Srinivasan et al., 2025; Chen, 2018).

Psychological Distress in Palliative Care

Psychological distress in patients arises from their illness and feelings of fear, anxiety, sadness, and hopelessness, as well as uncertainty about death (Kissane & Yates, 2018). Psychological distress can increase in various forms, such as:

- Physical illness causes patients to suffer from the loss of independence.
- Patients worry about their family and finances, which may leave their responsibilities unfinished.
- Ill patients face fear and a sense of burden regarding their health conditions.

This kind of distress is experienced by patients during treatment and can be reduced through various strategic plans that enhance patient health and well-being. These plans provide treatment adherence support, identify symptoms, and offer overall well-being support services (Deshields et al., 2021). Palliative care support involves various human resources, especially medical practitioners such as doctors, nurses, psychologists, and social workers, to provide counseling services, emotional support, and coping strategies to reduce stress levels (Rodin et al., 2020).

The Caregiving Process

Caregivers in non-institutional settings include family members, relatives, and close friends, who play a vital role in supporting the patient's health and well-being through palliative care (Lalani et al., 2018). Support services are provided in various ways, such as daily care, medical treatment adherence support and decision-making, and psychological support, including emotional support services (El-Mallakh& Findlay, 2015). Caregiving can involve various factors such as emotional exhaustion, financial strain, and caregiver burnout. Caregivers may experience anxiety, grief, guilt, and depression, which can affect the patient's emotional well-being (Gérain, P., & Zech, 2019). Patients recognizes the caregiving support in health aspects. Part of palliative care is to provide a "unit of care," offering various training, respite care services, and counseling support for groups of affected individuals (Alam et al., 2020; Dev et al., 2025).

Patient well-being and psychological distress are closely interconnected, and caregiving support plays a critical role for affected patients (Abdallah et al., 2025). When patients receive support through palliative care services—physically, emotionally, and psychologically—their stress levels can be reduced with the help of caregivers. Caregivers play a vital role in providing better care services, which can enhance patient well-being (Greer et al., 2020).

Research Gaps

The research study mainly emphasizes those who are affected by morbidity and co-morbidity illnesses. Many studies have been conducted on palliative care and support for affected patients. This research primarily focuses on the most effective ways to provide caregiving to the affected community. It also aims to address the research gap regarding how assistive technology supports caregiving and recovery for ill patients.

Research Objectives

1. To assess the role of palliative care in managing patient illness.
2. To understand the psychological distress experienced by patients.
3. To explore how palliative caregivers provide care to affected individuals.
4. To assess the role of assistive technology in supporting palliative care for patients.

Research Questions

Q1. What is the impact of palliative care treatment on patients' illnesses?
Q2. What are the strategic plans to address psychological distress?
Q3. What challenges do caregivers face while providing palliative care to patients?
Q4. What innovative technologies support and benefit palliative care?

BACKGROUND OF THE RESEARCH

Illness on patients' lives and their burden from non-communicable and chronic infectious diseases. The study mainly focused on Dehradun, Uttarakhand's administrative hub, which combines rapid development with characteristics of an urbanizing city. The palliative care services in hill stations create disparities for affected patients, and they influence the quality of life and supportive care services (Carey et al., 2016). The palliative care centers are located in various locations in Dehradun city to conduct interviews at particular centers and to assess psychological distress, anxiety, and depression levels. To identify demoralization from caregiver strain and how it anticipates grief when under-detected. The study mainly emphasizes screening, providing counseling services, and highlights that culturally sensitive psychosocial interventions for patients are uneven. This can be constrained by workforce shortages, stigma, and fragmented referral pathways (Ahmad, 2025).

Digital health tools played a vital role in extending palliative care services. Technology provides tele-consultation, identifies symptoms, and offers remote monitoring services, which increase the documentation of symptom reporting (Stummer et al., 2025). Digital technology is utilized during COVID-19 through SMS/MMS, phone-based regular follow-ups, treatment adherence reminder support services, and the maintenance of electronic health records (Acar & Oskay, 2021). Technology supports virtual consultations and caregiver support groups. Through Google Meet, it provides mentor support and peer-group services, enhancing health and well-being and increasing confidence levels (Heidelburg et al., 2024). Technology services also reduce travel and shorten the time required for managing uncontrolled symptoms.

Technology provides access to services for patients in hard-to-reach areas (Martins & Pinto, 2023). Evidence-based activities promote global adoption and increase the impact of palliative care erability across health settings, hospitals, and home-based care, thereby supporting potential gains (Hassan, 2020; Tian et al., 2024).

There is some backdrop for the study: it only emphasizes the Dehradun palliative care system. The map shows existing services provided by public, private, and community-based providers. This study was unable to focus on palliative care in other districts, which can be planned for in future research. The study estimates the burden and correlates psychological distress among individual patients and caregivers. The feasibility of the study adds value by assessing the cost of technological integration to identify patients, conduct screenings and follow-ups, and provide counseling support. The study focused on psychosocial care within palliative care pathways to enhance patient health and well-being at palliative care centers in Dehradun.

Contextualizing Dehradun's Unique Challenges in India

In India, palliative care faces barriers such as limited awareness, trained professionals, and uneven service distribution. These issues are more pronounced in Dehradun, where hilly terrain, semi-urban settings, and resource constraints hinder access to continuous and specialized care. Most patients rely on untrained family caregivers, leading to emotional strain and inconsistent support. Digital health adoption remains limited due to cost, low digital literacy, and connectivity gaps. These challenges heighten patient distress and caregiver burden. Strengthening community-based networks, caregiver training, and affordable tele-palliative services can help align Dehradun's care system with India's goal of equitable, patient-centered healthcare.

LITERATURE REVIEW

The literature provides a comprehensive understanding for the proposed research and highlights existing research gaps to address in the current study. The current research contributes to broader academic discussion and emphasizes the wider aspects. Psychosocial care within palliative pathways to enhance patient health and well-being at palliative care centers in Dehradun. Palliative care model approach provides various stages of support to protect and care for affected individuals throughout their illness, up to end-of-life care (Srinivasan & Praba Lama, 2025). This approach particularly focuses on patients, their treatment, and psychological distress.

The global aging trend is increasing, and older adults often face chronic illnesses, especially cancer, along with various forms of psychological distress. The need and demand for palliative care in the current scenario are tremendous, highlighting the situation nationwide (Yang et al., 2025). Worldwide, by 2060, nearly 48 million individuals are expected to be affected by severe illnesses and health complications, which will likely lead to an increase in deaths (Tan et al., 2024). It is alarming that traditional biomedical institutional and non-institutional healthcare services are insufficient to provide adequate palliative care support. Palliative care is not fully available, and not all services—such as physical, psychological, and counseling support—are consistently received (McLaughlan & Richards, 2023). Resources are limited and may vary by region. This can lead to individuals lacking essential care and support. There is a demand to implement palliative care within the medical community as well as institutional care, to reach patients and provide quality care services (Abel et al., 2018).

Psychological Distress

Psychological distress in palliative care refers to emotional suffering caused by illness, fear of death, and loss of independence, commonly presenting as anxiety, depression, or hopelessness (Gibson et al., 2006). In this study, 36.8% of patients found counseling effective, 63.5% valued emotional support from healthcare staff and caregivers, and 58.7% benefited from stress-reduction activities, while only 38.1% reported reduced distress from family involvement (Oladehinde-Omodona & Okusi, 2025). These findings emphasize the importance of strengthening psychosocial interventions, including consistent counseling, emotional support, and family-centered care, to enhance patient well-being.

Caregiver Burden

Caregiver burden involves physical, emotional, and financial strain faced by those providing continuous patient care. The study found that 43% of caregivers face financial challenges, 55.5% received adequate training, and 53.9% struggle to balance personal and caregiving duties (Hailu et al., 2025). Many feel emotionally exhausted and under-recognized by institutions. Structured support programs, including counseling, financial aid, and skill development, along with institutional acknowledgment and respite services, are essential to reduce caregiver stress and prevent burnout (Kasmaei et al., 2025).

Technological Integration in Palliative Care

Technology plays a key role in improving palliative care through tools like telemedicine, mobile apps, wearable sensors, and AI systems. These tools enable remote consultations, symptom monitoring, and virtual counseling, enhancing care quality and reducing caregiver burden (Rath et al., 2024). However, high costs, limited digital literacy, and inadequate training remain challenges. Sustainable integration requires capacity building, affordable digital tools, and culturally appropriate platforms to ensure equitable and effective palliative care delivery (Dilhani et al., 2024).

Digital tools create new innovative ideas to develop advanced technology in palliative care. This digital technology enhances virtual reality (VR) based on computers, mobile devices, and wearables to promote the healthcare system (Mo et al., 2022). Social engagement through communication-based channels supports individuals affected by cancer and monitors their systems. These kinds of equipment provide real-time feedback to care service centers, helping to reduce symptoms and lower stress levels in affected individuals. Palliative care centers use immersive 360° (VR) interventions to improve monitoring and strengthen the system to protect affected individuals during emergency situations (Mulukuntla, 2025). This can be achieved through video calling, monitoring, camera systems, and medication alarms to reduce pain and prevent health complications. Technological advancements provide wearable devices for health system monitoring in centers to enhance the healthcare system (Mamdiwar et al., 2021). This can support patient health and well-being, affected by illnesses such as cancer and other non-communicable diseases. This can be implemented for individual treatment and decision-making adjustments to improve the health system and enhance symptom management (Leon & Xu, 2023).

Palliative care centers have limited access to technology due to high service costs. The majority of palliative care technologies do not have proper digital tools for assessment services (Mills et al., 2021). Patient services and a lack of technology utilization in health centers. Interventions must be provided specifically to improve patient health outcomes and address the challenges faced by affected individuals (Kruse et al., 2019). The advancement of technology helps maintain large database records and monitoring services, emergency alarms, 24-hour webcam monitoring, and patient records, ensuring the confidentiality of patient information in palliative care (Marshall et al., 2024). Technology enhances patient health outcomes and daily routine activities by planning and arranging interventions for affected individuals. In the future, comprehensive development of innovations should focus on patient-centered outcomes and approaches in palliative care centers (Thomas et al., 2025).

Socio-demographic aspects of individuals help determine the care and support needed, and care services should be provided based on multi-morbidity conditions. Palliative care may enhance individual end-of-life care and could significantly improve outcomes (Llop-Medina et al., 2022). Less manpower reduces the provision of care and services in an inappropriate way. This can limit healthcare services, potentially affecting the lives of affected individuals and increasing health risks and complications in palliative care centers (Etkind et al., 2020).

Technology devices are designed for the use of information and communication services, providing treatment support for patients and enabling health practitioners to monitor and manage health risk behaviors, thereby improving individual health and well-being (Papa et al., 2020). Healthcare services provide support for the day-to-day tasks of affected individuals, reducing their workload in palliative care centers and offering better healthcare support. To prevent patient health issues and complications, symptoms are identified and monitored through visual consultations, providing quality services in palliative care centers (Wentlandt et al., 2016).

The sensor system enhances palliative care centers by providing proper care and monitoring services through pre-clinical diagnostic support. Digital tools support continuous automated services, which can be used without human intervention and provide easily accessible benefits (Shaheen & Salim, 2025). This involves the use of digital devices to detect medical emergencies and various apps that utilize AI learning to identify risks and prevent health complications. The research provides a proper contact-free sensor support system to detect and monitor vital signs in health issues, especially for pathophysiological changes, which can be associated with end-of-life conditions (Seibel et al., 2024).

The technology system can be more useful in detecting symptoms and stress in patients themselves, especially those with dementia, psychological issues, cancer, or other types of cognitive impairment. Palliative care helps reduce stress and sadness by providing proper care services (Lee-Cheong et al., 2022). It supports individuals affected by depression, anxiety, and other related psychological distress and helps detect the symptoms of their illness. Palliative care addresses the range of sadness experienced by affected individuals, including depression and anxiety, which may be triggered by somatic symptoms such as pain, dyspnea, and agitation (Satsangi & Brugnoli, 2018). This support helps reduce psychological problems, as individuals can express their opinions and preferences regarding treatment, such as the medications they have the right to receive. Monitoring provides practical support to assist nurses in detecting distress beyond the current observer standard rate (Lloyd-Jukes et al., 2021).

Digital services benefiting institutional care providers offer improved service quality through innovation and technological support, enhancing health outcomes for beneficiaries (Al-Assaf et al., 2024). Palliative care provides a high-quality sensor system based on health preferences, allowing patients to make decisions regarding their treatment. The knowledge gained supports healthcare practitioners in palliative care centers and facilitates contact with the contact-free sensor system to enhance support services (Zhang et al., 2022). Palliative services involve providing patients with a green environment without any disturbances, ensuring contact-free care. This emphasizes the use of sensor systems to monitor distress and support patient care services (Ott et al., 2023).

As per review, palliative learning is particularly important for health practitioners to provide palliative treatment to affected individuals and their family members. In the 21st century, there is a growing demand for education in the health field. Health professionals receive palliative care training in medical institutions (Reis et al., 2013). These professionals learn care services in different ways, such as practicing how to provide emotional, physical, and psychological support to patients. This study ensures that medical professionals will be prepared to deliver high-quality care and life-care to patients (Riegel et al., 2021).

Due to its increasing importance, nursing education also acknowledges that the palliative care approach is very useful in building emotional confidence in patients to help them recover faster (Alodhialah et al., 2024). Therefore, nowadays nursing education incorporates innovative teaching methods such as interdisciplinary collaboration, simulation-based learning, and experiential learning. On the other hand, several palliative care, such as families, society trying to avoid adopting such care facilities due to orthodox thinking, feelings of shame, and psychological fear about "what society will think if we acknowledge and access palliative treatment" (Bandieri et al., 2023). These kinds of negative mindsets naturally create barriers to palliative education and treatment. However, researchers, medical staff, and healthcare professionals are trying to deliver positive messages and raise awareness in society regarding the benefits (Mallon et al., 2021). Moreover, in many countries, treatment are special subjects in the curricula for nursing, medical, and healthcare students. Therefore, developed countries continuously evaluate innovative tools and methods to enhance palliative education (Head et al., 2016).

Policy Frameworks

The chapter minimally addresses national palliative care policies or their integration into public health systems. While local practices in Dehradun are discussed, the formal policy context—guidelines, funding, training, and integration with health systems—is largely missing. In India, examples include the National Programme for Palliative Care (2012) and initiatives under the National Health Mission. Linking local practices to these frameworks would clarify whether services align with national goals or reveal gaps in implementation.

Cultural Dimensions

Cultural factors shape attitudes toward death, dying, and caregiving. These include:

Attitudes toward death: Taboo around discussing death can limit patient and family engagement.

Caregiving norms: Family structures and gender roles influence who provides care and how.
Religious and spiritual beliefs: Preferences for home-based care, rituals, or spiritual support affect acceptance of clinical interventions.
Social stigma: Illness or dependence may carry stigma, affecting utilization of services.

Incorporating cultural dimensions in Uttarakhand would explain why patients accept or resist palliative care and how services can be made culturally sensitive.

Policy frameworks: Connect local practices to national strategies and public health integration.
Cultural dimensions: Highlight local beliefs, caregiving norms, and attitudes toward death to enrich the narrative.

Cultural Attitudes

Beyond stigma, local cultural beliefs in Uttarakhand influence palliative care:

- **Attitudes toward death:** Avoiding discussions about death can limit engagement with services.
- **Caregiving norms:** Family roles, gender expectations, and community support shape who provides care and how.
- **Religious and spiritual beliefs:** Preferences for rituals, home care, or spiritual support affect acceptance of interventions.
- Understanding these factors provides context-sensitive insights into patient behavior and service use.

Training Models

Effective palliative care requires trained personnel at all levels:

- **Formal training:** Palliative care modules in medical, nursing, and allied health curricula.
- **In-service training:** Capacity building for hospital and community healthcare providers.
- **Community and caregiver training:** Educating family members and volunteers on symptom management and emotional support.
- **Integration with public health:** Aligning training with national guidelines ensures consistent, quality care.

Discussing training models highlights how workforce development supports service delivery and links policy with practice.

Training Models – Gap

The chapter mentions training but lacks details on curriculum content, practical skills, and institutional initiatives, including the roles of hospitals, medical colleges, NGOs, and government programs. It also does not address alignment with national guidelines to ensure standardized, high-quality care. Including these aspects would clarify how workforce development supports palliative care delivery and bridges the gap between policy and practice.

Policy-Level Interventions and Government Schemes

Effective palliative care requires support through national policies and government programs. In India, the National Programme for Palliative Care (NPPC, 2012) provides a framework for service delivery, training, and integration with public health systems. Other initiatives under the National Health Mission aim to strengthen home-based care, capacity building, and accessibility in underserved areas. Policy-level interventions include standardizing care protocols, allocating funding, and promoting integration of palliative care into primary, secondary, and tertiary healthcare. Discussing these schemes would highlight how government support shapes service delivery, addresses gaps, and ensures equitable access to palliative care.

Nursing and Medical Education Models for Palliative Care

Education and training are essential for a competent palliative care workforce, covering undergraduate, postgraduate, and continuing professional development programs. Undergraduate training introduces core principles such as pain management, symptom control, communication, and ethical decision-making, often through lectures, case studies, and hospice/community exposure (Li et al., 2021). Postgraduate and specialized programs develop advanced clinical, research, and leadership skills. In-service training and CPD upskill providers via workshops, online modules, and certifications. Interdisciplinary and community-focused models train caregivers for home-based care, bridging hospital and community services. Alignment with national guidelines, such as the National Programme for Palliative Care (NPPC), ensures standardized competencies and quality care, fostering a skilled workforce capable of delivering compassionate, evidence-based, and culturally sensitive palliative care (Namisango et al., 2024).

Pain Management Protocols

The statement "Pain management protocols are mentioned but not explored in detail" indicates that while the chapter refers to pain management as part of palliative care, it lacks discussion of specific guidelines (e.g., WHO analgesic ladder, opioid and non-opioid use, dosing, and titration), management of different pain types (acute, chronic, neuropathic, cancer-related), clinical practices (non-pharmacological methods, pain assessment tools), and policy or institutional guidance (standardization of protocols and provider training). The reviewer suggests that a more detailed discussion of strategies, implementation, and supporting guidelines would strengthen the chapter.

Cultural and Spiritual Dimensions of Palliative Care Touched

The statement "Cultural and spiritual dimensions of palliative care are touched" indicates that the chapter briefly mentions these aspects but does not explore them in depth. Cultural dimensions include local beliefs, traditions, social norms, family structures, gender roles, and community expectations that influence caregiving and decision-making. Spiritual dimensions involve religious practices and preferences affecting coping, end-of-life decisions, and patient and caregiver well-being. The reviewer suggests a more detailed discussion to fully capture their impact on palliative care practices and experiences.

Pain Management Strategies and Ethical Dilemmas

Pain management is central to palliative care, aiming to improve quality of life. Pharmacological strategies include the WHO analgesic ladder (non-opioids to strong opioids), adjuvant medications for complex pain, and dose titration with monitoring. Non-pharmacological approaches involve physical therapies, relaxation, massage, acupuncture, psychosocial support, and mindfulness. Multidisciplinary care ensures collaboration among physicians, nurses, psychologists, and physiotherapists for holistic management.

Palliative care also involves ethical dilemmas, such as end-of-life decision-making (life-sustaining treatments vs. comfort care), balancing pain relief with potential side effects (principle of double effect), resource allocation, and conflicts between patient preferences, family expectations, and cultural or religious norms. Effective care requires evidence-based strategies that respect autonomy, minimize suffering, and account for social, cultural, and resource considerations.

Family-Centered Care Models and Psychological Impact

Family-centered care (FCC) in palliative care actively involves family members in planning, decision-making, and care delivery. Key aspects include collaborative decision-making, caregiver support through training, counseling, and respite services, and holistic care addressing emotional, social, and spiritual well-being while ensuring continuity between hospital, community, and home care. Psychologically, FCC can reduce caregiver stress, improve patient well-being, and strengthen family resilience, but high caregiving demands without adequate support may lead to burnout, depression, or conflicts among family members or with healthcare providers. Properly supported FCC enhances patient outcomes and caregiver mental health, while insufficient support can have negative effects.

Training and Education Models for Caregivers and Health Professionals

Caregivers and health professionals are vital to delivering high-quality palliative care. While briefly mentioned in the chapter, training deserves more emphasis as it directly affects patient outcomes, caregiver well-being, and care quality.

I. **Skill Development:** Equips caregivers with pain management, symptom monitoring, communication, and emotional support skills.
II. **Standardized Care:** Ensures consistent practices and adherence to guidelines.
III. **Psychological Support:** Helps manage stress, burnout, and ethical challenges.
IV. **Technology Use:** Improves telemedicine, digital health, and patient monitoring capabilities.
V. **Policy Implementation:** Facilitates application of regional and national palliative care protocols.

Common Models:

1. Formal workshops and certification programs
2. On-the-job training in hospitals, hospices, or communities
3. E-learning, webinars, and virtual mentoring
4. Peer mentorship programs

Focusing on training and education strengthens palliative care systems, enhances patient and family outcomes, and ensures sustainable, high-quality care.

DIGITAL HEALTH INTEGRATION

Digital health integration and caregiver burnout are well-articulated" means the chapter effectively highlights current developments and challenges in palliative care. Digital health integration refers to the use of telemedicine, electronic health records, remote symptom monitoring, mobile apps, and digital communication to improve access, efficiency, and quality of care. Caregiver burnout addresses the emotional, physical, and psychological stress faced by family or professional caregivers, emphasizing the need for support systems, training, and interventions. Overall, the chapter captures both technological innovations and human-centered challenges, demonstrating an understanding of contemporary palliative care trends.

Digital Health

Digital health uses technology and data-driven tools to improve healthcare delivery, patient outcomes, and system efficiency. Key applications include:

Telemedicine/Telehealth: Remote consultations via video, phone, or apps.

Mobile Health (mHealth): Apps for tracking health metrics, medication reminders, and patient education.

Wearables and Sensors: Devices monitoring vital signs, activity, or chronic conditions in real time.

Electronic Health Records (EHRs) and Data Analytics: Digital storage of patient information for better coordination and decision-making.

Artificial Intelligence (AI): Tools for diagnosis, predicting health risks, and personalizing treatment.

Benefits: Increased accessibility, improved patient monitoring, enhanced provider efficiency, and support for preventive care.

Post-COVID Care

Post-COVID care addresses long-term effects after COVID-19, such as fatigue, respiratory issues, cognitive problems, psychological distress, and cardiovascular complications.

Role of Digital Health

Remote Monitoring: Track vital signs and activity via wearables and apps.

Tele-Rehabilitation: Online physiotherapy, respiratory exercises, and mental health support.

Data Collection: EHRs and digital registries study long-COVID trends.

Patient Engagement: Apps guide symptom management, medication adherence, and lifestyle adjustments.

Significance: Combining digital health with post-COVID care ensures continuous, accessible, and personalized healthcare, especially in resource-limited settings.

RESEARCH METHODOLOGY

The research study endeavors to use quantitative methods to identify and capture the multi-dimensional nature of palliative center. This study allows for health professionals' outcomes and patient experiences regarding palliative care access. A descriptive design reviewed existing studies to identify gaps. Due to practical difficulties, the researcher used convenience sampling. The study will be conducted in Dehradun city, Uttarakhand State, as per the researcher's convenience.

Data will be collected from seven palliative care centers:

1. Max Super Speciality Hospital
2. Doon Cancer Pain and Palliative Care Center
3. Shri Mahant Indiresh Hospital
4. Cancer Research Institute, Swami Rama Himalayan University
5. American Care – Elderly Patient Care
6. Power Life Care Hospital
7. Emoha Elder Care

An equal sample distribution will be used for each palliative care center: 7 centers each center 9 samples = 63 samples selected in total.

Regarding secondary data, the research study will utilize national health surveys, electronic health records, and medical administrative data, which provide detailed information about patients' behavior, diagnoses, and reported outcomes related to palliative treatments. On the other hand, primary data will be collected using a self-prepared questionnaire focused on palliative care for patients who have utilized and benefited from palliative treatment. As per research ethics, approval will be obtained from a recognized authority before conducting the study, ensuring primary data security and confidentiality. The research findings will be analyzed using multivariate simple frequency analysis, T-test, and ANOVA, with the support of SPSS software.

Significance of the study

Traditional medical staff experienced that when a patient's disease became progressively incurable, their family members became uncontrollable and unsupportive (Stolberg et al., 2017). In such situations, bereavement counseling and palliative care were required to help stabilize family members, control emotions, and help them return to normal life (Bergstraesser, 2013). Over time, a holistic approach evolved where patients and family members receive physical, mental, and emotional support through the entire paramedical staff, providing care and therapy across the world in Europe, the USA, the UK, Canada, and other countries (Feerick et al., 2025).

In the early 1990s, the significance of academic study on palliative care became a key subject in medical curricula. The recognition of palliative care became an integral part of cancer patient management, and specific guidelines were introduced by WHO (Wright et al., 2008). Therefore, its importance in the 21st century is indispensable. This study highlights the expanding significance of palliative care due to various innovative approaches that enhance palliative care facilities (Tziraki et al., 2020). Furthermore, it addresses how the ethical and cultural background of society impacts palliative care for individual patients. Apart from this, the role of family members and the challenges they face while providing palliative treatment to their relative patients are also discussed in this research study (Cain et al., 2018). Overall, the study is important from different perspectives, contributing to the medical field. Most commercial hospitals in metropolitan cities like Delhi, Bangalore, Mumbai, Ahmedabad, and Chennai provide palliative care (Vijay & Monin, 2018).

LIMITATION OF THE STUDY

The research study takes samples only from patients aged above 40 years, affected by communicable and non-communicable diseases, and those having morbidities and co-morbidities in the specific area of Dehradun city, Uttarakhand state, India. Moreover, the samples will be taken from Max Super Speciality Hospital, Doon Cancer Pain and Palliative Care Center, Shri Mahant Indiresh Hospital, Cancer Research Institute, Swami Rama Himalayan University, American Care – Elderly Patient Care, Power Life Care Hospital, Emoha Elder Care.

Result

Figure 1. Age

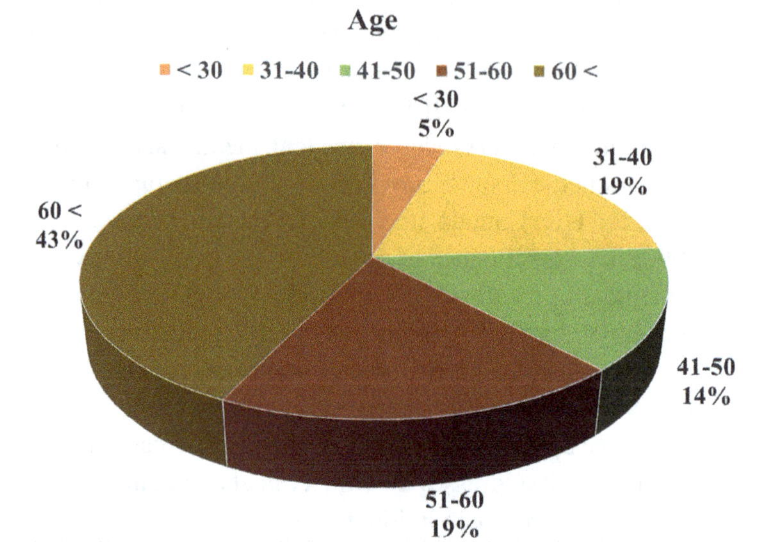

The age profile of 63 respondents shows that 42.9% are above 60 years, forming the largest group. Respondents aged 31–40 and 51–60 years each constitute 19%, while 14.3% fall in the 41–50 years category. Only 4.8% are below 30 years. Thus, the study population is predominantly older, with findings more reflective of senior citizens than younger groups.

Table 1. Demographic and Service Profile of Respondents in Palliative Care

Descriptions	Options	Frequency	Valid Percent
Gender	Male	42	66.7
	Female	21	33.3
	Total	63	100

continued on following page

Table 1. Continued

Descriptions	Options	Frequency	Valid Percent
Name of the Palliative Care	Max Super Speciality Hospital	9	14.3
	Doon Cancer Pain and Palliative Care Center	9	14.3
	Shri Mahant Indiresh Hospital	9	14.3
	Cancer Research Institute, Swami Rama Himalayan University	9	14.3
	American Care – Elderly Patient Care	9	14.3
	Power Life Care Hospital	9	14.3
	Emoha Elder Care	9	14.3
	Total	63	100
Service Received	Caregiver	45	71.4
	Healthcare Provider	18	28.6
	Total	63	100
Years of experience in palliative care	<1 year	5	7.9
	2 - 3 years	20	31.7
	4 - 6 years	33	52.4
	7 <	5	7.9
	Total	63	100

Among the 63 respondents, 66.7% were male and 33.3% female. The sample was evenly distributed across seven palliative care institutions (14.3% each). Most respondents were caregivers (71.4%), while 28.6% were healthcare providers. Over half (52.4%) had 4–6 years of experience, followed by 31.7% with 2–3 years, and smaller groups (7.9% each) with less than 1 year or more than 7 years. This shows the respondents are mainly male caregivers with moderate experience (2–6 years), drawn equally from multiple institutions.

Table 2. Role of Palliative Care in Managing Patient Illness

Options	Strongly Disagree	%	Disagree	%	Neutral	%	Agree	%	Strongly Agree	%	Total	%
Palliative care has improved patients' overall quality of life.	6	9.5	7	11.1	11	17.5	25	39.7	14	22.2	63	100
Palliative care helps in controlling pain and physical symptoms effectively.	11	17.5	15	23.8	14	22.2	12	19	11	17.5	63	100
Palliative care improves patients' ability to perform daily activities	3	4.8	10	15.9	20	31.7	15	23.8	15	23.8	63	100
Palliative care ensures better communication between patients, families, and doctors	6	9.5	7	11.1	7	11.1	17	27	26	41.3	63	100

The findings highlight the role of palliative care in managing patient illness. A majority of respondents (61.9%) agreed or strongly agreed that palliative care improved patients' overall quality of life, although 20.6% expressed disagreement. Perceptions were mixed regarding pain and symptom control, with only 36.5% agreeing or strongly agreeing to its effectiveness, while 41.3% disagreed. Nearly half of the respondents (47.6%) agreed or strongly agreed that palliative care improves patients' ability to perform daily activities, though 31.7% remained neutral. The strongest positive response was observed in terms of communication, where 68.3% agreed or strongly agreed that palliative care ensures better communication between patients, families, and doctors.

Table 3. Psychological Distress in Patients

Options	Strongly Disagree	%	Disagree	%	Neutral	%	Agree	%	Strongly Agree	%	Total	100
Counseling services are available and effective for patients	5	7.9	13	20.6	13	20.6	14	22.2	18	28.6	63	100
Patients receive emotional support from healthcare staff and caregivers	7	11.1	6	9.5	10	15.9	22	34.9	18	28.6	63	100
Stress-reduction activities	4	6.3	9	14.3	13	20.6	17	27	20	31.7	63	100
Family involvement reduces psychological distress of patients	11	17.5	16	25.4	12	19	17	27	7	11.1	63	100
Psychological well-being is regularly assessed as part of care	6	9.5	7	11.1	12	19	15	23.8	23	36.5	63	100

The study indicates that patients' perceptions of psychological care vary across different aspects. While 36.8% of patients agreed or strongly agreed that counseling services are available and effective, a similar proportion felt neutral or disagreed, highlighting the need to strengthen these services. Emotional support from healthcare staff and caregivers was viewed more positively, with 63.5% reporting adequate support, though about one-fifth of patients still felt it was lacking. Stress-reduction activities were moderately effective for most patients (58.7%), but nearly 1 in 5 considered them inadequate, suggesting scope for enhancement. Family involvement appeared less impactful, with only 38.1% agreeing it helped reduce distress, indicating gaps in family-centered care practices. Regular assessment of psychological well-being was reported by 60.3% of patients, showing that mental health monitoring is incorporated into care, but consistency needs improvement. Overall, while patients generally express moderate satisfaction with psychological care, improvements in counseling availability, family engagement, and individualized support could further alleviate psychological distress.

Table 4. Caregiver Experiences

Options	Strongly Disagree	%	Disagree	%	Neutral	%	Agree	%	Strongly Agree	%	Total	100
Caregivers provide high emotional stress support reduction while providing care	7	11.1	6	9.5	11	17.5	17	27	22	34.9	63	100
Financial and resource-related challenges affect caregivers' ability to provide care	11	17.5	16	25.4	13	20.6	16	25.4	7	11.1	63	100
Caregivers receive sufficient training and support to handle patients	5	7.9	6	9.5	17	27	15	23.8	20	31.7	63	100
Caregivers feel adequately recognized and valued by healthcare institutions	9	14.3	10	15.9	16	25.4	17	27	11	17.5	63	100
Caregivers face difficulties in balancing personal and caregiving responsibilities	7	11.1	11	17.5	11	17.5	15	23.8	19	30.2	63	100

Caregivers play a vital role in patient care but face multiple challenges. While 61.9% provide effective emotional support, nearly 43% report that financial and resource constraints hinder their caregiving. About 55.5% feel adequately trained and supported, yet only 44.5% feel recognized by healthcare institutions. Balancing personal and caregiving responsibilities is difficult for over half of caregivers (53.9%). These findings highlight the need for better training, recognition, and institutional support to enhance caregiver effectiveness and well-being.

The findings indicate that patients generally perceive psychological care as moderately effective. About 36.8% agreed or strongly agreed that counseling services are available and effective, though an equal proportion were neutral or disagreed, suggesting room for improvement. Emotional support from healthcare staff and caregivers was positively viewed by 63.5% of patients, indicating its crucial role in alleviating distress. Stress-reduction activities were considered helpful by 58.7% of patients, but nearly one-fifth felt they were insufficient. Family involvement appeared less effective, with only 38.1% reporting it reduces psychological distress, highlighting potential gaps in family-centered care. Regular assessment of psychological well-being was acknowledged by 60.3% of patients, showing that mental health monitoring is generally incorporated, though consistency could be improved. Overall, while patients report moderate satisfaction with psychological care, enhancing counseling, family engagement, and individualized support could further reduce distress.

Perceptions of Palliative Care: Insights from a One-Sample t-Test Analysis

The one-sample t-test (63 respondents, df = 62, test value = 0) shows all items are highly significant ($p = .000$), indicating positive perceptions of palliative care. The sample is predominantly older (mean age difference = 3.76). Respondents report improvements in quality of life (mean = 3.54), daily activities (3.46), and communication between patients, families, and doctors (3.79). Emotional and psychological support, including counseling (3.43), staff support (3.60), and stress-reduction activities (3.63), is valued, while family involvement moderately reduces distress (2.89). Psychological well-being assessment (3.67) and caregiver training/support (3.62–3.65) are recognized, though financial challenges (2.87) and institutional recognition (3.17) remain concerns. Technological interventions—assistive devices (3.25), telemedicine (3.38), mobile apps (3.67), and AI tools (3.52)—enhance care and ease caregiver burden. Overall, palliative care is effective, with strong impact on communication, stress reduction, caregiver support, and technology, while pain management and family involvement need improvement.

Consistency of Perceptions on Palliative Care: ANOVA Findings

The ANOVA results for palliative care-related variables show that all between-group differences are not statistically significant ($p > 0.05$), indicating that respondents' perceptions do not differ meaningfully across the groups analyzed. Variables such as overall quality of life, pain and symptom control, daily activities, communication, counseling services, emotional support, stress-reduction activities, family involvement, psychological well-being assessment, caregiver support, financial challenges, recognition, and technological interventions all show consistent perceptions across groups. This suggests a general agreement among respondents regarding the effectiveness of palliative care services, caregiver support, and technology in enhancing patient care, reducing caregiver burden, and improving overall well-being, regardless of the subgroup considered.

DISCUSSION

Palliative care supports patients with physical, mental, and life-threatening conditions, addressing medical, emotional, psychological, and spiritual needs. Despite an estimated global demand of 25.7 million people in 2024, only a fraction receive adequate services, reflecting gaps in awareness and accessibility. It reduces reliance on opioids, lowers hospitalization, and improves patient well-being, with caregivers providing crucial emotional and practical support. Technology—such as telemedicine, mobile apps, wearable devices, and sensors—enhances access, symptom monitoring, and caregiver efficiency. Evidence shows palliative care reduces anxiety and depression, improves quality of life, and strengthens family engagement. End-of-life ICU care and technology-intensive interventions balance dignity with medical support, though low-resource settings face challenges. Digital tools facilitate psychosocial support, treatment adherence, and real-time decisions. Training healthcare professionals through interdisciplinary and simulation-based methods is essential, yet social stigma, cultural barriers, and limited awareness continue to restrict uptake, underscoring the need for awareness campaigns and policy support.

The study of 63 respondents, predominantly older adults (42.9% above 60 years) and mainly male caregivers (66.7%), highlights the role of palliative care in managing patient illness. Most respondents had moderate experience (2–6 years) and were drawn equally from seven palliative care institutions. A majority (61.9%) reported that palliative care improved patients' overall quality of life, with communication between patients, families, and doctors receiving the highest positive response (68.3%). Perceptions varied regarding pain and symptom control (36.5% positive), daily activity improvement (47.6% positive), and psychological support. Counseling services were considered effective by 36.8%, emotional support by 63.5%, and stress-reduction activities by 58.7%, whereas family involvement was less impactful (38.1%). Regular assessment of psychological well-being was acknowledged by 60.3% of patients. Caregivers play a critical role but face challenges including financial constraints (43%), limited recognition (44.5%), and difficulty balancing responsibilities (53.9%), although 55.5% felt adequately trained. Overall, while patients report moderate satisfaction with psychological care, strengthening counseling, family engagement, and caregiver support could further reduce distress and improve outcomes.

The one-sample t-test and ANOVA analyses indicate that respondents hold positive and consistent perceptions of palliative care. Palliative care is seen to improve quality of life, daily activities, and communication, while providing emotional and psychological support through counseling, staff engagement, and stress-reduction activities. Caregivers are recognized for their training and support, though financial constraints (mean = 2.87) and limited institutional recognition (mean = 3.17) remain concerns. Technological interventions—assistive devices, telemedicine, mobile apps, and AI tools—enhance care and reduce caregiver burden. ANOVA results show no significant differences across groups ($p > 0.05$), reflecting broad agreement on the effectiveness of palliative care, caregiver support, and technology. Overall, palliative care is effective, but areas such as pain management, family involvement, and caregiver recognition require further improvement.

FUTURE OUTCOMES

Palliative care in hospitals focuses on overall well-being, not only end-of-life needs. It is a comprehensive approach applied throughout serious illness, addressing physical, emotional, and spiritual aspects. Care is undergoing a major shift with technological innovation, personalized medicine, and patient-centered approaches. Tele-palliative care expands access by enabling home-based consultations, reducing hospital visits, and ensuring continuity. Artificial intelligence enhances treatment by predicting pain, tailoring care plans, and minimizing unnecessary interventions. Personalized medicine, supported by genomic insights, aligns treatments with individual profiles, while integrative therapies such as acupuncture, massage, and mindfulness provide holistic support. AI and digital tools are easing transitions from hospital to home, lowering re-hospitalization risks. However, challenges remain in ensuring equitable access.

CONCLUSION

Palliative care stands at a transformative juncture, embracing innovations that enable symptom management from the comfort of home. Digital tools are streamlining care coordination, ensuring personalized treatment plans and smooth transitions from hospital to home. The incorporation of virtual reality therapies offers new avenues for psychological support, providing immersive experiences that can reduce anxiety and enhance emotional well-being. Community-based initiatives are also gaining traction, emphasizing the importance of extending care beyond institutional settings. In conclusion, the future of palliative care is set to become more accessible, personalized, and holistic, leveraging technology and community engagement to meet evolving patient needs.

REFERENCES

Abdallah, H. M. M., Amin, S. M., Hammouda, E. Y., Atta, M. H. R., El-Monshed, A. H., & Hamad, N. I. M. (2025). Family Intensive Care Unit Syndrome: Investigating the Mediating Role of Healthcare Communication in Psychological Well-Being Among Family Members. *Nursing in Critical Care, 30*(4), e70119. DOI: 10.1111/nicc.70119 PMID: 40726324

Abel, J., Kellehear, A., & Karapliagou, A. (2018). Palliative care—The new essentials. *Annals of Palliative Medicine, 7*(S2, Suppl 2), S3–S14. DOI: 10.21037/apm.2018.03.04 PMID: 29764169

Acar, Z., & Oskay, Ü. (2021). Mobile Health Applications Used in Perinatal Period and Nursing Roles. *Journal of Education & Research in Nursing/Hemşirelikte Eğitim ve Araştırma Dergisi, 18*(4). DOI: 10.5152/jern.2021.60343

Agarwal, V., & L, G. (2020). Standards of human rights to palliative care: Gaps and trends. *International Journal of Human Rights in Healthcare, 13*(4), 293–298. DOI: 10.1108/IJHRH-02-2020-0013

Ahmad, I. A. (2025). A scoping review of barriers within the cancer care continuum: Addressing screening, diagnosis, and treatment disparities for an equitable future. *Advances in Medicine, Psychology, and Public Health, 2*(2), 96–106.

Al-Assaf, K., Bahroun, Z., & Ahmed, V. (2024). Transforming service quality in healthcare: A comprehensive review of healthcare 4.0 and its impact on healthcare service quality. In *Informatics* (Vol. 11, No. 4, p. 96). MDPI. DOI: 10.3390/informatics11040096

Alam, S., Hannon, B., & Zimmermann, C. (2020). Palliative care for family caregivers. *Journal of Clinical Oncology, 38*(9), 926–936. DOI: 10.1200/JCO.19.00018 PMID: 32023152

Alhazmi, J. D. (2024). Nursing strategies to improve the quality of life for terminally ill patients. *Gland Surgery, 9*(2), 111–117.

Almada, A. L., Casquinha, P., Cotovio, V., Santos, M. H. D., & Caixeiro, A. (2018). The potential role of psychosocial rehabilitation in palliative care. *Journal of the Royal College of Physicians of Edinburgh, 48*(4), 311–317. DOI: 10.4997/jrcpe.2018.405 PMID: 30488884

Alodhialah, A. M., Almutairi, A. A., & Almutairi, M. (2024). Exploring nurses' emotional resilience and coping strategies in palliative and End-of-Life care settings in Saudi Arabia: A qualitative study. In *Healthcare* (Vol. 12, No. 16, p. 1647). MDPI. DOI: 10.3390/healthcare12161647

Aminabee, S. (2024). The future of healthcare and patient-centric care: Digital innovations, trends, and predictions. In *Emerging technologies for health literacy and medical practice* (pp. 240–262). IGI Global Scientific Publishing., DOI: 10.4018/979-8-3693-1214-8.ch012

Anandarajah, G., Mennillo, H. A., Rachu, G., Harder, T., & Ghosh, J. (2020). Lifestyle medicine interventions in patients with advanced disease receiving palliative or hospice care. *American Journal of Lifestyle Medicine*, *14*(3), 243–257. DOI: 10.1177/1559827619830049 PMID: 32477022

Bandieri, E., Borelli, E., Gilioli, F., Bigi, S., Mucciarini, C., Ferrari, U., Eliardo, S., Pinto, L., Porro, C. A., Efficace, F., Luppi, M., & Potenza, L. (2023). Stigma of palliative care among patients with advanced cancer and their caregivers on early palliative care. *Cancers (Basel)*, *15*(14), 3656. DOI: 10.3390/cancers15143656 PMID: 37509317

Bergstraesser, E. (2013). Pediatric palliative care—When quality of life becomes the main focus of treatment. *European Journal of Pediatrics*, *172*(2), 139–150. DOI: 10.1007/s00431-012-1710-z PMID: 22476440

Cain, C. L., Surbone, A., Elk, R., & Kagawa-Singer, M. (2018). Culture and palliative care: Preferences, communication, meaning, and mutual decision making. *Journal of Pain and Symptom Management*, *55*(5), 1408–1419. DOI: 10.1016/j.jpainsymman.2018.01.007 PMID: 29366913

Carey, T. A., Schouten, K., Wakerman, J., Humphreys, J. S., Miegel, F., Murphy, S., & Arundell, M. (2016). Improving the quality of life of palliative and chronic disease patients and carers in remote Australia with the establishment of a day respite facility. *BMC Palliative Care*, *15*(1), 62. DOI: 10.1186/s12904-016-0136-1 PMID: 27430257

Chen, J., Lin, Y., Yan, J., Wu, Y., & Hu, R. (2018). The effects of spiritual care on quality of life and spiritual well-being among patients with terminal illness: A systematic review. *Palliative Medicine*, *32*(7), 1167–1179. DOI: 10.1177/0269216318772267 PMID: 29708010

Chiaramonte, D. R., & Adler, S. R. (2020). Integrative palliative care: A new transformative field to alleviate suffering. *Journal of Alternative and Complementary Medicine (New York, N.Y.)*, *26*(9), 761–765. DOI: 10.1089/acm.2020.0366 PMID: 32924551

Deshields, T. L., Wells-Di Gregorio, S., Flowers, S. R., Irwin, K. E., Nipp, R., Padgett, L., & Zebrack, B. (2021). Addressing distress management challenges: Recommendations from the consensus panel of the American Psychosocial Oncology Society and the Association of Oncology Social Work. *CA: a Cancer Journal for Clinicians*, *71*(5), 407–436. DOI: 10.3322/caac.21672 PMID: 34028809

Dev, P. S., Eljo, J. J. G., & Srinivasan, S. (2025). Intergenerational Caregiving on Grandparents Health: A Case Study. In *Perspectives on the Economics of Aging* (pp. 205-236). IGI Global Scientific Publishing. DOI: 10.4018/979-8-3693-7753-6.ch008

Dev, P. S., Eljo, J. J. G., & Srinivasan, S. (2025). Navigating Mental Health Challenges in the Care of Elderly With Disabilities in Kerala: A Gerontological Social Work Perspective. In *Modern Digital Approaches to Care Technologies for Individuals With Disabilities* (pp. 33-56). IGI Global Scientific Publishing. DOI: 10.4018/979-8-3693-7560-0.ch003

Dilhani, W. N. S., Mitchell, S., Dale, J., Toor, K., Javaid, M., & MacArtney, J. I. (2024). A mixed-methods systematic review investigating the use of digital health interventions to provide palliative and end-of-life care for patients in low-and middle-income countries. *Palliative Care and Social Practice*, *18*, 26323524241236965. DOI: 10.1177/26323524241236965 PMID: 38617095

Dos Santos, F. C., Snigurska, U. A., Keenan, G. M., Lucero, R. J., & Modave, F. (2023). Clinical decision support systems for palliative care management: A scoping review. *Journal of Pain and Symptom Management*, *66*(2), e205–e218. DOI: 10.1016/j.jpainsymman.2023.03.006 PMID: 36933748

El-Mallakh, P., & Findlay, J. (2015). Strategies to improve medication adherence in patients with schizophrenia: The role of support services. *Neuropsychiatric Disease and Treatment*, ●●●, 1077–1090. DOI: 10.2147/NDT.S56107 PMID: 25931823

Etkind, S. N., Bone, A. E., Lovell, N., Cripps, R. L., Harding, R., Higginson, I. J., & Sleeman, K. E. (2020). The role and response of palliative care and hospice services in epidemics and pandemics: A rapid review to inform practice during the COVID-19 pandemic. *Journal of Pain and Symptom Management*, *60*(1), e31–e40. DOI: 10.1016/j.jpainsymman.2020.03.029 PMID: 32278097

Fan, S. Y., Lin, I. M., Hsieh, J. G., & Chang, C. J. (2017). Psychosocial care provided by physicians and nurses in palliative care: A mixed methods study. *Journal of Pain and Symptom Management, 53*(2), 216–223. DOI: 10.1016/j.jpainsymman.2016.08.019 PMID: 27756622

Feerick, F., Coughlan, E., Knox, S., Murphy, A., Grady, I. O., & Deasy, C. (2025). Barriers to paramedic professionalisation: A qualitative enquiry across the UK, Canada, Australia, USA and the republic of Ireland. *BMC Health Services Research, 25*(1), 993. DOI: 10.1186/s12913-025-13196-5 PMID: 40734170

Flieger, S. P., Chui, K., & Koch-Weser, S. (2020). Lack of awareness and common misconceptions about palliative care among adults: Insights from a national survey. *Journal of General Internal Medicine, 35*(7), 2059–2064. DOI: 10.1007/s11606-020-05730-4 PMID: 32157652

Gérain, P., & Zech, E. (2019). Informal caregiver burnout? Development of a theoretical framework to understand the impact of caregiving. *Frontiers in Psychology, 10*, 466359. DOI: 10.3389/fpsyg.2019.01748 PMID: 31428015

Gibson, C. A., Lichtenthal, W., Berg, A., & Breitbart, W. (2006). Psychologic issues in palliative care. *Anesthesiology Clinics of North America, 24*(1), 61–80. DOI: 10.1016/j.atc.2005.12.001 PMID: 16487896

Glajchen, M. (2012). Physical well-being of oncology caregivers: an important quality-of-life domain. In *Seminars in oncology nursing* (Vol. 28, No. 4, pp. 226-235). WB Saunders. DOI: 10.1016/j.soncn.2012.09.005

Greer, J. A., Applebaum, A. J., Jacobsen, J. C., Temel, J. S., & Jackson, V. A. (2020). Understanding and addressing the role of coping in palliative care for patients with advanced cancer. *Journal of Clinical Oncology, 38*(9), 915–925. DOI: 10.1200/JCO.19.00013 PMID: 32023161

Hailu, G. N., Gebru, H. B., Hagos, G. G., Weldemariam, A. H., Tadesse, D. B., & Mebrahtom, G. (2025). The role of family caregivers in supporting older adults in Africa: Systematic review. *BMC Geriatrics, 25*(1), 1–15. DOI: 10.1186/s12877-025-06154-7 PMID: 40610950

Hassan, A. Y. I. (2020). Challenges and recommendations for the deployment of information and communication technology solutions for informal caregivers: Scoping review. *JMIR Aging, 3*(2), e20310. DOI: 10.2196/20310 PMID: 32723720

Head, B. A., Schapmire, T. J., Earnshaw, L., Chenault, J., Pfeifer, M., Sawning, S., & Shaw, M. A. (2016). Improving medical graduates' training in palliative care: Advancing education and practice. *Advances in Medical Education and Practice*, ●●●, 99–113. DOI: 10.2147/AMEP.S94550 PMID: 26955298

Heidelburg, K., Parker, J., & Casella, J. (2024). Strategies for using technology to develop novice school psychology consultants' multicultural consultation skills. *Journal of Educational & Psychological Consultation*, *34*(4), 350–372. DOI: 10.1080/10474412.2024.2315092

Hui, D., Heung, Y., & Bruera, E. (2022). Timely palliative care: Personalizing the process of referral. *Cancers (Basel)*, *14*(4), 1047. DOI: 10.3390/cancers14041047 PMID: 35205793

Jaiswal, R., Alici, Y., & Breitbart, W. (2014). A comprehensive review of palliative care in patients with cancer. *International Review of Psychiatry (Abingdon, England)*, *26*(1), 87–101. DOI: 10.3109/09540261.2013.868788 PMID: 24716503

Kasmaei, M. S., Freeman, S., Banner, D., Klassen-Ross, T., & Martin-Khan, M. (2025). The Impact of the COVID-19 Pandemic on Care Aides' Job Satisfaction in Long-Term Care Facilities in Northern British Columbia: A Qualitative Study. *COVID*, *5*(9), 157. DOI: 10.3390/covid5090157

Kissane, D., & Yates, P. (2018). Psychological and existential distress. *Palliative care nursing*, 229-243.

Knaul, F. M., Arreola-Ornelas, H., Kwete, X. J., Bhadelia, A., Rosa, W. E., Touchton, M., Méndez-Carniado, O., Enciso, V. V., Pastrana, T., Friedman, J. R., Connor, S. R., Downing, J., Jamison, D. T., Krakauer, E. L., Watkins, D., Anyosa, R. C., Garcia-Santisteban, R., Nargund, R. S., Cleary, J., & Radbruch, L. (2025). The evolution of serious health-related suffering from 1990 to 2021: An update to The Lancet Commission on global access to palliative care and pain relief. *The Lancet. Global Health*, *13*(3), e422–e436. https://www.thelancet.com/journals/langlo/article/PIIS2214-109X(24)00476-5/fulltext. DOI: 10.1016/S2214-109X(24)00476-5 PMID: 40021301

Kruse, C., Betancourt, J., Ortiz, S., Luna, S. M. V., Bamrah, I. K., & Segovia, N. (2019). Barriers to the use of mobile health in improving health outcomes in developing countries: Systematic review. *Journal of Medical Internet Research*, *21*(10), e13263. DOI: 10.2196/13263 PMID: 31593543

Lalani, N., Duggleby, W., & Olson, J. (2018). Spirituality among family caregivers in palliative care: An integrative literature review. *International Journal of Palliative Nursing*, *24*(2), 80–91. DOI: 10.12968/ijpn.2018.24.2.80 PMID: 29469645

Lee-Cheong, S., Amanullah, S., & Jardine, M. (2022). New assistive technologies in dementia and mild cognitive impairment care: A PubMed review. *Asian Journal of Psychiatry, 73*, 103135. DOI: 10.1016/j.ajp.2022.103135 PMID: 35569363

Leon, N., & Xu, H. (2023). Implementation considerations for non-communicable disease-related integration in primary health care: A rapid review of qualitative evidence. *BMC Health Services Research, 23*(1), 169. DOI: 10.1186/s12913-023-09151-x PMID: 36803143

Li, W. W., Chhabra, J., & Singh, S. (2021). Palliative care education and its effectiveness: A systematic review. *Public Health, 194*, 9. DOI: 10.1016/j.puhe.2021.02.033 PMID: 33873061

Llop-Medina, L., Fu, Y., Garcés-Ferrer, J., & Doñate-Martínez, A. (2022). Palliative care in older people with multimorbidities: A scoping review on the palliative care needs of patients, carers, and health professionals. *International Journal of Environmental Research and Public Health, 19*(6), 3195. DOI: 10.3390/ijerph19063195 PMID: 35328881

Lloyd-Jukes, H., Gibson, O. J., Wrench, T., Odunlade, A., & Tarassenko, L. (2021). Vision-based patient monitoring and management in mental health settings. *Journal of Clinical Engineering, 46*(1), 36–43. DOI: 10.1097/JCE.0000000000000447

Maguraushe, K., & Ndlovu, B. M. (2024). The use of smart technologies for enhancing palliative care: A systematic review. *Digital Health, 10*, 20552076241271835. DOI: 10.1177/20552076241271835 PMID: 39493628

Mahmood, A. (2024). Integrating Palliative Care into Non-Communicable Disease Management: A Holistic Approach. *Non-Communicable Diseases and Care, 1*(2), 53-65. https://researchcorridor.org/index.php/ncdc/article/view/381

Mallon, A., Hasson, F., Casson, K., Slater, P., & McIlfatrick, S. (2021). Young adults understanding and readiness to engage with palliative care: extending the reach of palliative care through a public health approach: a qualitative study. *BMC Palliative Care, 20*(1), 120. DOI: 10.1186/s12904-021-00808-0 PMID: 34320961

Mamdiwar, S. D., R, A., Shakruwala, Z., Chadha, U., Srinivasan, K., & Chang, C.-Y. (2021). Recent advances on IoT-assisted wearable sensor systems for healthcare monitoring. *Biosensors (Basel), 11*(10), 372. DOI: 10.3390/bios11100372 PMID: 34677328

Mani, R. K., Bhatnagar, S., Butola, S., Gursahani, R., Mehta, D., Simha, S., Divatia, J. V., Kumar, A., Iyer, S. K., Deodhar, J., Bhat, R. S., Salins, N., Thota, R. S., Mathur, R., Iyer, R. K., Gupta, S., Kulkarni, P., Murugan, S., Nasa, P., & Myatra, S. N. (2024). Indian society of critical care medicine and Indian association of palliative care expert consensus and position statements for end-of-life and palliative care in the intensive care unit. *Indian Journal of Critical Care Medicine : Peer-Reviewed, Official Publication of Indian Society of Critical Care Medicine*, *28*(3), 200–250. DOI: 10.5005/jp-journals-10071-24661 PMID: 38477011

Marshall, C., Virdun, C., & Phillips, J. L. (2024). Patient and family perspectives on rural palliative care models: A systematic review and meta-synthesis. *Palliative Medicine*, *38*(9), 935–950. DOI: 10.1177/02692163241269796 PMID: 39254116

Martins, M. D. L. D. C., & Pinto, S. (2023). Analysis of a telephone hotline for palliative care patients at home and their families. *International Journal of Palliative Nursing*, *29*(12), 571–577. DOI: 10.12968/ijpn.2023.29.12.571 PMID: 38085617

McCauley, R., McQuillan, R., Ryan, K., & Foley, G. (2021). Mutual support between patients and family caregivers in palliative care: A systematic review and narrative synthesis. *Palliative Medicine*, *35*(5), 875–885. DOI: 10.1177/0269216321999962 PMID: 33794713

McLaughlan, R., & Richards, K. (2023). Realizing homeliness in palliative care: Inpatient and family perspectives on designing the built environment. *Design for Health (Abingdon, England)*, *7*(2), 138–157. DOI: 10.1080/24735132.2023.2228599

Micco, A., Carpentieri, E., Di Sorbo, A., Chetta, A., & Del Donno, M. (2023). Palliative care and end of life management in patients with idiopathic pulmonary fibrosis. *Multidisciplinary Respiratory Medicine*, *18*, 896. DOI: 10.4081/mrm.2023.896 PMID: 36909932

Mills, J., Fox, J., Damarell, R., Tieman, J., & Yates, P. (2021). Palliative care providers' use of digital health and perspectives on technological innovation: A national study. *BMC Palliative Care*, *20*(1), 124. DOI: 10.1186/s12904-021-00822-2 PMID: 34364379

Mo, J., Vickerstaff, V., Minton, O., Tavabie, S., Taubert, M., Stone, P., & White, N. (2022). How effective is virtual reality technology in palliative care? A systematic review and meta-analysis. *Palliative Medicine*, *36*(7), 1047–1058. DOI: 10.1177/02692163221099584 PMID: 35635018

Montesi, L., & Calestani, M. (2021). *Managing chronicity in unequal states: ethnographic perspectives on caring*. UCL Press., DOI: 10.14324/111.9781800080287

Mulukuntla, S. (2025). Monitoring and Remote Patient Management with Immersive Technologies. In *Augmented Wellness: Exploring the Power of VR and AR in Healthcare* (pp. 197-218). Singapore: Springer Nature Singapore. DOI: 10.1007/978-981-96-2952-7_9

Namisango, E., Onyeka, T., Esther, N., Luyirika, E. B., Ali, Z., & Powell, R. A. (2024). Creating the evidence base for palliative care in cancer–models and strategies to build research capacity. *ecancermedicalscience, 18*, 1819. DOI: 10.3332/ecancer.2024.1819

Nicholson, C. J., Combes, S., Mold, F., King, H., & Green, R. (2023). Addressing inequity in palliative care provision for older people living with multimorbidity. Perspectives of community-dwelling older people on their palliative care needs: A scoping review. *Palliative Medicine*, *37*(4), 475–497. DOI: 10.1177/02692163221118230 PMID: 36002975

Northouse, L. L., Katapodi, M. C., Schafenacker, A. M., & Weiss, D. (2012). The impact of caregiving on the psychological well-being of family caregivers and cancer patients. In *Seminars in oncology nursing* (Vol. 28, No. 4, pp. 236-245). WB Saunders. DOI: 10.1016/j.soncn.2012.09.006

Oechsle, K. (2019). Current advances in palliative & hospice care: Problems and needs of relatives and family caregivers during palliative and hospice care—An overview of current literature. *Medical Science*, *7*(3), 43. DOI: 10.3390/medsci7030043 PMID: 30871105

Oladehinde-Omodona, B., & Okusi, O. (2025). Stress mangement on professional health care givers. https://www.theseus.fi/handle/10024/886095

Ott, T., Heckel, M., Öhl, N., Steigleder, T., Albrecht, N. C., Ostgathe, C., & Dabrock, P. (2023). Palliative care and new technologies. The use of smart sensor technologies and its impact on the Total Care principle. *BMC Palliative Care*, *22*(1), 50. DOI: 10.1186/s12904-023-01174-9 PMID: 37101258

Papa, A., Mital, M., Pisano, P., & Del Giudice, M. (2020). E-health and wellbeing monitoring using smart healthcare devices: An empirical investigation. *Technological Forecasting and Social Change*, *153*, 119226. DOI: 10.1016/j.techfore.2018.02.018

Peeler, A., Afolabi, O., Adcock, M., Evans, C., Nkhoma, K., van Breevoort, D., Farrant, L., & Harding, R. (2024). Primary palliative care in low-and middle-income countries: A systematic review and thematic synthesis of the evidence for models and outcomes. *Palliative Medicine*, *38*(8), 776–789. DOI: 10.1177/02692163241248324 PMID: 38693716

Perpiñá-Galvañ, J., Orts-Beneito, N., Fernández-Alcántara, M., García-Sanjuán, S., García-Caro, M. P., & Cabañero-Martínez, M. J. (2019). Level of burden and health-related quality of life in caregivers of palliative care patients. *International Journal of Environmental Research and Public Health, 16*(23), 4806. DOI: 10.3390/ijerph16234806 PMID: 31795461

Petrovic, M., & Gaggioli, A. (2020). Digital mental health tools for caregivers of older adults—a scoping review. *Frontiers in Public Health, 8*, 128. Petrovic, M., & Gaggioli, A. (2020). Digital mental health tools for caregivers of older adults—a scoping review. *Frontiers in Public Health, 8*, 128. DOI: 10.3389/fpubh.2020.00128 PMID: 32411643

Rabow, M. W., Hauser, J. M., & Adams, J. (2004). Supporting family caregivers at the end of life: They don't know what they don't know. *Journal of the American Medical Association, 291*(4), 483–491. DOI: 10.1001/jama.291.4.483 PMID: 14747506

Rao, S. R., Salins, N., Joshi, U., Patel, J., Remawi, B. N., Simha, S., Preston, N., & Walshe, C. (2022). Palliative and end-of-life care in intensive care units in low-and middle-income countries: A systematically constructed scoping review. *Journal of Critical Care, 71*, 154115. DOI: 10.1016/j.jcrc.2022.154115 PMID: 35907272

Rath, K. C., Khang, A., Rath, S. K., Satapathy, N., Satapathy, S. K., & Kar, S. (2024). Artificial intelligence (AI)-enabled technology in medicine-advancing holistic healthcare monitoring and control systems. In *Computer vision and AI-integrated IoT technologies in the medical ecosystem* (pp. 87–108). CRC Press. DOI: 10.1201/9781003429609-6

Reis, A., Pedrosa, A., Dourado, M., & Reis, C. (2013). Information and communication technologies in long-term and palliative care. *Procedia Technology, 9*, 1303–1312. DOI: 10.1016/j.protcy.2013.12.146

Riegel, M., Randall, S., Ranse, K., & Buckley, T. (2021). Healthcare professionals' values about and experience with facilitating end-of-life care in the adult intensive care unit. *Intensive & Critical Care Nursing, 65*, 103057. DOI: 10.1016/j.iccn.2021.103057 PMID: 33888382

Rodin, G., An, E., Shnall, J., & Malfitano, C. (2020). Psychological interventions for patients with advanced disease: Implications for oncology and palliative care. *Journal of Clinical Oncology, 38*(9), 885–904. DOI: 10.1200/JCO.19.00058 PMID: 32023159

Rumbold, B., & Aoun, S. M. (2021). Palliative and end-of-life care service models: To what extent are consumer perspectives considered? In *Healthcare* (Vol. 9, No. 10, p. 1286). MDPI. DOI: 10.3390/healthcare9101286

Sarmento, V. P., Higginson, I. J., Ferreira, P. L., & Gomes, B. (2016). Past trends and projections of hospital deaths to inform the integration of palliative care in one of the most ageing countries in the world. *Palliative Medicine, 30*(4), 363–373. DOI: 10.1177/0269216315594974 PMID: 26163531

Satsangi, A. K., & Brugnoli, M. P. (2018). Anxiety and psychosomatic symptoms in palliative care: From neuro-psychobiological response to stress, to symptoms' management with clinical hypnosis and meditative states. *Annals of Palliative Medicine, 7*(1), 7511–7111. DOI: 10.21037/apm.2017.07.01 PMID: 28866901

Schweighoffer, R., Reeves, E., & Liebig, B. (2020). Collaborative networks in primary and specialized palliative care in Switzerland-Perspectives of doctors and nurses. *The Open Public Health Journal, 13*(1), 36–43. Advance online publication. DOI: 10.2174/1874944502013010036

Seibel, K., Rios, C. L. O., Sparna, T., Becker, C., Gaertner, J., Becker, G., & Boehlke, C. (2024). Implementation of a digital distress detection system in palliative care: Qualitative data on perspectives of a multiprofessional palliative care team. *BMC Palliative Care, 23*(1), 203. DOI: 10.1186/s12904-024-01530-3 PMID: 39113031

Sengupta, J., & Chatterjee, S. C. (2017). Dying in intensive care units of India: Commentaries on policies and position papers on palliative and end-of-life care. *Journal of Critical Care, 39*, 11–17. DOI: 10.1016/j.jcrc.2016.12.017 PMID: 28104546

Shaheen, R., & Salim, H. (2025). Role of artificial intelligence in healthcare. In *Intersection of Human Rights and AI in Healthcare* (pp. 173–200). IGI Global Scientific Publishing., DOI: 10.4018/979-8-3693-7051-3.ch007

Sharma, S. (2025). Enhancing patient satisfaction and care. In *Exploration of Transformative Technologies in Healthcare 6.0* (pp. 421–442). IGI Global Scientific Publishing., DOI: 10.4018/979-8-3693-7210-4.ch015

Srinivasan, S. (2025). Patient-Centric Care in Tuberculosis Management: Addressing Challenges and Improving Health Outcomes. In *Convergence of Population Health Management, Pharmacogenomics, and Patient-Centered Care* (pp. 265-282). IGI Global. DOI: 10.4018/979-8-3693-3260-3.ch012

Srinivasan, S., & Praba Lama (2025). Patient-Centered Care for TB Patients: An Effective Approach to Corporate Social Responsibility. In Corporate Social Responsibility in Health and Social Care (pp. 183-218).IGI Global. DOI: 10.4018/979-8-3693-5991-4.ch008

Srinivasan, S., Vallipriya, R., & Singh, A. K. (2025). Spiritual Well-Being Index for Incarcerated Populations: An Exploratory Study. In *Sustainable Development Goals (SDG) and Its Intersection With Health and Well-Being* (pp. 425-460). IGI Global Scientific Publishing. DOI: 10.4018/979-8-3693-9755-8.ch015

Srivastava, M., & Ghosh, A. (2024). Societal impact of death anxiety and mental health among nurses in India. *Societal Impacts*, *4*, 100095. DOI: 10.1016/j.socimp.2024.100095

Stolberg, M., Kennedy, L., & Unglaub, L. (2017). *History of palliative care, 1500-1970* (Vol. 123). Springer., DOI: 10.1007/978-3-319-54178-5

Stummer, F. O., Mayrhofer, M., Szabo, N., & Hoffmann, K. (2025). Barriers to and potential of remote consultations in general practice: Insights from the SARS-CoV-2 pandemic in Austria. *BMC Digital Health*, *3*(1), 33. DOI: 10.1186/s44247-025-00176-2

Sultana, A., Tasnim, S., Sharma, R., Pawar, P., Bhattcharya, S., & Hossain, M. M. (2021). Psychosocial challenges in palliative care: Bridging the gaps using digital health. *Indian Journal of Palliative Care*, *27*(3), 442–447. DOI: 10.25259/IJPC_381_20 PMID: 34898939

Sun, X., Zhang, G., Yu, Z., Li, K., & Fan, L. (2024). The meaning of respect and dignity for intensive care unit patients: A meta-synthesis of qualitative research. *Nursing Ethics*, *31*(4), 652–669. DOI: 10.1177/09697330231222598 PMID: 38147009

Tan, Y., Liang, X., Ming, W., Xing, H., Wang, Y., & Gao, Y. (2024). A scoping review of digital technology applications in palliative care. *BMC Palliative Care*, *23*(1), 290. DOI: 10.1186/s12904-024-01626-w PMID: 39707313

Thomas, A., Denis, A., Robert, W., Kabiito, S. P., Morish, Z., Samuel, A., Sallam, M., & Adamopoulos, I. (2025). Artificial Intelligence-Powered Robotic Technology for Transforming Palliative Care. *Mesopotamian Journal of Artificial Intelligence in Healthcare*, *2025*, 58–84. DOI: 10.58496/MJAIH/2025/007

Thomas, J. (2007). Optimizing opioid management in palliative care. *Journal of Palliative Medicine*, *10*(Supplement_1), S-1–S-18. DOI: 10.1089/jpm.2007.9828 PMID: 18052750

Tian, Y. J., Felber, N. A., Pageau, F., Schwab, D. R., & Wangmo, T. (2024). Benefits and barriers associated with the use of smart home health technologies in the care of older persons: A systematic review. *BMC Geriatrics*, *24*(1), 152. DOI: 10.1186/s12877-024-04702-1 PMID: 38355464

Tziraki, C., Grimes, C., Ventura, F., O'Caoimh, R., Santana, S., Zavagli, V., Varani, S., Tramontano, D., Apóstolo, J., Geurden, B., Luca, V. D., Tramontano, G., Romano, M. R., Anastasaki, M., Lionis, C., Rodríguez-Acuña, R., Capelas, M. L., & Afonso, T. (2020). Rethinking palliative care in a public health context: Addressing the needs of persons with non-communicable chronic diseases. *Primary Health Care Research and Development, 21*, e32. DOI: 10.1017/S1463423620000328 PMID: 32928334

Ullrich, A., Ascherfeld, L., Marx, G., Bokemeyer, C., Bergelt, C., & Oechsle, K. (2017). Quality of life, psychological burden, needs, and satisfaction during specialized inpatient palliative care in family caregivers of advanced cancer patients. *BMC Palliative Care, 16*(1), 31. DOI: 10.1186/s12904-017-0206-z PMID: 28486962

Vélez-López, A., Carmona-Torres, J. M., López-González, Á., Laredo-Aguilera, J. A., Callado-Pérez, D., & Rabanales-Sotos, J. (2024). Community-based interventions in people with palliative care needs: an integrative review of studies from 2017 to 2022. In *Healthcare* (Vol. 12, No. 15, p. 1477). MDPI. DOI: 10.3390/healthcare12151477

Vijay, D., & Monin, P. (2018). Poisedness for social innovation: The genesis and propagation of community-based palliative care in Kerala (India). *M@ n@ gement, 21*(4), 1329-1356. DOI: 10.3917/mana.214.1329

Wang, M., & Ding, X. (2025). Integrated palliative care improves the quality of life of advanced cancer patients. *BMC Palliative Care, 24*(1), 162. DOI: 10.1186/s12904-025-01800-8 PMID: 40483417

Wentlandt, K., Seccareccia, D., Kevork, N., Workentin, K., Blacker, S., Grossman, D., & Zimmermann, C. (2016). Quality of care and satisfaction with care on palliative care units. *Journal of Pain and Symptom Management, 51*(2), 184–192. DOI: 10.1016/j.jpainsymman.2015.10.006 PMID: 26598036

Wright, M., Wood, J., Lynch, T., & Clark, D. (2008). Mapping levels of palliative care development: A global view. *Journal of Pain and Symptom Management, 35*(5), 469–485. DOI: 10.1016/j.jpainsymman.2007.06.006 PMID: 18243637

Yang, Y., Liang, X., Liu, Q., & Liu, J. (2025). Navigating limited resources: Experiences of caregivers for elderly terminal cancer patients in a region with limited palliative care services. *Supportive Care in Cancer, 33*(3), 207. DOI: 10.1007/s00520-025-09270-7 PMID: 39971822

Yao, H., Jingyue, W., Rui, Z., Hou, Y., & Hui, Y. (2025). E-CARE as core competencies for palliative social workers: A systematic review. *BMC Palliative Care, 24*(1), 163. DOI: 10.1186/s12904-025-01735-0 PMID: 40490802

Zhang, K., Yuan, H., & Fang, Y. (2022). Evaluation of smart agitation prediction and management for dementia care and novel universal village oriented solution for integration, resilience, inclusiveness and sustainability. In *2022 6th International Conference on Universal Village (UV)* (pp. 1-34). IEEE. DOI: 10.1109/UV56588.2022.10185497

Chapter 7
Laughter Yoga for Parkinson's Disease:
A Mind-Body Nursing Intervention to Support Home Care

Ecem Özgül
https://orcid.org/0000-0002-1294-9446
Independent Researcher, Turkey

Burcu Akpınar Söylemez
Independent Researcher, Turkey

ABSTRACT

Parkinson's disease (PD) is a progressive neurodegenerative disorder impairing motor function, profoundly affecting patients and their caregivers. PD is characterized by motor impairments as well as various health-related quality of life, including well-being, anxiety, apathy, cognitive deficits, sleep disturbances, depression, and autonomic dysfunction. Studies indicate that mind-body interventions can complement PD medications and enhance patients' quality of life. Among mind-body interventions, Laughter Yoga (LY) has gained popularity, with evidence suggesting its potential for management of PD symptoms. LY has been shown to reduce stress, pain, tension, depression, anxiety, and sleep problems. The benefits of LY may inform evidence-based nursing interventions to enhance the psychological well-being of individuals with PD and their caregivers. Nurses should receive training in LY or refer patients and caregivers to LY sessions during secondary care. Future research should investigate the use and effectiveness of LY as a nursing intervention for PD patients and their caregivers.

DOI: 10.4018/979-8-3373-4094-4.ch007

INTRODUCTION

Parkinson's disease (PD) is a chronic, progressive, neurodegenerative syndrome characterized by the degeneration of dopaminergic neurons in the substantia nigra (Kouli, Torsney, Kuan, 2018). This neurodegeneration characterized by the presence of abnormal protein mass and reduced levels of dopamine, a crucial neurotransmitter responsible for regulating smooth and coordinated motor functions (Tolosa, Garrido, Scholz, Poewe, 2021; Kalia and Lang, 2015). Therefore, individuals with PD experience a range of motor symptoms, including rigidity, tremors, bradykinesia, and postural weakness (Tolosa, Garrido, Scholz, Poewe, 2021; German PD's Guidelines Committee, 2024). PD negatively affects health-related quality of life factors such as well-being, anxiety, apathy, cognitive impairment, sleep disorders, depression and autonomic dysfunction, as well as problems related to motor impairment (Tosin, Goetz, and Stebbins, 2024; Angelopoulou et al., 2024). The literature reports that pharmacological treatments for PD are inadequate for some motor and non-motor symptoms (Höglinger et al., 2024; Church, 2021; Muleiro Alvarez et al., 2024; Zhang et al., 2024). In this regard, studies have emphasized that mind-body health interventions in PD can improve the quality of life (Yang et al., 2022; Blard et al., 2024; Harris, O'Bryan, and Latella, 2024). Among mind-body health interventions, Laughter Yoga (LY) has become increasingly popular, with some studies suggesting that it is useful for PD symptom management (Memarian, Sanatkaran, and Bahari, 2017; Bressington et al., 2019; Kumar, Singh, and Sharma, 2024, Meier et al., 2021).

LY is an extended form of intentional laughter that incorporates deep breathing and concludes with meditation and relaxation. There are three primary principles for achieving positive health outcomes: laugh with or without a reason, laugh regularly to boost happy hormones and laugh to oxygenate the body and brain (Cheung and Leung, 2020). LY is a non-invasive and non-pharmacological technique. It involves yoga breathing exercises and laughter practices (Kuru Alici and Arikan Dönmez, 2020). Research supports numerous psychological and physiological impacts on body systems. The findings on the health benefits of LY can be summarized as follows: laughter activates and relaxes muscles, increases respiratory rate, enhances circulation and boosts oxygen levels, reduces stress hormones (e.g., adrenaline, noradrenaline, cortisol), (elevates beta endorphin levels and relieves pain, enhances mental functioning (Ozturk and Tezel, 2021; Kuru Alici and Arikan Dönmez, 2020; Heo et al., 2016; Cheung and Leung, 2020). Furthermore, it can enhance neurotransmitter activity, including dopamine, leading to better memory, focus, concentration, and interpersonal interactions (Ozturk and Tezel, 2021). The positive effects of LY may be important in developing evidence-based nursing interventions that can increase the psychological and physiological well-being of individuals with PD and caregivers. Additionally, involving family caregivers in LY sessions may support their own psychosocial health, reduce stress, and enhance their ability to provide care. Accordingly, this chapter aims to discuss the effects of LY on PD and their caregivers its potential benefits and limitations. This chapter also aims to highlight the potential of LY to improve the quality of life of individuals with PD and their caregivers, serving as a guide for both patients and caregivers.

HISTORICAL DEVELOPMENT OF LAUGHTER YOGA

LY is defined as a laughter experience within the domain of complementary and alternative therapies, involving interactive participation and therapeutic discussions, with physiological, psychological, and behavioral health outcomes (Mora-Ripoll, 2010). Since the 1980s, it has been reported that laughter has positive physiological and psychological effects on the human body. Norman Cousins, in his 1979 book "Anatomy of an Illness as Perceived by the Patient: Reflections on Healing and Regeneration", highlighted how watching humorous videos and laughing regularly alleviated his pain and facilitated better sleep (Savage et al., 2017). The connection between laughter and the vascular system was first identified by researchers at the Maryland Medical Center in 2005. It was reported that laughter induces dilation of the endothelium lining the blood vessels and increases blood flow (Ruch and Raskin, 2008). William Fry (Stanford University) and Dr. Michael Miller (University of Maryland) discovered that beta-endorphins released from the hypothalamus activate receptors on the endothelial surface, leading to the secretion of nitric oxide and subsequent vasodilation (Ruch and Raskin, 2008). Cousins was the first to describe laughter as a therapeutic intervention based on his personal experiences, suggesting that 10 minutes of laughter could provide a pain-relieving effect comparable to that of analgesics for twelve hours (Ruch and Raskin, 2008). The historical development of LY reveals that Dr. Madan Kataria was the first to utilize it as a therapeutic approach. Dr. Kataria, a physician from Mumbai, India, published his research titled "Laughter – The Best Medicine" in 1995 for a health magazine. In this study, Kataria described LY and noted that laughter could initially be simulated but quickly transform into genuine laughter. He emphasized that this transformation enhances the oxygen saturation of the brain and body. The reason Dr. Kataria named this innovative method "Laughter Yoga" was due to the integration of yoga breathing exercises with laughter exercises (Kataria, 2018).

The Benefits of Laughter Yoga

LY sessions typically begin with light warming techniques including stretching, clapping, singing, and body movements. These activities foster a sense of playful engagement while preparing the lungs for subsequent laughter exercises (Si and Kılınç, 2022). Participants often feel healthier, less stressed, more positive, youthful, and calm while laughing (Hatzipapas et al., 2017; El-Sayed et al., 2024; Ozturk and Tezel, 2021; Kuru Alici and Arikan Dönmez, 2020; Li et al., 2024; Li et al., 2024). These positive emotions can have a beneficial impact on daily life and prevent social withdrawal (Ozturk and Tezel, 2021). Laughter involves the opening of the trachea, the narrowing of the larynx by the epiglottis, and the vibration of the vocal cords, with the tear glands reflexively moistening the eyes (Noureldein and Eid, 2018). Imaging studies have shown that various brain regions, including the amygdala, hypothalamus, temporal, and cerebellar areas, are active during laughter (Cheung and Leung, 2020). The limbic system, including the hippocampus and amygdala, is also involved in laughter. The Neuroscience Society has divided the neural control of laughter into three components: the cognitive domain, which processes various stimuli; the motor domain, which produces the muscle movements necessary for laughter; and the emotional domain, particularly the nucleus accumbens which mediates feelings of happiness (Mohajer et al., 2022). Laughter has been shown to positively affect the musculoskeletal, cardiovascular, respiratory, endocrine, immune, and central nervous systems (Ozturk and Tezel, 2021; Kuru Alici and Arikan Dönmez, 2020; Heo et al., 2016; Cheung and Leung, 2020). LY, has been linked to heightened self-efficacy, including better mood and increased productivity (Ozturk and Tezel, 2021). Randomized controlled trial have evaluated the impact of LY on elderly women suffering from depression, showing increased life satisfaction and reduced depressive symptoms (Armat et al., 2022). Controlled studies in the medical field have used both physiological and psychosocial measures, revealing that LY enhanced positive emotions in patients awaiting organ transplants, regulated blood glucose levels, reduced stress in individuals with type 2 diabetes, and enhanced biopsychosocial functioning in stroke survivors (Van der Wal and Kok, 2019; Rouhi, Etemadi ve Pooraghajan, 2020). In a systematic review by Li et al., it was stated that LY improved health functions such as quality of life, pain intensity, sleep quality, well-being, mood, depression, and blood pressure in patients undergoing hemodialysis treatment (Li et al., 2024). In the study by Rouhi et al., it was suggested that the use of LY as a complementary intervention to control the stress and anxiety experienced by patients with coronary heart disease during the treatment process is effective, and that more research should be done on the subject (Rouhi, Etemadi ve Pooraghajan, 2020). In the systematic review conducted by Gonot-Schoupinsky and Garip, five studies representing a total sample of 369 participants who received LY intervention were included. In the conclusion and recommendations section, it was concluded that LY is an important intervention that increases the well-being of older individuals and it was recommended that more studies be conducted in this field (Gonot-Schoupinsky and Garip, 2018).

Laughter Yoga on Parkinson's disease and Nursing Interventions

Neurodegenerative disorders are an increasing public health concern and a significant contributor to the global burden of disease (Huang, Pan and Han, 2023). PD is recognized as the second most prevalent neurodegenerative disorder after Alzheimer's disease which mostly affects elderly individuals (Ciurea et al., 2023). Over the past 25 years, the prevalence of PD has doubled, and more than 10 million people worldwide are currently living with the condition (Wang et al., 2023; Chaudhuri et al., 2024). The risk of developing PD is multifactorial, with studies identifying genetic modifiers of environmental risk factors (Wang et al., 2023; Chaudhuri et al., 2024). The contribution of genetics to PD is suggested by the increased risk of disease associated with a family history. Age is the most significant risk factor for PD, with both prevalence and incidence rising nearly exponentially with advancing age, peaking after 80 years. Men are 1.5 times more likely to develop PD than women. Additional risk factors for PD include environmental exposures such as pesticide exposure, prior head injury, rural living, beta-blocker use, and agricultural occupation (Wang et al., 2023; Chaudhuri et al., 2024).

Fundamentally, in PD's disease, the brain is unable to produce dopamine, a neurotransmitter that controls muscle activities. This condition typically arises due to the reduction or loss of a significant portion of the dopamine-producing nerve cells in the substantia nigra region of the brain (Thomas, Edwards and Kobylecki, 2024). Without dopamine, the brain cannot transmit motor messages, leading to symptoms such as bradykinesia, tremors, cognitive decline, and other autonomic nervous system dysfunctions (Wang et al., 2023; Chaudhuri et al., 2024). Furthermore, PD can result in psychological issues such as depression, anxiety, low self-esteem, sleep disturbances, fear, and shame (Thomas, Edwards and Kobylecki, 2024). These symptoms are prevalent in the early stages of PD and are associated with diminished health-related quality of life. The progression of PD is characterized by a worsening of motor symptoms, which initially can be managed with symptomatic therapies. However, as PD progresses, symptoms including both motor and non-motor fluctuations, become increasingly evident (Wang et al., 2023; Chaudhuri et al., 2024; Thomas, Edwards and Kobylecki, 2024). These symptoms present significant challenges in the clinical management of advanced PD's disease. This situation progressively deteriorates the quality of life for individuals with PD's disease (Thomas, Edwards and Kobylecki, 2024). The literature highlights the significance of incorporating non-pharmacological methods alongside pharmacological approaches to enhance the quality of life for those with PD (Höglinger et al., 2024; Church, 2021; Muleiro Alvarez et al., 2024; Zhang et al., 2024). In this regard, studies have emphasized that mind-body health interventions can serve as effective complementary treatments to pharmacological therapies (Yang et al., 2022; Blard et al., 2024; Harris, O'Bryan, and Latella, 2024). Among such interventions, LY has gained increasing popularity, with some studies suggesting that it may be beneficial for managing PD symptoms (Memarian, Sanatkaran, and Bahari, 2017; Bressington et al., 2019; Kumar, Singh, and Sharma, 2024, Meier et al., 2021).

Laughter enhances both physical and psychological health outcomes across various diseases and populations. Research focusing on psychological benefits frequently indicates that laughter can alleviate stress, improve mood, boost memory, strengthen interpersonal relationships, enhance psychological well-being, and increase overall quality of life (Ozturk and Tezel, 2021; Kuru Alici and Arikan Dönmez, 2020; Heo et al., 2016; Cheung and Leung, 2020; Armat et al., 2022;Li et al., 2024). Laughter activates the amygdala, which could be beneficial for adults with PD, as impairments in amygdala functions have been associated with PD symptoms (Klingbeil et al., 2021). The link between laughter-induced increases in dopamine and improvements in mood among adults with PD has not yet been thoroughly investigated in randomized clinical trials, despite anecdotal evidence supporting laughter's positive effects on mood (Manninen et al., 2017; Huang et al., 2018). Laughter may present a viable intervention for adults with PD experiencing psychosocial symptoms, potentially offering positive physical benefits similar to those achieved through physical exercise (Memarian, Sanatkaran, and Bahari, 2017; Bressington et al., 2019; Kumar, Singh, and Sharma, 2024, Meier et al., 2021). In the study conducted by Memarian et al. in 2017, including 24 individuals with PD, the effect of LY on PD's symptoms was examined, and as a result of the study, it was found that LY exercises can reduce anxiety and improve sleep quality in individuals with PD (Memarian, Sanatkaran, and Bahari, 2017). In the recommendation of the study, LY be used as a complementary treatment in the treatment process of individuals with PD. In the study of Keykhahoseinpoor et al., the effect of LY on motor functions of PD was examined and it was concluded that LY had a positive effect on motor function and flexibility in individuals with PD after 8 weeks of LY intervention, and LY sessions were recommended to improve balance, motor function and activities of daily living for individuals with PD (Keykhahoseinpoor, Rahnama and Chitsaz, 2013). In the study of Kumar et al. 64 individuals with PD who were also diagnosed with type 2 diabetes mellitus were included and this sample was applied LY sessions lasting 30 minutes and 5 sessions per week for 3 months. After the intervention, it was concluded that LY contributed positively to the improvement of stress level, motor and non-motor symptoms and positively affected the quality of life of individuals with PD (Kumar, Singh and Sharma, 2024). As a result of the study conducted by Tanaka et al. in 2018, regular LY can likely be applied safely to healthy adults and that it can be effective in improving mood and stress (Tanaka, Tokuda and Ichihara, 2018). In the systematic review meta-analysis conducted by Suarez-Iglesias et al., the effect of yoga on PD was investigated, and it was concluded that yoga interventions are promising for the management of motor and non-motor symptoms of patients with PD in places where yoga is safe for individuals with PD's disease (Suarez-Iglesias et al., 2022). As highlighted by other studies examining the effects of LY on PD's disease, LY can enhance muscle strength in the face, chest, and abdomen, which is particularly advantageous for hospitalized patients and elderly individuals using wheelchairs (Legault et al., 2021; Bressington et al., 2019). It also helps in reducing muscle tension by lowering stress hormones such as epinephrine and cortisol (Li et al., 2024). Furthermore, LY positively impacts the respiratory system by exercising the lungs and chest muscles, leading to improved vital capacity and breathing. It increases ventilation, aids in mucus removal, and boosts oxygen levels in the blood (Legault et al., 2021; Bressington et al., 2019). During laughter, air is expelled from the lungs, and carbon dioxide and water vapor are released, subsequently increasing oxygen intake (Ozturk and Tezel, 2021). Thus, considering the benefits of LY including pain relief, muscle relaxation, reduced anxiety and depression, and enhanced respiratory function it can be concluded that LY significantly improves sleep quality in patients with PD's disease, both directly and indirectly (Hatzipapas et al., 2017; El-Sayed et al., 2024; Ozturk and Tezel, 2021; Kuru Alici and Arikan Dönmez, 2020; Li et al., 2024). The effects of LY on PD are summarized in Table 1.

Table 1. The Impact of Laughter Yoga on Parkinson

Impacts	Description
Enhanced Muscle Strength	Improves strength in face, chest, and abdomen
Reduction in Muscle Tension	Lowers stress hormones and eases muscle tension
Improved Respiratory Function	Enhances lung and chest muscle function
Increased Oxygenation	Boosts blood oxygen levels and ventilation
Pain Relief	Relieves pain through muscle relaxation
Enhanced Mood	Elevates mood and psychological well-being
Reduced Anxiety and Depression	Alleviates anxiety and depression symptoms
Improved Sleep Quality	Enhances sleep quality directly and indirectly
Boosted Cognitive Function	Improves mental clarity and cognitive function
Strengthened Social Connections	Fosters social interaction and reduces isolation
Increased Dopamine Levels	Boosting dopamine levels, improving motor and mood symptoms
Enhanced Quality of Life	Contributes to a more positive outlook on life

The use of LY in nursing has gained prominence in recent literature and is recognized as a significant nursing intervention (Ozturk and Tezel, 2021). LY can serve as a method for managing stress for healthy individuals, patients, caregivers, and nurses themselves (Özer and Ateş, 2021). A study involving nurses caring for psychiatric patients reported that LY, when used appropriately, helps in building a trusting relationship with patients (Bag, 2020). Another study with nurses working in intensive care units found that LY was utilized among patients, their families, and the nurses themselves, especially during patient visits and handovers, proving beneficial (Menekli, and Doğan, 2021). Oncology nurses have noted that LY can be useful for reducing pain and managing the fear of death in oncology patients (Chelly et al., 2022). Pediatric nurses have highlighted the effectiveness of LY in helping children cope with illness and the stress associated with hospitalization (Sánchez et al., 2017). Interest in LY within the field of nursing began with doctoral theses, and it is recognized as an intervention that can be applied to both healthy and ill individuals, offering health benefits and enhancing nurse-patient interactions (Ozturk and Tezel, 2021). Systematic reviews indicate that laughter therapies are applicable in a variety of settings and for diverse patient groups (Bressington et al., 2019; Gonot-Schoupinsky and Garip, 2018). Laughter-inducing therapies should preferably be conducted in group and individual settings under the guidance of an experienced instructor in group dynamics and laughter exercises. It is noted that implementing LY in clinical practice requires a certified instructor (Bressington et al., 2019). Health professionals can either apply the intervention after obtaining the necessary certification or refer patients to specialists in this field (Ozturk and Tezel, 2021; Özer and Ateş, 2021). In the context of rising healthcare costs and an aging population, LY demonstrates potential as a low-cost, simple intervention that can be applied by healthcare professionals (Bressington et al., 2019; Li et al., 2024). The application of LY in nursing approaches for PD is particularly promising. Research into LY's effects on PD has highlighted its potential benefits in managing symptoms associated with this condition (Bressington et al., 2019; Gonot-Schoupinsky and Garip, 2018).

Laughter Yoga for Caregivers

LY has emerged as a complementary therapeutic approach that can benefit not only patients but also their family caregivers (DeCaro and Constantine Brown, 2016). Caregivers of PD frequently experience high levels of stress, emotional burden, and decreased well-being due to the chronic nature of the disease and its impact on daily functioning (Geerlings et al., 2023; Schrag et al., 2006; D'Amelio et al., 2009). Including caregivers in LY sessions may enhance patient engagement while simultaneously alleviating caregiver stress and enhancing psychosocial well-being (Yim, 2016). Involving caregivers in the sessions is critical for ensuring safety and maximizing therapeutic effectiveness (DeCaro and Constantine Brown, 2016). This engagement strengthens social interaction and fosters caregivers' self-efficacy, thereby supporting their psychosocial well-being. Moreover, observations and feedback collected during the sessions further reinforce caregivers' active participation and deepen their interaction with the patient (Van der Wal and Kok, 2019). It is therefore anticipated that including caregivers in LY interventions could positively influence the overall quality of life of both the caregiver and the patient. Such an approach is considered an important strategy for sustaining the therapeutic process and enhancing the effectiveness of LY in home settings (Akimbekov and Razzaque, 2021). Studies investigating LY and similar psychosocial interventions have consistently demonstrated improvements in patients' psychological and physiological states (Kim et al., 2015; Bressington et al., 2019; Tavakoli et al., 2019; DeCaro and Constantine Brown, 2016). However, the majority of the existing literature has focused primarily on patients, rather than family caregivers. Consequently, inferences regarding caregiver outcomes are largely indirect. For instance, Kim et al. (2015) reported that four LY sessions in cancer patients led to reductions in anxiety, depression, and stress (Kim et al., 2015). These findings suggest that improvements in patients' psychological well-being may indirectly reduce caregivers' mental burden. Similarly, Özer and Ateş (2021) found that 16 LY sessions in hemodialysis patients decreased pain levels and improved sleep quality (Özer & Ateş, 2021), which may facilitate caregivers' daily responsibilities and alleviate emotional strain. In a study of patients with depression, Bressington et al. (2019) observed that eight LY sessions led to enhancements in both physical and mental functioning (Bressington et al., 2019). Despite variability in anxiety, depression, and stress outcomes, improvements in patients' quality of life have the potential to ease caregiver burden. Likewise, Tavakoli et al. (2019) reported that seven LY sessions in IBS patients resulted in reduced symptom severity and anxiety, which could decrease the time and effort caregivers must devote, thereby reducing stress (Tavakoli et al., 2019). Together, these findings indicate that improvements in patients' psychological and physiological well-being may indirectly alleviate caregiver burden. A recent pre-experimental study examined the effects of a 45-minute LY session on adults with PD (n = 47) and their caregivers (n = 38) across six support groups in Southern California. Participants completed the "How Do You Feel?" questionnaire, which assessed ten domains of well-being, including mood, energy, optimism, stress, social connectedness, muscle and mental relaxation, and the ability to laugh without a reason. This study revealed statistically significant improvements in all measured domains for both patients and caregivers, suggesting that LY can effectively enhance overall well-being (DeCaro and Constantine Brown, 2016). The literature indicates that, in addition to its positive effects on patients, including caregivers in LY sessions may enhance caregivers' psychosocial well-being. However, to evaluate the sustained impact of LY on caregiver burden and quality of life, well-designed studies that directly assess caregivers are needed. Given the accessibility of certified LY training programs and online courses, caregivers have the opportunity to engage in LY themselves, which may provide practical benefits in stress reduction and overall well-being. Future research should explore the effectiveness of caregiver-led LY sessions as a sustainable strategy for supporting both patients and family caregivers.

Practical Implementation of Laughter Yoga at Home

Home-based LY has been identified as a significant intervention for improving quality of life and overall well-being in both patients and healthy individuals (Akimbekov & Razzaque, 2021; Han et al., 2023; Heidari et al., 2020; Qu et al., 2025). LY can be implemented either individually or in groups under the guidance of certified instructors, and healthcare professionals may apply it at home after appropriate training or refer patients to specialists as needed (Bressington et al., 2019; Ozturk & Tezel, 2021). Home-based LY offers advantages in terms of accessibility, continuity, and personalization (Akimbekov & Razzaque, 2021). Practicing regularly in the comfort of one's home reduces barriers such as transportation difficulties, mobility limitations, or scheduling conflicts, thereby enhancing participation and engagement (Heidari et al., 2020). Additionally, home-based practice facilitates the active involvement of caregivers or family members, strengthening the patient's surrounding psychosocial support system (Han et al., 2023; Heidari et al., 2020). For safe and effective implementation at home, careful planning and adaptation to the individual's functional capacity are essential. LY, as a low-cost and simple intervention, has the potential to enhance both patient and healthcare provider interaction and can serve as a motivational adjunct to conventional therapeutic approaches (Li et al., 2024; Bressington et al., 2019). Establishing a consistent routine, implementing safety measures, and creating an enjoyable environment increase the sustainability of home-based LY practice (Heidari et al., 2020).

Safety and Implementation Recommendations

The effectiveness and safety of home-based LY are closely linked to a structured session flow (Heidari et al., 2020; Qu et al., 2025). For example, sessions are recommended to include a 5-minute warm-up, 15-minute laughter exercises, and a 5-minute relaxation phase. This structure allows participants to prepare both physically and mentally while promoting post-session relaxation (Akimbekov & Razzaque, 2021). Safety measures are particularly critical for older adults or individuals with limited mobility (Heidari et al., 2020). Recommendations include ensuring adequate space, avoiding slippery surfaces, and using supportive equipment when necessary. Moreover, certain medical conditions, such as advanced heart failure, severe respiratory disorders, or acute illnesses, require prior consultation with a healthcare professional before commencing LY practice (Akimbekov & Razzaque, 2021).

Following these safety considerations, the stages of home-based LY practice are outlined below (Akimbekov & Razzaque, 2021; Shahidi et al., 2011):

1-Preparation and Environment Arrangement

Effective implementation of LY at home first requires identifying an appropriate setting. Selecting a quiet, safe, and comfortable room is recommended, as it provides an environment supports participants and facilitates a positive experience during the sessions. External distractions, noise, or uncomfortable surroundings can diminish the effectiveness of the intervention and impede participants' focus. Therefore, a calm and secure environment serves as a supportive foundation both physically and psychologically. Promoting social interaction among participants is also a critical component of LY sessions. Arranging chairs in close proximity is particularly recommended, as it enables eye contact and fosters interpersonal communication. This setup is especially beneficial for older adults, as it strengthens social bonds, reduces feelings of loneliness, and enhances motivation. Eye contact and close seating arrangements also help participants feel included and secure, thereby encouraging active engagement throughout the session. Environmental factors further contribute to the effectiveness of LY practice. Access to natural light or the presence of brightly colored objects can help maintain participants' attention and increase engagement. Visual stimulation and adequate lighting enhance cognitive alertness, preventing attention lapses that may occur in monotonous settings. This consideration is particularly relevant for older adults, for whom cognitive stimulation is crucial. Regarding session duration, a period of 20–30 minutes is recommended. This timeframe is both achievable and sustainable for participants. Longer sessions may induce fatigue or attention decline, while excessively short sessions may not allow sufficient therapeutic benefit. Establishing this duration facilitates the creation of a consistent daily or weekly routine, which helps build habits and maximizes the cognitive, emotional, and social benefits of LY practice over time. In conclusion, the effective implementation of LY at home depends on selecting an appropriate space, arranging seating to support social interaction, optimizing environmental conditions, and defining suitable session durations. The combination of these factors ensures that LY practice can be both enjoyable and therapeutically effective for participants.

2-Warm-up and Rhythm Exercises

LY sessions typically commence with hand-clapping and gentle body movements. This initial phase is essential for boosting participant motivation and physically preparing the body for subsequent laughter exercises. Simple vocalizations, such as the phrase "Ho-Ho-Ha-Ha-Ha," combined with slow and controlled breathing exercises, have been reported to yield positive effects at the beginning of the session. Warm-up and rhythm exercises facilitate participants' physical, cognitive, and emotional engagement. Hand-clapping and gentle body movements help to increase body temperature and promote physical readiness, while rhythmic, coordinated actions within the group foster a sense of unity and social connection. These practices promote relaxation, reduce tension, and enhance active participation throughout the session. Furthermore, incorporating vocal exercises and controlled breathing allows participants to regulate their respiratory patterns and increase energy levels through vocal expression. Slow, mindful breathing helps to balance heart rate, reduce stress, and ease the transition into laughter exercises. This combination ensures that participants are prepared both physically and vocally, ensuring a smooth and effective transition to the core components of the LY session. In conclusion, warm-up and rhythm exercises form a foundational component of LY sessions. This phase not only promotes physical, cognitive, and emotional readiness but also enhances group cohesion and participant motivation, ultimately making the subsequent laughter exercises more effective and enjoyable.

3-Deep Breathing Exercises

Deep breathing exercises are recognized as a fundamental practice for promoting both mental and physical relaxation. In this stage, participants are encouraged to inhale deeply through the nose, hold the breath for several seconds, and then exhale through the mouth while while lightly laughing. This practice not only increases oxygen intake but also triggers physiological mechanisms. Deep breathing exercises enhance participants' mental focus and help alleviate feelings of tension or anxiety. For older adults or individuals with limited mobility, these exercises should be performed more slowly and gently to ensure safety. Careful adaptation minimizes the risk of dizziness, breathlessness, or other discomforts, while supporting a safe and effective practice. Controlled breathing also helps regulate heart rate and promotes an overall state of calm and relaxation.

Exhaling in conjunction with light laughter prepares participants both physically and emotionally for the subsequent components of the session. This technique activates the respiratory muscles, supports lung capacity, and enhances the flow of energy within the body. Additionally, performing these exercises in a group setting fosters a shared experience and strengthens social bonds among participants. In conclusion, deep breathing exercises constitute a core element of LY sessions. This practice facilitates physical relaxation, mental focus, and emotional calm, thereby enabling a safe and effective transition into the following stages of the session. Adaptations for age and physical capacity ensure that the exercises are both accessible and safe, allowing participants to derive maximum benefit from the practice.

4-Childlike Acting and Play

In the later stages of the session, participants are encouraged to engage in activities that foster a childlike spirit. This phase typically includes simple games, singing, or movement imitation, which the literature indicates can trigger spontaneous and genuine laughter. Childlike acting and play exercises support emotional relaxation by helping participants reduce stress experienced in daily life. These activities allow individuals to express themselves freely, explore their creativity, and interact more comfortably in a social context. Simple games and movement imitation activate both physical and cognitive engagement, naturally promoting laughter production. Additionally, activities such as singing or movement imitation create shared experiences within the group, enhancing social interaction and cohesion among participants. This social connection can reduce feelings of loneliness and increase engagement with the session. Childlike acting allows participants to express themselves without fear of judgment, thereby fostering self-confidence and emotional security. In conclusion, the childlike acting and play stage constitutes one of the most emotionally impactful components of LY sessions. It facilitates stress reduction, promotes spontaneous laughter, and strengthens social bonds, contributing to an enjoyable and therapeutically valuable experience for participants.

5-Laughter Exercises

Laughter exercises can be implemented in a variety of forms. Physical laughter exercises, often combined with arm and leg movements, have been reported in the literature to contribute to enhanced mobility. When integrated with breathing techniques and meditation, these exercises are emphasized as supporting mental relaxation and overall well-being. Cheerful laughter exercises, supplemented with simple jokes or animated activities, enhance the enjoyment and participant-centered nature of the session. The literature indicates that laughter initiated artificially can, within a short period, evolve into genuine and contagious laughter. This transformation encourages participants to engage both physically and emotionally, fostering active participation and interaction within the group. Laughter exercises also strengthen social bonds and promote group cohesion. Physical engagement during laughter contributes to regulating heart rate, reducing stress, and increasing energy levels. Additionally, allowing participants to express themselves freely through laughter supports emotional relaxation and the emergence of positive affect. In conclusion, laughter exercises constitute a core and highly effective component of LY sessions.

This stage provides benefits for physical health as well as mental and emotional well-being. Even laughter initiated artificially can quickly develop into genuine and contagious laughter, enhancing the energy of the session and providing participants with an enjoyable and therapeutically valuable experience.

6-Session Closure and Feedback

The session is concluded with gentle stretching and relaxation exercises. This phase is important for allowing participants to release muscle tension, promote physical relaxation, and integrate the effects of the activities performed during the session. Stretching and relaxation exercises support both physical calmness and mental tranquility, enabling participants to continue the remainder of their day in a more balanced and energized state. Observing and documenting participants' post-session experiences is emphasized as a critical component for evaluating the therapeutic process. Monitoring participants' emotional states, attention levels, energy, and responses to laughter and play activities provides valuable data for understanding the session's effects and planning future interventions. When conducted at home with a partner or family member, reciprocal feedback and brief discussion are reported to enhance social bonding. Participants have the opportunity to express their experiences, share reflections, and strengthen relational connections. This process not only encourages social interaction but also reduces feelings of isolation, thereby reinforcing the positive outcomes of the session. In conclusion, session closure and feedback constitute a complementary and essential component of LY sessions. This phase facilitates physical and emotional relaxation, supports the assessment of therapeutic progress, and promotes the strengthening of social bonds. Regular observation and feedback enhance the effectiveness of the session and ensure that participants derive maximum benefit from the practice.

Limitations of Laughter Yoga for Parkinson's disease

LY has been recognized as a cost-effective, safe, and accessible intervention with positive impacts on quality of life, sleep quality, and both physical and mental symptoms, including depression, pain, anxiety, and stress (Hatzipapas et al., 2017; El-Sayed et al., 2024; Ozturk & Tezel, 2021; Kuru Alici & Arikan Dönmez, 2020; Li et al., 2024). Research findings are generally consistent with international studies, highlighting its potential benefits (Bressington et al., 2019; Gonot-Schoupinsky & Garip, 2018). However, several limitations in the current literature must be noted. Firstly, there is a low level of evidence supporting the effectiveness of LY for PD and their caregivers, primarily due to the insufficient quality of the studies conducted (Bressington et al., 2019; Van der Wal & Kok, 2019). While the intervention shows promise, the current body of evidence is inadequate compared to other group-based interventions. To enhance the validity of LY as a treatment for PD, there is a need for randomized controlled trials involving larger participant groups and more rigorous study designs (Bressington et al., 2019; Van der Wal & Kok, 2019). Although LY can be delivered individually or in group settings under the guidance of certified instructors, and healthcare professionals may administer it after receiving appropriate training or refer patients to qualified specialists, a key limitation is that access to trained instructors and adequately trained healthcare providers is often limited. This scarcity may restrict the widespread implementation of LY for patients with PD and caregivers, hindering its integration into routine care (Bressington et al., 2019; Ozturk & Tezel, 2021). Despite its potential, the absence of standardized clinical guidelines for LY introduces uncertainties regarding its implementation (Gonot-Schoupinsky & Garip, 2018). This may lead to variability in how healthcare professionals, including nurses, apply LY in patient care. Furthermore, the lack of LY training in nursing education represents a critical limitation, as it prevents nurses from integrating this potentially beneficial intervention into routine care. Incorporating LY training into nursing curricula could enable nurses to apply the intervention effectively, thereby enhancing both patient outcomes and caregiver engagement (Ozturk & Tezel, 2021; Özer & Ateş, 2021). Moreover, LY has the potential to strengthen interactions between patients and caregivers, providing psychosocial support and improving adherence to home-based exercises. Including caregivers in LY sessions can foster active participation, facilitate motivation, and enhance the overall therapeutic effect for patients with PD but there is a low level of evidence supporting this knowledge (Li et al., 2024; Bressington et al., 2019). Overall, these limitations underscore the necessity for further observational and experimental research to establish LY as an evidence-based intervention. Improving the quality of evidence, strengthening study methodologies, developing standardized clinical guidelines, and integrating LY training into healthcare education are crucial steps for validating LY's effectiveness and guiding its implementation in PD management and nursing practice (Bressington et al., 2019).

CONCLUSION AND RECOMMENDATIONS

Current literature suggests that LY has potential benefits for symptom management, psychosocial support, and quality of life in patients with PD and their caregivers. LY is a low-cost, safe, and feasible intervention that may improve both physical and psychological symptoms, including depression, anxiety, stress, pain, and sleep disturbances (Hatzipapas et al., 2017; El-Sayed et al., 2024; Ozturk & Tezel, 2021; Kuru Alici & Arikan Dönmez, 2020; Li et al., 2024). However, the current body of evidence is limited in quality and consistency, preventing reliable comparisons of LY with other group-based interventions. This limitation arises from heterogeneous findings, insufficiently detailed intervention protocols, inadequate descriptions of group facilitators and study populations, high risk of bias, and overall methodological shortcomings in the available studies.

To establish LY as an evidence-based intervention for PD symptom management, rigorously designed and thoroughly reported randomized controlled trials are essential. Future studies should prioritize symptom management as a primary outcome, include adequately powered sample sizes, employ long-term follow-up, comprehensively describe population characteristics and contextual factors influencing implementation, and standardize interventions through a manual or protocol to ensure replicability. Moreover, LY has the potential to strengthen interactions between patients and caregivers, providing psychosocial support and improving adherence to home-based exercises. Including caregivers in LY sessions can promote active participation, enhance motivation, and amplify the overall therapeutic effect (Li et al., 2024; Bressington et al., 2019). However, the evidence supporting these benefits remains limited, underscoring the need for additional studies that evaluate caregiver involvement and its impact on patient outcomes. Expanding this research will allow LY to be recommended more reliably for both PD patients and caregivers, increasing its feasibility and effectiveness in home-based interventions. Additionally, LY can be implemented individually or in group settings under the guidance of certified instructors, and healthcare professionals may administer the intervention following appropriate training or refer patients to qualified specialists (Bressington et al., 2019; Ozturk & Tezel, 2021). However, the scarcity of trained personnel and structured programs may restrict the widespread implementation of LY and hinder its integration into routine care. Consequently, incorporating LY and similar non-pharmacological therapeutic approaches into undergraduate, graduate, and clinical in-service nursing curricula is recommended. This integration would allow nursing professionals to acquire competence in these alternative interventions, enhancing patient care and expanding therapeutic options for symptom management in PD. In conclusion, LY represents a promising intervention for PD management and caregiver support. Nonetheless, given the current limitations and gaps in evidence, further high-quality research is required to support its widespread clinical application and educational integration. Improving study methodology, standardizing intervention protocols, and including caregivers in evaluations will strengthen the reliability of LY as an evidence-based approach, ultimately improving quality of life and clinical outcomes for both patients and their caregivers.

REFERENCES

Akimbekov, N. S., & Razzaque, M. S. (2021). Laughter therapy: A humor-induced hormonal intervention to reduce stress and anxiety. *Current Research in Physiology, 4*, 135–138. DOI: 10.1016/j.crphys.2021.04.002 PMID: 34642668

Angelopoulou, E., Bougea, A., Hatzimanolis, A., Stefanis, L., Scarmeas, N., & Papageorgiou, S. (2024). Mild Behavioral Impairment in Parkinson's Disease: An Updated Review on the Clinical, Genetic, Neuroanatomical, and Pathophysiological Aspects. *Medicina (Kaunas, Lithuania), 60*(1), 115. DOI: 10.3390/medicina60010115 PMID: 38256375

Armat, M. R., Emami Zeydi, A., Mokarami, H., Nakhlband, A., & Hojjat, S. K. (2022). The impact of laughter yoga on depression and anxiety among retired women: A randomized controlled clinical trial. *Journal of Women & Aging, 34*(1), 31–42. DOI: 10.1080/08952841.2020.1774225 PMID: 32552530

Bag, B. (2020). Therapeutic Use of Humor in Psychiatric Care. *Psikiyatride Güncel Yaklasimlar, 12*(4), 519–533. DOI: 10.18863/pgy.689943

Blard, F., Erraud, J., Bonnet, M., Auzou, N., & Tison, F. (2024). Mindfulness in Parkinson's disease: A French national survey and a pilot intervention feasibility trial using the MBSR program (M-Park). Revue neurologique, S0035-3787(24)00521-6. Advance online publication. https://doi.org/DOI: 10.1016/j.neurol.2024.03.013

Bressington, D., Mui, J., Yu, C., Leung, S. F., Cheung, K., Wu, C. S. T., Bollard, M., & Chien, W. T. (2019). Feasibility of a group-based laughter yoga intervention as an adjunctive treatment for residual symptoms of depression, anxiety and stress in people with depression. *Journal of Affective Disorders, 248*, 42–51. DOI: 10.1016/j.jad.2019.01.030 PMID: 30711868

Chaudhuri, K. R., Azulay, J. P., Odin, P., Lindvall, S., Domingos, J., Alobaidi, A., Kandukuri, P. L., Chaudhari, V. S., Parra, J. C., Yamazaki, T., Oddsdottir, J., Wright, J., & Martinez-Martin, P. (2024). Economic Burden of Parkinson's Disease: A Multinational, Real-World, Cost-of-Illness Study. *Drugs - Real World Outcomes, 11*(1), 1–11. DOI: 10.1007/s40801-023-00410-1 PMID: 38193999

Chelly, F., Kacem, I., Moussa, A., Ghenim, A., Krifa, I., Methamem, F., Chouachane, A., Aloui, A., Brahem, A., Kalboussi, H., El Maalel, O., Chatti, S., Maoua, M., Bannanou, S., & Mrizak, N. (2022). Healing humor: The use of humor in the nurse-patient relationship. *Occupational Diseases and Environmental Medicine, 10*(3), 217–231. DOI: 10.4236/odem.2022.103017

Cheung, M., & Leung, C. A. (2020). LYas a social work intervention. *Smith College Studies in Social Work, 90*(4), 288–301. DOI: 10.1080/00377317.2020.1819938

Church, F. C. (2021). Treatment Options for Motor and Non-Motor Symptoms of Parkinson's Disease. *Biomolecules, 11*(4), 612. DOI: 10.3390/biom11040612 PMID: 33924103

Ciurea, A. V., Mohan, A. G., Covache-Busuioc, R. A., Costin, H. P., Glavan, L. A., Corlatescu, A. D., & Saceleanu, V. M. (2023). Unraveling Molecular and Genetic Insights into Neurodegenerative Diseases: Advances in Understanding Alzheimer's, Parkinson's, and Huntington's Diseases and Amyotrophic Lateral Sclerosis. *International Journal of Molecular Sciences, 24*(13), 10809. DOI: 10.3390/ijms241310809 PMID: 37445986

D'Amelio, M., Terruso, V., Palmeri, B., Di Benedetto, N., Famoso, G., Cottone, P., Aridon, P., Ragonese, P., & Savettieri, G. (2009). Predictors of caregiver burden in partners of patients with Parkinson's disease. Neurological sciences: official journal of the Italian Neurological Society and of the Italian Society of Clinical Neurophysiology, 30(2), 171–174. https://doi.org/DOI: 10.1007/s10072-009-0024-z

DeCaro, D. S., & Constantine Brown, J. L. (2016). Laughter Yoga, Adults Living With Parkinson s Disease, and Caregivers: A Pilot Study. *Explore (New York, N.Y.), 12*(3), 196–199. DOI: 10.1016/j.explore.2016.02.005 PMID: 27033323

El-Sayed, M. M., Hafez, S. A., Nashwan, A. J., Khedr, M. A., & El-Ashry, A. M. (2024). Feasibility of a group-based laughter yoga therapy on anxiety and happiness among community-dwelling older adults: A quasi-experimental study. *International Journal of Africa Nursing Sciences, 20*, 100675. DOI: 10.1016/j.ijans.2024.100675

Geerlings, A. D., Kapelle, W. M., Sederel, C. J., Tenison, E., Wijngaards-Berenbroek, H., Meinders, M. J., Munneke, M., Ben-Shlomo, Y., Bloem, B. R., & Darweesh, S. K. L. (2023). Caregiver burden in Parkinson's disease: A mixed-methods study. *BMC Medicine, 21*(1), 247. DOI: 10.1186/s12916-023-02933-4 PMID: 37424022

Gonot-Schoupinsky, F. N., & Garip, G. (2018). Laughter and humour interventions for well-being in older adults: A systematic review and intervention classification. *Complementary Therapies in Medicine, 38*, 85–91. DOI: 10.1016/j.ctim.2018.04.009 PMID: 29857886

Han, S., Zhang, L., Li, Q., Wang, X., & Lian, S. (2023). The Effects of Laughter Yoga on Perceived Stress, Positive Psychological Capital, and Exercise Capacity in Lung Cancer Chemotherapy Patients: A Pilot Randomized Trial. *Integrative Cancer Therapies, 22*, 15347354231218271. DOI: 10.1177/15347354231218271 PMID: 38102816

Harris, D. M., O'Bryan, S. J., & Latella, C. (2024). Non-invasive brain stimulation as treatment for motor impairment in people with Parkinson's disease: Protocol for an umbrella review. *PLoS One*, *19*(6), e0304717. DOI: 10.1371/journal.pone.0304717 PMID: 38870241

Hatzipapas, I., Visser, M. J., & Janse van Rensburg, E. (2017). Laughter therapy as an intervention to promote psychological well-being of volunteer community care workers working with HIV-affected families. *SAHARA J : Journal of Social Aspects of HIV/AIDS Research Alliance*, *14*(1), 202–212. DOI: 10.1080/17290376.2017.1402696 PMID: 29169302

Heidari, M., Ghodusi Borujeni, M., Rezaei, P., Kabirian Abyaneh, S., & Heidari, K. (2020). Effect of Laughter Therapy on Depression and Quality of Life of the Elderly Living in Nursing Homes. *The Malaysian Journal of Medical Sciences : MJMS*, *27*(4), 119–129. DOI: 10.21315/mjms2020.27.4.11 PMID: 32863751

Heo, E. H., Kim, S., Park, H. J., & Kil, S. Y. (2016). The effects of a simulated laughter programme on mood, cortisol levels, and health-related quality of life among haemodialysis patients. *Complementary Therapies in Clinical Practice*, *25*, 1–7. DOI: 10.1016/j.ctcp.2016.07.001 PMID: 27863598

Höglinger, G., Bähr, M., Becktepe, J., Berg, D., Brockmann, K., Buhmann, C., Ceballos-Baumann, A., Claßen, J., Deuschl, C., Deuschl, G., Dodel, R., Ebersbach, G., Eggers, C., van Eimeren, T., Fanciulli, A., Fimm, B., Folkerts, A.-K., Gausepohl, M., Hasan, A., & Trenkwalder, C.German Parkinson's Guidelines Committee. (2024). Diagnosis and treatment of Parkinson's disease (guideline of the German Society for Neurology). *Neurological Research and Practice*, *6*(1), 30. DOI: 10.1186/s42466-024-00325-4 PMID: 38845028

Huang, Y., Aronson, J. P., Pilitsis, J. G., Gee, L., Durphy, J., Molho, E. S., & Ramirez-Zamora, A. (2018). Anatomical Correlates of Uncontrollable Laughter With Unilateral Subthalamic Deep Brain Stimulation in Parkinson's Disease. *Frontiers in Neurology*, *9*, 341. DOI: 10.3389/fneur.2018.00341 PMID: 29887826

Huang, Y., Li, Y., Pan, H., & Han, L. (2023). Global, regional, and national burden of neurological disorders in 204 countries and territories worldwide. *Journal of Global Health*, *13*, 04160. DOI: 10.7189/jogh.13.04160 PMID: 38018250

Kalia, L. V., & Lang, A. E. (2015). Parkinson's disease. *Lancet*, *386*(9996), 896–912. DOI: 10.1016/S0140-6736(14)61393-3 PMID: 25904081

Kataria, M. (2018). *Laughter yoga: Daily laughter practices for health and happiness*. Penguin Random House India Private Limited.

Keykhahoseinpoor, A., Rahnama, N., & Chitsaz, A. (2013). Effects of eight weeks LYtraining on motor function, balance, and flexibility in subjects with PD's disease. Journal of research in rehabilitation sciences, 9(1), 39-47. https://doi.org/DOI: 10.22122/jrrs.v9i1.856

Kim, S. H., Kim, Y. H., & Kim, H. J. (2015). Laughter and stress relief in cancer patients: A pilot study. *Evidence-Based Complementary and Alternative Medicine : eCAM*, *2015*, 1–6. DOI: 10.1155/2015/864739 PMID: 26064177

Klingbeil, J., Wawrzyniak, M., Stockert, A., Brandt, M. L., Schneider, H. R., Metelmann, M., & Saur, D. (2021). Pathological laughter and crying: Insights from lesion network-symptom-mapping. *Brain*, *144*(10), 3264–3276. DOI: 10.1093/brain/awab224 PMID: 34142117

Kouli, A., Torsney, K. M., & Kuan, W. L. (2018). Parkinson's Disease: Etiology, Neuropathology, and Pathogenesis. In T. B. Stoker (Eds.) et al., Parkinson's Disease: Pathogenesis and Clinical Aspects. Codon Publications. DOI: 10.15586/codonpublications.parkinsonsdisease.2018.ch1

Kumar, R., Singh, R., & Sharma, V. (2024). Protective potential of LYand clapping exercises on stress level and motor functions in PD patients with type 2 diabetes. *PDism & Related Disorders*, *122*. Advance online publication. DOI: 10.1016/j.parkreldis.2024.106915

Kuru Alici, N., & Arikan Dönmez, A. (2020). A systematic review of the effect of laughter yoga on physical function and psychosocial outcomes in older adults. *Complementary Therapies in Clinical Practice*, *41*, 101252. DOI: 10.1016/j.ctcp.2020.101252 PMID: 33217706

Legault, Z., Znaty, A., Smith, S., & Boudrias, M. H. (2021). Yoga Interventions Used for the Rehabilitation of Stroke, Parkinson's Disease, and Multiple Sclerosis: A Scoping Review of Clinical Research. *Journal of Alternative and Complementary Medicine (New York, N.Y.)*, *27*(12), 1023–1057. DOI: 10.1089/acm.2021.0003 PMID: 34185577

Li, J., Liao, Y., Zhang, S. Y., Jin, L., Congdon, N., Fan, Z., Zeng, Y., Zheng, Y., Liu, Z., Liu, Y., & Liang, L. (2024). Effect of laughter exercise versus 0.1% sodium hyaluronic acid on ocular surface discomfort in dry eye disease: Non-inferiority randomised controlled trial. *BMJ (Clinical Research Ed.)*, *386*, e080474. DOI: 10.1136/bmj-2024-080474 PMID: 39260878

Li, T., Soh, K. L., Zakaria, N. F., Pang, Y., Wang, P., & Hu, N. (2024). Effects of LYon Patients Receiving Hemodialysis: A Systematic Review. *Holistic Nursing Practice*, *38*(4), 202–212. DOI: 10.1097/HNP.0000000000000650 PMID: 38900006

Manninen, S., Tuominen, L., Dunbar, R. I., Karjalainen, T., Hirvonen, J., Arponen, E., Hari, R., Jääskeläinen, I. P., Sams, M., & Nummenmaa, L. (2017). Social Laughter Triggers Endogenous Opioid Release in Humans. *The Journal of Neuroscience : The Official Journal of the Society for Neuroscience*, *37*(25), 6125–6131. DOI: 10.1523/JNEUROSCI.0688-16.2017 PMID: 28536272

Meier, M., Wirz, L., Dickinson, P., & Pruessner, J. C. (2021). Laughter yoga reduces the cortisol response to acute stress in healthy individuals. *Stress (Amsterdam, Netherlands)*, *24*(1), 44–52. DOI: 10.1080/10253890.2020.1766018 PMID: 32393092

Memarian, A., Sanatkaran, A., & Bahari, S. M. (2017). The effect of LYexercises on anxiety and sleep quality in patients suffering from PD's disease. *Biomedical Research and Therapy*, *4*(07), 1463–1479. DOI: 10.15419/bmrat.v4i07.200

Menekli, T., & Doğan, R. (2021). The relationship between humor style and death anxiety of palliative care patients. *International Journal of Health Services Research and Policy*, *6*(3), 369–379. DOI: 10.33457/ijhsrp.996104

Mohajer, S., Mazlum, S. R., Rajabzadeh, M., & Namazinia, M. (2022). The effect of laughter yoga on depression in cancer patients undergoing chemotherapy: A randomized clinical trial. *Hayat (Tihran)*, *28*(3), 284–295. DOI: 10.30699/hayat.28.3.284

Muleiro Alvarez, M., Cano-Herrera, G., Osorio Martínez, M. F., Vega Gonzales-Portillo, J., Monroy, G. R., Murguiondo Pérez, R., Torres-Ríos, J. A., van Tienhoven, X. A., Garibaldi Bernot, E. M., Esparza Salazar, F., & Ibarra, A. (2024). A Comprehensive Approach to Parkinson's Disease: Addressing Its Molecular, Clinical, and Therapeutic Aspects. *International Journal of Molecular Sciences*, *25*(13), 7183. DOI: 10.3390/ijms25137183 PMID: 39000288

Noureldein, M. H., & Eid, A. A. (2018). Homeostatic effect of laughter on diabetic cardiovascular complications: The myth turned to fact. *Diabetes Research and Clinical Practice*, *135*, 111–119. DOI: 10.1016/j.diabres.2017.11.014 PMID: 29162513

Özer, Z., & Ateş, S. (2021). Effects of laughter yoga on hemodialysis patients' plasma-beta endorphin levels, pain levels and sleep quality: A randomized controlled trial. *Complementary Therapies in Clinical Practice*, *43*, 101382. DOI: 10.1016/j.ctcp.2021.101382 PMID: 33831803

Ozturk, F. O., & Tezel, A. (2021). Effect of laughter yoga on mental symptoms and salivary cortisol levels in first-year nursing students: A randomized controlled trial. *International Journal of Nursing Practice*, *27*(2), e12924. DOI: 10.1111/ijn.12924 PMID: 33580606

Qu, L., Cao, Y., Wang, M., Song, D., & Huang, G. (2025). Effects of laughter therapy on improving physical and psychological symptoms among cancer patients: a systematic review and meta-analysis. Supportive care in cancer: official journal of the Multinational Association of Supportive Care in Cancer, 33(3), 230. https://doi.org/1DOI: 10.1007/s00520-025-09276-

Rouhi, S., Etemadi, S., & Pooraghajan, M. (2020). Laughter in combination with yoga exercises: Changes in psychological distress and quality of life in patients with coronary heart disease (CHD). *The Open Psychology Journal*, *13*(1), 144–150. Advance online publication. DOI: 10.2174/1874350102013010144

Ruch, W., & Raskin, V. (2008). Psychology of humor (No. 8, pp. 17-100). Mouton de Gruyter.

Sánchez, J. C., Echeverri, L. F., Londoño, M. J., Ochoa, S. A., Quiroz, A. F., Romero, C. R., & Ruiz, J. O. (2017). Effects of a Humor Therapy Program on Stress Levels in Pediatric Inpatients. *Hospital Pediatrics*, *7*(1), 46–53. DOI: 10.1542/hpeds.2016-0128 PMID: 27908974

Savage, B. M., Lujan, H. L., Thipparthi, R. R., & DiCarlo, S. E. (2017). Humor, laughter, learning, and health! A brief review. *Advances in Physiology Education*, *41*(3), 341–347. DOI: 10.1152/advan.00030.2017 PMID: 28679569

Schrag, A., Hovris, A., Morley, D., Quinn, N., & Jahanshahi, M. (2006). Caregiver-burden in parkinson's disease is closely associated with psychiatric symptoms, falls, and disability. *Parkinsonism & Related Disorders*, *12*(1), 35–41. DOI: 10.1016/j.parkreldis.2005.06.011 PMID: 16271496

Shahidi, M., Mojtahed, A., Modabbernia, A., Mojtahed, M., Shafiabady, A., Delavar, A., & Honari, H. (2011). Laughter yoga versus group exercise program in elderly depressed women: A randomized controlled trial. *International Journal of Geriatric Psychiatry*, *26*(3), 322–327. DOI: 10.1002/gps.2545 PMID: 20848578

Suarez-Iglesias, D., Santos, L., Sanchez-Lastra, M. A., & Ayan, C. (2022). Systematic review and meta-analysis of randomised controlled trials on the effects of yoga in people with PD's disease. *Disability and Rehabilitation*, *44*(21), 6210–6229. DOI: 10.1080/09638288.2021.1966522 PMID: 34533097

Tanaka, A., Tokuda, N., & Ichihara, K. (2018). Psychological and physiological effects of LYsessions in Japan: A pilot study. *Nursing & Health Sciences*, *20*(3), 304–312. DOI: 10.1111/nhs.12562 PMID: 30156373

Tavakoli, T., Davoodi, N., Jafar Tabatabaee, T. S., Rostami, Z., Mollaei, H., Salmani, F., Ayati, S., & Tabrizi, S. (2019). Comparison of Laughter Yoga and Anti-Anxiety Medication on Anxiety and Gastrointestinal Symptoms of Patients with Irritable Bowel Syndrome. *Middle East Journal of Digestive Diseases*, *11*(4), 211–217. DOI: 10.15171/mejdd.2019.151 PMID: 31824624

Thomas, S., Edwards, E., & Kobylecki, C. (2024, August 13). (2024). Parkinson's Nurses Are Crucial for the Management of Parkinson's Disease: 2007-2024. *Journal of Parkinson's Disease*, *14*(s1), S209–S217. Advance online publication. DOI: 10.3233/JPD-230224 PMID: 38578901

Tolosa, E., Garrido, A., Scholz, S. W., & Poewe, W. (2021). Challenges in the diagnosis of Parkinson's disease. *Lancet Neurology*, *20*(5), 385–397. DOI: 10.1016/S1474-4422(21)00030-2 PMID: 33894193

Tosin, M. H., Goetz, C. G., & Stebbins, G. T. (2024). Patient With Parkinson Disease and Care Partner Perceptions of Key Domains Affecting Health-Related Quality of Life: Systematic Review. *Neurology*, *102*(3), e208028. DOI: 10.1212/WNL.0000000000208028 PMID: 38215353

Van der Wal, C. N., & Kok, R. N. (2019). Laughter-inducing therapies: Systematic review and meta-analysis. *Social Science & Medicine*, *232*, 473–488. DOI: 10.1016/j.socscimed.2019.02.018 PMID: 31029483

Wang, Y., Liang, J., Fang, Y., Yao, D., Zhang, L., Zhou, Y., Wang, Y., Hu, L., Lu, Z., Wang, Y., & Xiao, Z. (2023). Burden of common neurologic diseases in Asian countries, 1990–2019: An analysis for the Global Burden of Disease Study 2019. *Neurology*, *100*(21), e2141–e2154. DOI: 10.1212/WNL.0000000000207218 PMID: 37015823

Yang, Y., Wang, G., Zhang, S., Wang, H., Zhou, W., Ren, F., Liang, H., Wu, D., Ji, X., Hashimoto, M., & Wei, J. (2022). Efficacy and evaluation of therapeutic exercises on adults with Parkinson's disease: A systematic review and network meta-analysis. *BMC Geriatrics*, *22*(1), 813. DOI: 10.1186/s12877-022-03510-9 PMID: 36271367

Yim, J. (2016). Therapeutic Benefits of Laughter in Mental Health: A Theoretical Review. *The Tohoku Journal of Experimental Medicine*, *239*(3), 243–249. DOI: 10.1620/tjem.239.243 PMID: 27439375

Zhang, Y., Liu, S., Xu, K., Zhou, Y., Shen, Y., Liu, Z., Bai, Y., & Wang, S. (2024). Non-pharmacological therapies for treating non-motor symptoms in patients with Parkinson's disease: A systematic review and meta-analysis. *Frontiers in Aging Neuroscience*, *16*, 1363115. DOI: 10.3389/fnagi.2024.1363115 PMID: 38737585

Chapter 8
What Works Best?
Comparing Music Therapy Approaches in Home Care

Matthew A. Ward
School of Media and Applied Arts, University of Management and Technology Ho Chi Minh City, Vietnam

Tuong-Minh Ly-Le
https://orcid.org/0000-0001-8203-7357
School of Media and Applied Arts, University of Management and Technology Ho Chi Minh City, Vietnam

ABSTRACT

There has been growing interest in music therapy as a non-pharmacological home care treatment that decreases pain symptoms, anxiety, and emotional distress. Even though there exists evidence supporting its general efficacy, there remains little investigation into the relative efficacy of different music therapy modalities and the influence of intervention frequency and duration on outcomes. The aim of this study is to perform a systematic review of RCTs and compare the differential effectiveness of music therapy interventions in adult palliative care populations. The main outcomes are pain, anxiety, depression, and quality of life, as measured by validated instruments. Studies were included and were sought through systematic searches of a number of databases for publications up to 2015-2025. The study is expected to identify the most effective forms of music therapy, whether frequency and duration impact effectiveness, and thus inform evidence-based practice recommendations for the integration of music interventions into home care.

DOI: 10.4018/979-8-3373-4094-4.ch008

1. INTRODUCTION

Over the last twenty years, music therapy has emerged as a viable option for non-pharmacological intervention in palliative or holistic care which focuses on providing relief for the symptoms and stresses resulting from serious and life-limiting illnesses, improving quality of life for the patients as well as their families and caretakers. The setting for palliative care involves treatment focusing on quality of life rather than "curative intent" which may be administered alongside or mutually exclusively from the holistic approach in which music therapy has become a tenable option. The field of music therapy and the efficacy of this approach is supported by an ever-growing body of research, randomized controlled trials (RCTs), and systematic reviews (Li et al., 2025; Boyde et al., 2024).

Despite the sizeable body of research conducted in the field of palliative music therapy, the field lacks robust comparative evaluations of different therapeutic modalities. Passive receptive listening, guided imagery and music (GIM), vibroacoustic interventions, and active participatory sessions (e.g., singing, playing instruments, composing/songwriting) are often generalized and grouped under the umbrella term "music therapy," yet they may operate through distinct mechanisms and offer benefits which may be best sourced in different ways, at different times, and different contexts for individuals. For example, receptive listening may be particularly effective for rapid relaxation and symptom management in bedridden patients, whereas active engagement may better enhance mood, self-expression, and social interaction depending on the individual/s. Even vibroacoustic music therapy, which combines auditory and tactile stimulation, has demonstrated short-term effects on subjective well-being and perception of body warmth (S. Bieligmeyer et al., 2018). Not all benefits in this area are exclusively restricted to auditory channels, which in one way exemplifies the diversity of these benefits.

An important factor in the examination of this multi-dimensional study is the amount or "dosage" of music therapy and to what degree it is useful and effective for given circumstances and stages of illness and healing. Session length, intervention frequency, and overall program duration can influence clinical outcomes as suggested by research data. One from a meta-analysis of lung cancer patients (Li et al., 2025) indicates that engaging in music therapy for 30 minutes, one to two times per day, over two to twelve weeks, was associated with significantly greater reductions in anxiety and depression compared to less frequent or shorter intervention. These effects are associated with the physiology and psychology of the patients. These parameters may vary depending on individual patient conditions, modalities, and the targeted outcomes.

This chapter addresses the variances and gaps in the quantitative research by comparing results, "dosage," conditions, and modalities from RCTs in recent years for adult palliative care populations. Primary aims:

1. Comparative and relative effectiveness of various musical therapy modalities. Including but not limited to active participation, receptive listening, vibroacoustic interventions, guided music/imagery, and/or hybrid approaches with focus on key clinical outcomes such as pain, anxiety, sleep quality, depression, and quality of life.
2. Assess "dosage" interventions and influence, particularly the frequency, duration, and overall length of therapy programs (long-term vs short-term), on treatment effectiveness.
3. Identify practical relative implications of data and evidence-based music-therapy integration into multidisciplinary palliative care.

This chapter seeks to synthesize, compare, and contrast recent evidence from data-sourced research in multiple palliative care contexts to gain further understanding about the application of music therapy as a means for better qualitative healing. Researchers, clinicians, caregivers, and policy makers may make more informed and well-guided intervention decisions and strategies going forward for those suffering from serious life-altering illnesses and provide a more nuanced understanding of quality-of-life improvements both for those on the path to full recovery as well as for patients at the end of life.

The World Health Organization (WHO, 2020) recognizes music therapy as a viable and complementary practice based on supportive evidence within palliative and supportive care, and emphasizing its role in addressing the physical, emotional, and spiritual needs of individuals facing life-limiting illness. Also, the American Music Therapy Association (AMTA, 2020) identifies music therapy as a clinical discipline rooted in empirical research and a key component for interdisciplinary care teams. Both organizations support that music therapy alleviates pain and psychological distress and also enhances quality of life and family communication. These endorsements provide theoretical justification for the integration of music therapy as a viable option of service in palliative care frameworks, aligning with international standards for holistic, person-centered health interventions. (WHO, 2020; AMTA, 2020).

2. BACKGROUND AND THEORETICAL FRAMEWORK

Music therapy as defined by the American Music Therapy Association (AMTA) is the clinical and evidence-based use of music interventions to accomplish individualized goals within a therapeutic relationship by a credentialed professional who has completed an approved music therapy program or the "systematic use of music within a therapeutic relationship which aims at restoring, maintaining and furthering emotional, physical and mental health." (Warth et al., 2015). Interventions in music therapy can address a variety of healthcare & educational goals. These goals include but are not limited to promoting wellness, managing stress, alleviating pain, expressing feelings, enhancing memory, improving communication, and promoting physical rehabilitation. In palliative care, music therapy involves the deliberate use of musical experience (live and/or recorded) tailored to the physical, emotional, cognitive, and spiritual needs of patients facing life-limiting illness.

The purpose of holistic and palliative care is to approach treatment and healing with the aim of improving the quality of care and life of the patient and families affected by the illness. This approach is designed to address symptom relief, psychosocial support, and spiritual care, regardless of prognosis or stage of disease. Music therapy fits within the framework of palliative care in that the desired results are virtually identical. Notable qualitative improvements such as coping with stresses, enhancing communication, and maintaining a sense of agency and identity are key components in complementing pharmacological and psychosocial interventions as well. Music therapy compliments other treatments and fits within individual contexts of care, delivered in multiple and diverse modalities in the literature of the discipline including:

- Active participation - patients engage in singing, playing instruments, or improvisation, fostering self-expression and agency (Boyde et al., 2024).
- Receptive listening - patients listen to live or recorded music, often selected for relaxation or emotional resonance; the most foundational and universally recognized modality (Warth et al., 2015).
- Guided imagery and music (GIM) - patients explore personal imagery evoked by music under therapist guidance, often to process emotions and memories (Papanikolaou et al., 2023).
- Vibroacoustic therapy - combines music or sound with low-frequency vibrations to provide both auditory and tactile stimulation (Bieligmeyer et al. 2018).
- Hybrid or integrative approaches - music therapy combined with techniques such as biofeedback, mindfulness, or psychotherapy (Sumneangsanor et al., 2022).

Music therapy has foundational principles defined within these frameworks, but in the application may have more dynamic and diversity in approach.

2.1 Methods and Mechanisms of Action

The pathways by which music therapy operates are neurophysiological and psychosocial. These pathways are deeply relevant to palliative care and can be categorized and defined as such:

1. Autonomic nervous system regulation - The sympathetic and parasympathetic nervous systems are two branches of the autonomic nervous system that work in opposition to maintain homeostasis within the body. The sympathetic nervous system (SNS) is activated during times of stress or perceived danger, triggering the "fight-or-flight" response, while the parasympathetic nervous system (PNS) promotes "rest-and-digest" functions, returning the body to a relaxed state. Music can reduce sympathetic activity and promote parasympathetic dominance, lowering heart rate, blood pressure, and cortisol levels. This stress-reducing effect is central to alleviating anxiety and promoting relaxation (Li et al., 2025).
2. Neurochemical modulation - Listening to or making music may stimulate the release of endorphins, dopamine and oxytocin, contributing to mood elevation, pain modulation, and bonding (Li et al., 2025).
3. Emotional expression and processing - Music provides a non-verbal channel for expressing complex emotions which might be difficult to articulate, supporting psychological processing and help foster meaning and closure at the end of life.
4. Distraction and attention redirection – Engagement in musical activities and/or focused listening can divert attention away from pain, distress, and other symptoms, enhancing perception of control and agency over a patient's environment.
5. Physiological entrainment - Music with specific tempos and rhythms can entrain or "sync" breathing and/or heart rate, the synchronization of two or more oscillating systems, where one system's rhythm influences or matches the rhythm of the other, promoting physical relaxation and internal coherence.
6. Social and relational engagement – Interaction is key in these modalities, especially those involving family or caregivers, strengthening social bonds, improving communication, and supporting positive shared experiences.

These mechanisms for data-driven quality of life improvements are effective as a means of creating strategies for implementation in palliative care dependent upon individual patient needs and response. Evidence of the effectiveness of these strategies has been documented in studies over the last twenty years. These mechanisms will be revisited later through the lens of integration.

2.2 Existing Evidence of Effectiveness

Within the last two decades, many systematic reviews and meta-analyses have documented the benefits of music therapy in palliative and oncological care. Primarily qualitative data has shown positive results in the pursuit of quality-of-life improvements.

Key findings include:

- Pain management - Music therapy has been shown to significantly reduce perceived pain intensity in patients with advanced cancer, particularly when personalized or live music is used (Li et al., 2025).
- Fatigue and relaxation - Short-term interventions, such as vibroacoustic therapy, have been associated with immediate improvements in relaxation and perceived well-being (Bieligmeyer et al. 2018).
- Sleep quality - Receptive music therapy, especially with slow-tempo, calming music, has been shown to improve sleep in cancer patients undergoing chemotherapy or radiotherapy (Vinayak et al., 2017).
- Psychological distress - Reductions in anxiety and depression have been consistently observed, with some evidence suggesting that active participation yields greater psychological benefit than receptive listening.
- Social and familial outcomes - Interaction-focused music therapy involving patients and significant others enhances family bonding, mutual coping, and social integration.

Despite this growing evidence base, gaps remain in understanding the comparative efficacy of different modalities, the optimal "dose" of therapy, and the sustainability of benefits over time. Palliative healthcare is often tailored specifically for the individual patient's needs and context of treatment, diagnosis, and care. Addressing these gaps is essential to developing evidence-based guidelines that may be implemented in varied cultural and healthcare contexts.

2.3 Recent Developments in Music Therapy and Palliative Care (2020 – 2025)

1. Reducing Pain and Anxiety

Music therapy continues to demonstrate strong benefits in reducing pain and anxiety for patients in palliative care. A large meta-analysis of thirty controlled trials with adult oncology patients found significant improvements in psychological well-being, quality of life, and physical symptom distress (Koehler et al., 2020).

Similarly, the *Harmonising Hope* study (Jethva et al., 2025) reported measurable decreases in pain intensity and anxiety after short bedside sessions, together with improvements in mood and motivation. These findings indicate that live and receptive music therapy may complement pharmacological management, and may offer a safe and immediately effective means of emotional stability within multidisciplinary care.

2. Physiological and Psychoneuroendocrine Mechanisms

Recent studies have expanded biological explanations for these effects. Within the neuro-psycho-endocrine-immunological (NPEI) model, music activates neural and hormonal pathways that modulate stress responses (Terzoni et al., 2025). Controlled trials show reduced cortisol, stabilized heart rate, and improved parasympathetic activity during and after sessions (Koehler et al., 2021; Terzoni et al., 2025). Some autonomic and cortisol changes have also been observed under other supportive conditions, so effect sizes vary depending on comparator and protocol. Overall, these data reinforce that music therapy is a biologically grounded, evidence-based intervention rather than a purely emotional comfort measure.

3. Spiritual and Existential Well-Being

Beyond symptom relief, recent research highlights music therapy's role in fostering spiritual and existential peace. Biographical songwriting and legacy-creation interventions have been linked to higher spiritual well-being and ego integrity compared with mindfulness or relaxation alone (Koehler et al., 2020). Patients describe these sessions as opportunities to express identity, reconcile life narratives, and experience continuity of self (Terzoni et al., 2025). Such outcomes affirm that music provides a language for meaning-making when verbal communication or cognitive strength is diminished at the end of life.

4. Enhancing Caregiver Support and Dyadic Coping

The family context has become a major focus in newer studies. Music therapy sessions involving caregivers have been shown to reduce anxiety, ease anticipatory grief, and improve communication (Terzoni et al., 2025). In pediatric "hospital-at-home" programs, parents report that shared music-making fosters connection and restores a sense of normalcy (Steinhardt et al., 2021). These dyadic approaches emphasize that music therapy strengthens both patients and caregivers, functioning as an emotionally restorative practice that sustains family resilience under stress.

5. Comparing Home-Based and Facility-Based Care

Different settings shape the therapeutic experience. In hospital environments, programs such as *Harmonising Hope* frequently emphasize immediate pain and anxiety management through structured sessions integrated with standard care (Jethva et al., 2025). Home-based models, by contrast, highlight relational and contextual benefits—continuity of care, family participation, and integration into daily routines (Steinhardt et al., 2021). Both demonstrate that music therapy is most effective when embedded within the interdisciplinary framework of palliative care rather than delivered as a stand-alone service.

Synthesis and Transition

Taken together, studies from 2020 to 2025 show that music therapy alleviates pain and anxiety (Koehler et al., 2020; Jethva et al., 2025), regulates physiological stress systems (Koehler et al., 2021; Terzoni et al., 2025), enhances spiritual well-being (Koehler et al., 2020), and strengthens caregiver resilience (Steinhardt et al., 2021). Around 30 minutes per session often appears optimal for sustained symptom relief, though timing and format vary by context. Collectively, these findings justify continued research into music therapy's integration within home-based and hybrid palliative models—providing the rationale for the methodological framework presented in the next section.

Table 1. International Overview of Recent Music Therapy Research in Palliative Care (2020–2025)

Year	Country	Sample / Participants	Type of Intervention	Outcomes
2025	**India**	43 adult oncology in-patients (*Harmoniing Hope*)	Individualized live music therapy (voice + instrument) integrated with pharmacological pain management	Significant reductions in pain and anxiety; improved mood and motivation (Jethva et al., 2025).
2025	**Italy**	Narrative review synthesizing 30+ studies on end-of-life care	Multi-modal MT approaches (active + receptive) emphasizing neuro-psycho-endocrine-immunological pathways	Lower cortisol, slower HR/BP, improved immune modulation and caregiver well-being (Terzoni et al., 2025).
2022	**Germany**	104 adult palliative in-patients	Biographical music therapy with physiological monitoring	Decreased salivary cortisol and mean heart rate; reduced distress; greater emotional regulation (Koehler et al., 2021).

continued on following page

Table 1. Continued

Year	Country	Sample / Participants	Type of Intervention	Outcomes
2021	**Norway**	10 pediatric palliative "hospital-at-home" families	Home-based MT delivered 1–2 sessions/week (45 min each)	Enhanced family connection, emotional stability, and parental coping (Steinhardt et al., 2021).
2021	**Australia / UK**	120 palliative patients across community hospices	Recorded music and guided imagery sessions	Decreased anxiety and fatigue; improved relaxation and quality of life (Boyde et al., 2024).
2020	**Germany / Switzerland**	Meta-analysis of 30 RCTs (adult cancer)	Various MT formats: active, receptive, songwriting, listening	Significant gains in QoL and psychological well-being; reduced symptom distress (Koehler et al., 2020).
2020	**Spain**	Protocol for multicenter RCT (home palliative care)	Complementary MT for cancer patients and caregivers (home visits)	Feasibility and cost-utility framework; expected outcomes: QoL, anxiety, caregiver strain (Valero-Cantero et al., 2020).
2020	**United States**	85 hospice patients across 3 states	Live bedside MT (voice/ guitar, receptive listening)	Reduced symptom burden; higher satisfaction with spiritual care and emotional peace (Huda et al., 2020).

3. METHODOLOGY

We conducted a systematic search for studies evaluating structured music therapy (MT) in oncology and palliative/hospice care, including both adult and pediatric populations, published 2015–2025. Randomized and other controlled clinical trials were prioritized for quantitative effect estimates; quasi-experimental and single-arm pre–post studies were included as supportive evidence, and qualitative studies informed feasibility, acceptability, and experience. Systematic reviews and meta-analyses were treated as contextual evidence and were not pooled with primary trials. Screening, data extraction, and synthesis followed established systematic-review procedures. Searches covered PubMed, CINAHL, PsycINFO, the Cochrane Central Register of Controlled Trials (CENTRAL), Scopus, and Web of Science, supplemented by regional databases (CNKI and Wanfang) to capture non-English literature. Reference lists of relevant articles and reviews were checked manually. Search terms combined controlled vocabulary and free-text words related to music therapy, palliative care, and randomized controlled trials, for example:

("music therapy" OR "music intervention" OR "music-based therapy" OR "guided imagery and music" OR "vibroacoustic" OR "music listening" OR "songwriting")
AND
("palliative care" OR "end-of-life" OR "hospice" OR "advanced cancer")
AND
("randomized controlled trial" OR "RCT").

The search yielded 18 studies that met inclusion criteria, covering receptive, active, guided imagery, vibroacoustic, biofeedback-assisted, and online modalities.

3.1 Inclusion Criteria

Studies were considered if they:

- Enrolled adult or pediatric patients (≥5 years) with cancer receiving active treatment, palliative care, or hospice services.
- Used a structured music therapy protocol delivered by a credentialed therapist. Accepted modalities included receptive listening (live or recorded), active participation (singing, playing instruments, improvisation), guided imagery and music (GIM), vibroacoustic therapy, or hybrid formats such as biofeedback-assisted, mindfulness-integrated, or online MT.
- Compared MT against standard care, attention-control, or another non-music intervention.
- Reported at least one relevant outcome such as pain, anxiety, depression, fatigue, sleep quality, quality of life, physiological markers (e.g., HRV, cortisol), or family/social interaction.
- Employed an RCT or feasibility RCT design with quantitative outcomes.

We excluded studies in which music was used only as background or environmental enrichment without therapeutic intent, multi-component programs where MT effects could not be isolated, and non-randomized observational or qualitative-only reports.

3.2 Data Extraction and Analysis

For each study, we noted author, year, country, clinical setting, participant characteristics, cancer type, and palliative stage. Intervention details such as MT modality, delivery mode, frequency, session duration, overall treatment length, and any cultural adaptations were extracted. Control conditions (standard care, attention control, or alternative therapy) were documented.

Outcome measures included validated tools for symptoms, quality of life, and psychosocial domains, such as the Pittsburgh Sleep Quality Index (PSQI), Functional Assessment of Cancer Therapy – Fatigue (FACT-F), Hospital Anxiety and Depression Scale (HADS), State-Trait Anxiety Inventory (STAI), European Organization for Research and Treatment of Cancer Quality of Life Questionnaire – Core 30 (EORTC QLQ-C30), and the Assessment of Parent–Child Interaction (APCI). Primary and secondary outcomes, effect sizes, and significance levels were summarized.

Because of variation across study designs and measures, most results were synthesized narratively. Subgroup patterns—such as receptive versus active modalities, live versus recorded delivery, in-person versus online interventions, and different session frequencies or durations—were considered descriptively. Where designs were highly diverse or reported mainly feasibility indicators, the findings were summarized qualitatively, grouped by modality and outcome domain.

4. RESULTS - OVERVIEW OF INCLUDED STUDIES

These trials were conducted between 2015 and 2025, including the ~960 from the 17 RCTs + ~1,700 pooled in Li (2025) across 9 countries, representing a mix of adult oncology, palliative care, and pediatric oncology populations. Studies were conducted in Asia (China, India, Thailand, Iran), Europe (Germany, Denmark, Norway, Greece), North America (USA), South America (Brazil), and the Middle East (Israel), reflecting a broad cultural range in music selection and delivery. Cultural bias may be characterized as minimal in the approach to this study by way of the diversity in participants as well as setting: Hospital inpatient wards, outpatient chemotherapy suites, radiotherapy departments, perioperative units, palliative care facilities, online environments, and home-based eHealth programs.

Table 2. Characteristics of Included Studies

Study	Population	Intervention	Frequency & Duration	Main Outcomes
Alcântara-Silva et al., 2018	Women with breast/ gynecological cancer undergoing radiotherapy	Individual music therapy (receptive listening + relaxation) delivered by a trained music therapist	≈10 sessions across radiotherapy; 30–40 minutes each	Reduced radiotherapy-related fatigue (FACT-F/FACT-G/ TOI); improvements in depressive symptoms
Bieligmeyer et al., 2018	Adult oncology patients (mixed tumor types)	Vibroacoustic music via sound-bed (receptive intervention)	Single 10-minute session (randomized crossover)	Improved well-being, inner balance, and perceived warmth distribution immediately post-session
Boyde et al., 2024	Children with cancer and significant others (family dyads)	Interaction-focused, family-centered music therapy (active/ receptive as indicated)	Multiple sessions over treatment phase (dose varied by dyad)	Feasibility demonstrated; enhanced parent–child interaction/synchrony and shared meaning-making
Bro et al., 2019	Newly diagnosed lymphoma patients undergoing chemotherapy (n≈143)	Patient-preferred live music vs pre-recorded music vs standard care during chemotherapy	Up to 5 sessions; ~30 minutes per session	Borderline anxiety reduction with live music vs standard care; no consistent effects on secondary outcomes
Fleszar-Pavlovic et al., 2024	Allogeneic HSCT patients (pilot RCT protocol; planned n≈60)	eHealth mindfulness-based music therapy (eMBMT) vs eHealth mindfulness meditation	8 remote sessions; 60 minutes each	Protocol outcomes: feasibility/acceptability, HRQOL, symptom burden, biomarkers (no results yet)
Jethva et al., 2025	Oncology in-patients in palliative care (n=43; 102 total sessions)	Individualized, therapist-delivered music therapy: receptive listening, relaxation, lyric discussion, guided imagery, and active music-making	2–4 sessions per patient; ~30 minutes (20–45) each	Significant reductions in pain and anxiety; improved mood/ motivation ($p<0.01$)
Köhler et al., 2020	Adult cancer patients across multiple trials (systematic review & meta-analysis)	Therapist-delivered music therapy (active and receptive) across included studies	Varied across included trials (e.g., 1–10 sessions; 15–90 minutes)	Small but significant improvements in psychological well-being, symptom distress, and quality of life

continued on following page

Table 2. Continued

Study	Population	Intervention	Frequency & Duration	Main Outcomes
Köhler et al., 2022	Adult palliative in-patients (multicenter RCT; randomized N=104; biomarker subsample n≈89)	Biographical 'Song of Life' music therapy vs standardized mindfulness/relaxation (active control); S1 identify meaningful song; S2 lullaby-style live performance; S3 recording handover & reflection	3 sessions; 20–30 minutes each	Greater reduction in distress vs control (p=0.02); no between-group differences on cortisol/α-amylase/ HRV; cortisol and heart rate decreased over time in both groups
Li et al., 2025	Lung cancer patients (meta-analysis of RCTs; total n≈1,991)	Therapist-delivered music therapy (active/ receptive) across included trials	Typical dosing across trials: ~30 minutes, 1–2×/day for 2–12 weeks (varied)	Reduced anxiety, depression, and pain; improved sleep quality and quality of life
Mondanaro et al., 2021	Adults undergoing oncology infusion	Clinical music therapy improvisation (instrumental or vocal) delivered bedside	3 sessions; ~20 minutes each	Increased resiliency; immediate post-session reductions in pain; minimal change on anxiety/depression scales
Palmer et al., 2015	Women undergoing ambulatory breast surgery for cancer diagnosis/treatment (n≈207)	Live or recorded perioperative music vs usual care; brief preop song; intraop music/ earmuffs per arm	Single ~5-minute preoperative song; intraoperative exposure per protocol	Both music arms achieved larger preop anxiety reduction vs control; no propofol dose difference; live music showed shorter recovery than recorded
Papanikolaou et al., 2023	Breast and gynecologic cancer patients in supportive care	Guided Imagery and Music (short-GIM) protocol	6 sessions over 6 weeks	Reduced fatigue; improved hope and mood; significant gains on VAS measures
Rabinowitch et al., 2023	Adult cancer patients (online Zoom groups)	Balance-Space: 30-min group music listening + 30-min facilitated discussion	Single 60-minute online session	Reduced pain vs meditation control; positive group experience/connection
Steinhardt et al., 2021	Paediatric palliative care (hospital-at-home); 10 families enrolled (9 interviewed)	Home-based family-centred music therapy: songwriting, instrument training, improvisation, listening, relaxation, imagery	1–2 sessions/ week; up to 5 sessions; ~45 minutes each	Qualitative themes: 'isolated—yet connected'; valued joint music-making; strong MDT integration

continued on following page

Table 2. Continued

Study	Population	Intervention	Frequency & Duration	Main Outcomes
Sumneangsanor et al., 2022	Thai patients with cancer receiving palliative care	Biofeedback + music training program	Multi-session program (repeated measures across time)	Significant reductions in stress over time (multivariate tests)
Terzoni et al., 2025	End-of-life/palliative care (narrative review)	Synthesis of active/receptive music therapy within a neuro-psycho-endocrine-immunological (NPEI) framework	Not applicable	Physiological and psycho-emotional modulation; emphasizes individualized dosing and calls for standardization
Vinayak et al., 2017	Adult cancer patients receiving chemotherapy or radiotherapy	Active (group singing/ guitar) and receptive (preferred listening) music therapy	10 sessions of 20–30 minutes	Improved sleep quality (PSQI); active format favored on several subscales
Warth et al., 2015	Palliative care inpatients	Live music-based relaxation vs verbal relaxation (control)	Two sessions; ~30 minutes each; two days apart	Increased relaxation and well-being; HRV high-frequency power increased; fatigue decreased; no pain difference vs control

4.1 Types of Interventions

The modality, delivery mode, and degree of patient participation in these interventions varied on a wide spectrum:

1. Receptive Listening
    - Live music – Therapist performed live receptive MT during chemotherapy (Bro et al., 2019) and in palliative rooms (Warth et al., 2015).
    - Recorded music – Structured recorded listening during radiotherapy (Alcântara-Silva et al., 2018); culturally tailored selections (e.g., preferred Persian pop in Vinayak et al., 2017; Five-Element music reported within the included meta-analysis, Li et al., 2025).
    - Group singing and guitar playing (Vinayak et al., 2017); clinical improvisation and dyadic, interaction-focused work (Boyde et al., 2024); songwriting/improvisation in adult infusion settings (Mondanaro et al., 2021)
2. Guided Imagery and Music (GIM)

- Facilitated/guided and structured imagery with curated music in breast/gynecologic cancer (Papanikolaou et al., 2023).

3. Vibroacoustic Therapy
    - Low-frequency vibroacoustic sound-bed (Bieligmeyer et al., 2018).
4. Hybrid / Complementary Formats
    - Biofeedback-assisted MT (Sumneangsanor et al., 2022); online synchronous MT (Rabinowitch et al., 2023); eHealth mindfulness-based MT protocol for allo-SCT (allogeneic stem cell transplantation patients) (Fleszar-Pavlovic et al., 2024).

4.2 Intervention Parameters

- Frequency - Varied from single-session trial protocols (perioperative breast surgery, vibroacoustic MT) to daily sessions over 10 days (MT for Sleep Quality) or multi-week programs lasting 8-12 weeks (Interaction-Focused MT, GIM, Fleszar-Pavlovic et al., 2024).
- Session duration ranged from ~5 minutes (perioperative pre-op) to ~60 minutes (GIM/online). Throughout included trials and the meta-analysis, ~30 minutes was the most common target, but effects varied by setting and modality
- Total Intervention Period - Spanned from one day to up to several weeks, with cumulative exposure hypothesized to influence sustained effects.

4.3 Outcomes Assessed - Measurement Tools

Primary outcomes included in these studies:

- Physical symptoms - pain, fatigue, sleep quality, anesthesia drug requirements.
- Psychological distress - anxiety, depression, stress.
- Quality of life - general and disease-specific instruments.
- Physiological markers - heart rate variability (HRV), catecholamines levels, blood pressure.
- Family and relational outcomes - parent-child interaction measures.

Measurement tools included validated scales such as PSQI (Vinayak et al., 2017), FACT-F (Alcântara-Silva et al., 2018), STAI (Bro et al., 2019), EORTC QLQ-C30 (Bieligmeyer et al., 2018), and APCI (Boyde et al., 2024).

4.5 Summary of Effects

Details of comparative analyses are presented in Section 5, but an initial overview shows:

- Improvements were most consistent for situational anxiety (perioperative etc.) and sleep (daily programs etc.), while effects on pain and physiological markers were mixed and dependent upon modality; recorded-only conditions were mixed in their findings. (Alcântara-Silva et al., 2018; Bieligmeyer et al., 2018; Bro et al., 2019; Sumneangsanor et al., 2022; Bro et al., 2019; Li et al., 2025)
- Greater psychosocial benefits (family bonding, coping) from interactive/dyadic approaches compared to purely receptive listening (Mondanaro et al., 2021 Boyde et al. 2024).
- Short-term warmth and well-being effects with vibroacoustic MT (Bieligmeyer 2018); HRV improvements reported only with biofeedback-assisted MT (Sumneangsanor 2022).
- Online MT demonstrated feasibility and positive experiences (Rabinowitch 2023). An eHealth mindfulness-based MT protocol was developed for allo-SCT recipients' adherence and outcomes are pending trial results (Fleszar-Pavlovic 2024).

5. COMPARING EFFECTIVENESS OF MUSIC THERAPY MODALITIES

The 18 studies under review illustrate that "music therapy" does not mean one single approach. Instead, a range of modalities – receptive, active, guided imagery, vibroacoustic, and technology-based – were applied in different ways. Each had its own rhythm of delivery and tended to align with particular symptom targets.

5.1 Pain and Treatment-Related Discomfort

Patients receiving live music at the chemotherapy chair, for example, often reported feeling more comfortable and emotionally supported. In the lymphoma trial led by Bro and colleagues (2019), those who heard live bedside music showed better emotional well-being than those in standard care. Recorded music was less reliable. In radiotherapy, Alcântara-Silva et al. (2018) noted fatigue improvements, but pain reduction was inconsistent. By contrast, Li et al. (2025), pooling multiple lung cancer RCTs, concluded that patient-chosen receptive music was capable of reducing pain meaningfully across several datasets. For longer-term or existential discomfort, guided imagery and music sessions offered another pathway, helping women with breast or gynecologic cancer manage distress and strengthen coping resources (Papanikolaou et al., 2023).

5.2 Anxiety and Depression

The clearest findings come from settings where patients face acute stress. Palmer et al. (2015) showed that even five minutes of receptive listening before breast surgery was enough to reduce pre-operative anxiety. Anxiety and depression were also lowered when patients engaged in daily music listening during chemotherapy or radiotherapy (Vinayak et al., 2017). Li's (2025) meta-analysis reinforced these outcomes with striking pooled effect sizes for both anxiety and depression. Meanwhile, interactive approaches extended the impact beyond receptive listening. The INMUT feasibility trial with children and their parents (Boyde et al., 2024) documented better coping and improved mood, while Mondanaro et al. (2021) saw resilience benefits in adults undergoing infusion. Online formats, though newer, also showed promise: Rabinowitch et al. (2023) reported stress relief and stronger coping in their Balance-Space sessions, and Fleszar-Pavlovic et al. (2024) developed an eHealth program for patients preparing for stem cell transplantation.

5.3 Sleep Quality

Sleep disturbance is one of the more consistently improved outcomes. Vinayak et al. (2017) found that ten consecutive days of music therapy—including both active and receptive elements—improved PSQI sleep scores. Bedtime listening with slow-tempo music also proved useful, helping patients sustain sleep and reduce fatigue during radiotherapy (Vinayak et al., 2017; Alcântara-Silva et al., 2018). In this area, daily repetition seemed more important than the exact form of music chosen.

5.4 Stress Regulation and Physiological Markers

Not all stress-related measures responded in the same way. A biofeedback-based program in Thai palliative patients reduced stress and showed measurable changes in heart rate variability (Sumneangsanor et al., 2022). Vibroacoustic therapy, in contrast, gave immediate but short-lived effects: after a ten-minute session on a vibroacoustic sound-bed, patients felt warmer and more settled (Bieligmeyer et al., 2018). Fatigue during radiotherapy was also reduced by receptive listening (Alcântara-Silva et al., 2018), though autonomic markers generally improved only in the biofeedback trial.

5.5 Family, Social, and Relational Outcomes

Music therapy's impact was not limited to individuals. In the pediatric INMUT study, parents and children communicated more fluidly and seemed better attuned to each other (Boyde et al., 2024). Adults, by contrast, gained more from online group settings. The Balance-Space program, for example, provided a sense of shared experience and peer support, which many participants valued (Rabinowitch et al., 2023).

5.6 Considering Modality, Dose, and Personalization

Looking across trials, some patterns appear. Thirty minutes was a common session length and was often associated with better outcomes (Li et al., 2025), although shorter sessions could still reduce acute anxiety in surgical settings (Palmer et al., 2015). Daily use was particularly important for sleep and fatigue (Vinayak et al., 2017; Alcântara-Silva et al., 2018), whereas weekly formats were sufficient for guided imagery (Papanikolaou et al., 2023) or online groups (Rabinowitch et al., 2023). Multi-week programs tended to sustain improvements, as seen in both GIM and pediatric dyadic therapy (Boyde et al., 2024). Patient preference mattered: chosen music generally outperformed standardized playlists (Li et al., 2025). Interestingly, single-session studies sometimes showed more positive immediate effects on psychological well-being than higher-frequency programs—likely reflecting short-term, relaxation-focused aims and assessment timing, not a blanket superiority. (Koehler et al., 2021) And, not surprisingly, studies where trained therapists guided the process showed stronger effects than those without that involvement (Boyde et al., 2024; Papanikolaou et al., 2023; Warth et al., 2015).

5.7 Practical Guidance by Symptom

Although evidence is uneven, several practical lessons can be drawn. Acute preoperative anxiety can be eased with only a few minutes of receptive listening (Palmer et al., 2015). For ongoing anxiety and depression, daily 30-minute listening sessions show consistent benefits (Li et al., 2025). Pain and discomfort respond best to live receptive music during chemotherapy (Bro et al., 2019). Nightly listening and daily protocols support sleep quality (Vinayak et al., 2017; Alcântara-Silva et al., 2018). Stress and fatigue have been alleviated with biofeedback-based programs and, in the short term, vibroacoustic sessions (Sumneangsanor et al., 2022; Bieligmeyer et al., 2018). Finally, relational strain in pediatric settings was reduced through dyadic interaction-focused therapy (Boyde et al., 2024).

6. INFLUENCE OF FREQUENCY AND DURATION (DOSING EFFECTS)

6.1 Session Length

Several trials converged on a session duration of approximately 30 minutes as the most effective dose. In the lung cancer meta-analysis, 30-minute receptive listening sessions were associated with the largest reductions in anxiety, depression, and pain (Li et al., 2025). Similarly, daily recorded listening sessions of 30 minutes improved fatigue and HRV in women receiving radiotherapy. By contrast, ultra-brief sessions (5-10 minutes), such as peri-operative MT for breast surgery patients, reduced acute anxiety but produced limited physiological change (Palmer et al., 2015). Essentially, around 30 minutes per session appears optimal for sustained symptom relief, while ultra-brief formats are best suited for acute anxiety and short-term comfort. Ultra-brief forms seem best used in contexts where a short-term benefit suits the situation and purpose of its inclusion.

6.2 Frequency of Sessions

Evidence suggests that daily sessions enhance benefits. Ten consecutive days of daily MT significantly improved sleep quality in chemo/radiotherapy patients (Vinayak et al., 2017). Daily 30-minute listening sessions also improved fatigue outcomes during radiotherapy. By contrast, weekly sessions in guided imagery protocols (Papanikolaou et al., 2023) or in online Rabinowitch et al., 2023 were sufficient to improve mood and coping but produced more modest physiological changes. Daily MT sessions maximize physical and psychological outcomes, while weekly sessions remain effective for psychosocial interventions requiring less intensity.

6.3 Duration of Programs

Along with the frequency and length of the sessions, the length of the treatment program shaped outcomes as well. Eight- to twelve-week programs, such as GIM for gynecologic cancer survivors (Papanikolaou et al., 2023) and the INMUT dyadic MT with pediatric oncology families (Boyde et al., 2024), provided sustained improvements in coping and communication. By contrast, single-session interventions such as vibroacoustic MT offered immediate but short-lived benefits (Bieligmeyer et al., 2018). Two- to five-week programs, as in radiotherapy fatigue protocols, were effective in reducing physical symptoms but less impactful on psychosocial measures. The extended vs shorter intervention frequency, duration, and length of sessions share similar qualities in function of use. Extended multi-week MT programs yield durable psychosocial gains. Shorter interventions are most effective for acute symptom management.

7. DISCUSSION

The findings from these randomized controlled trials (RCTs), meta-analyses, and feasibility studies emphasize the versatility and clinical relevance of music therapy in oncology and palliative care. Interventions varied in scope and practice from receptive listening during chemotherapy and radiotherapy, to active and dyadic programs with children and families, to guided imagery, vibroacoustic treatments, and digitally mediated platforms. Results and outcomes may be varied according to frequency, modality, and duration; however, the collective evidence points to music therapy's unique capacity to address patients' physical symptoms, psychological distress, and social well-being in ways that complement medical treatment alongside palliative care. The following discussion section synthesizes these results, situating them within theoretical frameworks and clinical practice.

7.1 Integration of Findings

Across modalities, receptive MT was the most widely studied and found to be the most consistently effective intervention as well. In settings where patients received chemotherapy and radiotherapy, live or recorded receptive music was shown to reduced pain, fatigue, and anxiety (Vinayak et al., 2017; Alcântara-Silva et al., 2018). In the lung cancer meta-analysis, robust pooled effects on anxiety, depression, pain, and sleep quality were confirmed (Li et al., 2025). These findings show receptive formats as scalable and adaptable across clinical contexts and settings.

Active and interaction-focused MT demonstrated added psychosocial benefits. In pediatric oncology, dyadic interaction-focused sessions significantly improved parent-child communication and coping (Boyde et al., 2024). GIM facilitated results similarly with emotional processing and resilience in breast and gynecologic cancer survivors (Papanikolaou et al., 2023). These results suggest that receptive formats are effective for core symptoms, while active participation specifically offers unique benefits in terms of relationships and communication for patients and families while undergoing palliative care.

Emerging hybrid formats implementing technology and employing remote approaches extend accessibility for patients. This also provides caregivers versatility in implementation. BMT (biofeedback music therapy) improved stress regulation and directly affects brainwaves, which are transmitted to the muscular system and promote relaxation in Thai palliative care (Sumneangsanor et al., (2022). Additionally, MT online intervention and eHealth mindfulness approaches demonstrated feasibility for patients unable to attend in-person sessions (Rabinowitch et al., 2023). Though resulting effects were more modest than in therapist-guided in-person interventions, these approaches expand reach and support continuity of care.

Ultimately, taken together, these findings reinforce music therapy as a multi-modal, adaptable intervention which reliably alleviates physical as well as psychological symptoms, with active and hybrid modalities providing added psychosocial and relational benefits beyond receptive listening.

7.2 Considering Mechanisms of Action

Earlier in this chapter, mechanisms of action were listed through the framework of patient needs; now we will consider them in terms of results from implementation.

- Psychological mechanisms: Receptive listening engages the process of and ability to regulate attention and emotion by shifting focus away from stressors and thereby reducing anxiety. This was evident in peri-operative breast surgery, where a brief pre-surgical session produced immediate calming effects (Palmer et al., 2015). Guided Imagery and Music facilitated deeper cognitive-emotional processing, helping breast and gynecologic cancer survivors reframe distress and strengthen resilience (Papanikolaou et al., 2023)
- Physiological mechanisms: The body's automatic stress responses such as heart rate and breathing as well as stress control, relaxation, and energy levels are all shown to be affected by music. Biofeedback-assisted MT was shown to improve heart rate variability in Thai palliative care patients, and daily receptive listening during radiotherapy reduced fatigue. Vibroacoustic MT produced acute improvements in subjective warmth and vitality, likely mediated by somatosensory resonance (Bieligmeyer et al., 2018).
- Social and relational mechanisms: Active and dyadic (or involving two people) approaches create opportunities for communication and shared experience. The INMUT pediatric feasibility trial demonstrated how interaction-focused MT improved parent-child attunement and coping strategies (Boyde et al., 2024). Online intervention fostered peer connection and normalization among adults with cancer (Rabinowitch et al., 2023).
- Neurobiological framework: Despite lacking long-term clinical trials with larger samples, symptoms such as sleep, mood, and fatigue were improved by tracking biomarkers showing music therapy positively influences neuroendocrine stress pathways. Improvements in sleep quality after daily MT sessions (Vinayak et al., 2017) and reductions in depression in the lung cancer meta-

analysis (Li et al., 2025) indicate music's ability to regulate cortisol rhythms and serotonergic activity.

7.3 Clinical Implications and Practical Considerations

The evidence across these 18 studies underscores that music therapy (MT) is not only clinically effective but also feasible to implement across a variety of oncology and palliative care settings.

- Symptom-specific applications: Different modalities align with distinct clinical goals. Receptive MT consistently reduces procedural anxiety and treatment-related discomfort (Mondanaro et al., 2021; Palmer et al., 2015), while structured daily listening regimens also improve fatigue, sleep, and mood (Vinayak et al., 2017; Alcântara-Silva et al., 2018; Li et al., 2025). Resilience, communication, and coping are results directly supported by active and dyadic interventions, such as sessions focused on interaction with pediatric patients, parents, and caregivers. (Boyde et al., 2024).
- Dose and delivery: Frequency of sessions, length, and duration or the "dose" of MT is a critical factor in assessing the approach for MT caregivers. Delivered daily or several times weekly, sessions of about 30 minutes produce the most reliable improvements in anxiety, depression, and sleep quality (Li et al., 2025; Vinayak et al., 2017). "Ultra-brief" sessions of 5-10 minutes can be used more strategically for acute anxiety before procedures (Palmer et al., 2015) for example, but they should not be expected to create lasting effects. Extended programs lasting 8-12 weeks, such as GIM or pediatric dyadic MT, sustain psychosocial gains over time (Papanikolaou et al., 2023; Boyde et al., 2024)
- Practical and flexible implementation across settings: A great asset in MT is adaptability. It produces positive results in multiple environments: infusion suites, radiotherapy departments, surgical theaters (Palmer et al., 2015), pediatric oncology wards (Boyde et al., 2024), as well as patients' homes through online or eHealth platforms. This flexibility is essential and even critical in some circumstances for reaching patients whose physical condition or geographic distance might otherwise limit access to supportive care.
- Monitoring physiology and communication: Several studies demonstrate that MT influences measurable stress physiology, improving heart rate variability (HRV), lowering cortisol (the "stress" hormone), and reducing fatigue. Clinically, this reflects music's capacity to balance the body's stress and relaxation systems. Communicating these results in plain terms (e.g., "music

helps the body calm itself") can improve patient understanding and foster adoption by caregivers and clinicians.

- Cultural context and personalization: Trials note that patient-preferred and culturally congruent music consistently produce better results than standardized or generic playlists (Li et al., 2025; Vinayak et al., 2017). Giving patients the agency to choose meaningful music not only enhances outcomes but also supports engagement and adherence, which are practical considerations in high-burden palliative populations.

Ultimately, clinical MT is a flexible, evidence-based successful intervention that can be integrated into diverse modes of palliative care. Effective practice depends on coordinating and aligning modality, dose, and setting with patient needs while also ensuring personalization and therapist/clinician/care-giver guidance. Analysis of these diverse studies shows receptive MT is the most scalable for acute symptom relief, while active and dyadic approaches provide deeper psychosocial benefits.

7.4 Current Gaps and Limitations in Evidence

Despite the evidence driven by data for the benefits of music therapy (MT) in oncology and palliative care, several noticeable limitations and gaps exist in the research which may hinder the universal or standardized application of current findings.

- Heterogeneity of interventions: Studies included are starkly varied in design and range from single-session peri-operative interventions (Palmer et al., 2015; Bieligmeyer et al., 2018) to multi-week programs such as guided imagery (Papanikolaou et al., 2023) and pediatric dyadic MT (Boyde et al., 2024). Diversity may highlight MT's adaptability, but creates complications for direct comparison and meta-analytic pooling/grouping. Not all interventions share the same therapeutic intent, structure, or outcome measures, which may convolute application.
- Variability in outcome measurement: Different studies used different tools to assess anxiety, depression, sleep, and quality of life. For example, measures included the Hospital Anxiety and Depression Scale (HADS), the State-Trait Anxiety Inventory (STAI), the Pittsburgh Sleep Quality Index (PSQI), and the European Organisation for Research and Treatment of Cancer Quality of Life Questionnaire (EORTC QLQ-C30) (Li et al., 2025; Vinayak et al., 2017; Alcântara-Silva et al., 2018). This lack of standardization may limit cross-trial comparison and create challenges in synthesizing results into specific unified clinical guidelines.

- Small samples, scale, and feasibility: Several trials were small feasibility studies or pilot RCTs (Boyde et al., 2024; Rabinowitch et al., 2023; Fleszar-Pavlovic et al., 2024), which provided important evidence and proof of concept but were perhaps insufficient to detect subtle effects auxiliary outcomes. Larger confirmatory RCTs would be needed to validate efficacy across populations and cultural contexts for wider confirmation of results and more specific and/or nuanced findings.
- Placebo and blinding challenges: The practice of complete blinding for participants and therapists is inherently difficult in music therapy because patients know when they are hearing or making music, and therapists know when they are providing it. While some studies tried to use "attention controls" (for example, giving patients headphones with noise but no music), most could not fully prevent patients from expecting to feel better simply because they were receiving music (Palmer et al., 2015). This expectation, akin to the placebo effect, can unintentionally influence how patients rate their own symptoms. As a result, there is a risk of bias in self-reported outcomes such as anxiety, mood, and/or pain relief.
- Limited long-term follow-up: Few trials included follow-up beyond the intervention period. While extended programs (e.g., 8-12 weeks) showed durable psychosocial improvements (Papanikolaou et al., 2023; Boyde et al., 2024), most studies measured outcomes only during or immediately post-treatment. More data studies are needed to assess whether benefits persist after therapy ends, for how long, and whether treatment could be extended beyond initial intervention period (e.g. follow-up care related to trauma etc.).
- Under-resourced populations and homogeneous illnesses representation: These trials primarily focused on cancer patients in hospital settings with strong access to resources, lacking under-resourced settings. Evidence is scarce for non-cancer palliative populations (e.g., advanced heart failure, neurodegenerative conditions, etc.) and for patients in low-resource environments where access to certified music therapists may be limited.

Evidence currently and definitively supports MT's effectiveness, however, there are limitations in the variety or heterogeneity of intervention, measurement of outcome, sample size and diversity, blinding, and follow-up studies which restrict the ability to draw definitive conclusions. For these reasons, standardized approach is difficult to outline for caregivers. Addressing these gaps will be essential to strengthening clinical guidelines and broaden MT's reach in palliative care going forward.

7.5 Barriers and Implementation Challenges

Despite growing evidence for the therapeutic value of music therapy in palliative care, several implementation barriers persist. A major limitation is the shortage of credentialed music therapists, particularly in low- and middle-income regions, where programs often rely on volunteers or part-time practitioners. Financial constraints and the perceived non-essential status of creative therapies limit investment in specialized equipment and dedicated session time. Integration with interdisciplinary care teams also remains inconsistent, as clinical protocols frequently prioritize medical interventions over psychosocial care. Furthermore, limited awareness among policymakers and healthcare administrators reduces institutional support and referral pathways. Addressing these barriers requires coordinated strategies—expanding accredited training programs, embedding music therapy positions within palliative units, and including creative arts in health funding policies—to ensure that evidence-based music therapy becomes a sustainable, equitable component of holistic end-of-life care.

8. RECOMMENDATIONS FOR PRACTICE

8.1 Choosing the Right Modality

No single form of music therapy fits all patients. The choice depends on what the patient needs most and how much energy or interest they can bring to a session.

Receptive listening—whether someone is playing live at the bedside or the patient is given headphones with recorded tracks—has been the most straightforward and broadly useful. It is practical, easy to implement, and has shown good results for anxiety before surgery and for easing distress during chemotherapy (Bro et al., 2019; Palmer et al., 2015; Warth et al., 2015).

Active and dyadic work is different. It requires more engagement but offers benefits that go beyond symptom scores. Singing together, improvising, or even simple call-and-response exercises helped families and children in the INMUT study feel more connected (Boyde et al., 2024). Adults, too, have benefited from improvisation during infusions (Mondanaro et al., 2021).

Guided Imagery and Music has a special role for patients who are facing deeper psychological or existential struggles. In Papanikolaou's trial with breast and gynecologic cancer patients, GIM offered a way to process emotions that standard receptive listening did not.

Finally, hybrid and technology-based approaches are opening doors. Online group programs have already shown feasibility (Rabinowitch et al., 2023), and biofeedback-assisted interventions or eHealth mindfulness programs are being tested for patients who cannot attend in person (Sumneangsanor et al., 2022; Fleszar-Pavlovic et al., 2024).

8.2 Dosing Patterns

Across the literature, thirty minutes shows up again and again as a workable session length. That said, shorter bursts—just five or ten minutes—were still enough to calm pre-operative patients (Palmer et al., 2015). Daily or near-daily use seems best for sleep and fatigue (Vinayak et al., 2017; Alcântara-Silva et al., 2018). By contrast, weekly sessions are enough for GIM (Papanikolaou et al., 2023) and online Balance-Space groups (Rabinowitch et al., 2023). Multi-week programs, whether dyadic or guided imagery, tend to leave more durable psychosocial benefits than one-off exposures. Vibroacoustic sessions are useful but mainly for short-term relief (Bieligmeyer et al., 2018).

It's also worth remembering that "dose" must be adapted to the patient's condition. A fatigued patient may not tolerate half an hour, even if the evidence points to that as the sweet spot.

8.3 Intervention Settings and Approaches

Home-Based Music Therapy (HBMT) includes several complementary modalities that vary in structure, goal, and patient engagement. These approaches—receptive, active, and integrative—are adapted to individual needs, illness trajectory, and home context. Sessions may occur face-to-face or online, depending on mobility and family availability. The three major categories below summarize common applications in current practice.

Receptive Approach

Receptive HBMT centers on listening and emotional attunement. The therapist selects or co-creates music that reflects the patient's mood, physical condition, or preferred memories. This approach often uses personalized playlists or live acoustic performance to achieve relaxation, pain relief, or sleep regulation. Sessions typically last about 30 minutes, delivered daily or several times per week. Evidence from home and hospice contexts indicates that receptive listening stabilizes mood and reduces physiological arousal (Li et al., 2025; Vinayak et al., 2017).

Active Approach

Active HBMT engages patients and caregivers in musical creation through singing, instrument playing, improvisation, or songwriting. These methods restore a sense of agency and self-expression while promoting interpersonal connection. In family-centered programs, dyadic singing and creative participation foster emotional closeness and support coping among both patients and relatives (Boyde et al., 2024). Active sessions typically last 30–45 minutes and occur weekly or bi-weekly, balancing energy conservation with meaningful interaction.

Integrative Approach

Integrative HBMT combines music with mindfulness, movement, guided imagery, or relaxation exercises. This model engages both body and mind to regulate stress, enhance self-awareness, and promote acceptance. Variants include mindfulness-based MT and music-assisted biofeedback (Sumneangsanor et al., 2022; Fleszar-Pavlovic et al., 2024). Integrative sessions usually last 45–60 minutes once or twice per week, making them suitable for home-based or telehealth delivery. Across modalities, a session duration of around 30 minutes remains most sustainable for palliative patients, while continuity over several weeks enhances psychosocial gains (Li et al., 2025; Boyde et al., 2024).

Table 3. Common Approaches in Home-Based Music Therapy (HBMT)

Approach	Example Intervention	Application in Palliative Care
Receptive	Personalized playlists; guided listening with therapist or family participation	Reduces anxiety, pain, and insomnia; enhances relaxation and sleep quality (Li et al., 2025; Vinayak et al., 2017).
Active	Singing, songwriting, or instrument improvisation involving patient and caregiver	Strengthens emotional expression, family bonding, and communication (Boyde et al., 2024).
Integrative	Music combined with mindfulness, guided imagery, movement, or biofeedback	Regulates physiological stress responses and fosters holistic comfort (Sumneangsanor et al., 2022; Fleszar-Pavlovic et al., 2024).

8.3.1 Technology and Digital Delivery in Home-Based Music Therapy

Recent advances in telehealth and digital media have expanded the accessibility of music therapy for palliative care patients. Virtual music therapy sessions—delivered through video conferencing or streaming platforms—allow continuous engagement for homebound individuals and caregivers, particularly in remote or resource-limited areas. Streaming-based programs and curated therapeutic playlists have been shown to maintain emotional connection between patients and therapists while reducing logistical challenges of in-person visits. Emerging applications of artificial intelligence now enable the creation of adaptive playlists that respond to user mood, physiological signals, or therapeutic goals, offering new tools for personalized relaxation and emotional support. Integrating such technologies into home-based care enhances reach and continuity while complementing, rather than replacing, the relational dimension that defines the therapeutic process.

8.4 Integrating MT into Care

Music therapy should not stand apart from the rest of care. It works best when it is built into the team. Bedside sessions can run alongside pharmacological management (Warth et al., 2015). At home, online programs keep patients connected. And for families, dyadic or group-based formats can sit naturally beside counseling or other psychosocial services (Boyde et al., 2024).

9. CONCLUSION

Looking across 18 trials and feasibility studies, a few themes are clear. Receptive listening is reliable for immediate relief—whether for anxiety before surgery, discomfort during treatment, or fatigue during radiotherapy. Active and dyadic formats contribute something different: a sense of resilience and connection, especially for children and their parents. Guided imagery is powerful for patients needing to process deep psychological distress. Digital and hybrid formats make music therapy accessible to patients who cannot easily attend in person, though these are still early days.

The evidence base has limits. Most of the trials were small, ran at a single site, and varied in how they defined both interventions and outcomes. That makes broad generalizations risky. Long-term outcomes, cultural adaptation, and cost-effectiveness remain understudied.

Even so, the direction of findings is consistent. Music therapy—when personalized and delivered by trained therapists—can reduce suffering and improve quality of life. Sessions of around 30 minutes, offered daily or several times a week over a period of weeks, seem to provide the most stable benefits. While the field needs larger, more rigorous, and more diverse trials, the existing evidence already supports integrating music therapy into oncology and palliative care teams. At its best, MT not only eases pain and anxiety but also strengthens human connection and resilience in the most difficult stages of illness.

ACKNOWLEDGEMENT

The authors would like to thank the University of Management and Technology Ho Chi Minh City, Ho Chi Minh City, Vietnam for their continued support.

REFERENCES

Alcântara-Silva, T. R., Freitas-Junior, R., Freitas, N. M. A., Machado, G. D. S., Ribeiro, M. K. A., da Silva, D. J., de Paula, W.Junior, & Panobianco, M. S. (2018). Music therapy reduces radiotherapy-induced fatigue in patients with breast or gynecological cancer: A randomized trial. *Integrative Cancer Therapies*, *17*(3), 628–635. DOI: 10.1177/1534735418757349 PMID: 29633652

American Music Therapy Association. (2020). *Definition and Scope of Music Therapy Practice 2020*. AMTA.

Bieligmeyer, S., Kesselring, A., Kleinschmidt, R., & Bardenheuer, H. (2018). Feeling the sound – Short-term effect of a vibroacoustic music intervention on well-being and subjectively assessed warmth distribution in cancer patients. *Complementary Therapies in Medicine*, *40*, 171–178. DOI: 10.1016/j.ctim.2018.03.002 PMID: 30219444

Boyde, C., Thaut, M., Roeser, J., Riedl, A., Klein, P., & von Georgi, R. (2024). Interaction-focused music therapy with cancer-affected children and their significant others (INMUT). *Pilot and Feasibility Studies*, *10*(86), 1–15. PMID: 38807165

Bro, M. L., Johansen, C., Vuust, P., Enggaard, L., Himmelstrup, B., Mourits-Andersen, T., Brown, P., d'Amore, F., Andersen, E., Abildgaard, N., & Gram, J. (2019). Effects of live music during chemotherapy in lymphoma patients: A randomized controlled trial. *Supportive Care in Cancer*, *27*(10), 3887–3896. DOI: 10.1007/s00520-019-04666-8 PMID: 30762141

Fleszar-Pavlovic, S. E., McConnell, T., Schmid, W., & Pavlicevic, M. (2024). eHealth mindfulness-based music therapy for patients undergoing allogeneic stem cell transplantation: A pilot randomized controlled trial protocol. *Supportive Care in Cancer*, *31*(9), 4512–4522. PMID: 38763308

Jethva, D. D., Patel, B. C., Sundar, S., Patel, J. B., Vora, H. H., & Sanghavi, P. R. (2025). Harmonising hope: Impact of music therapy on cancer pain and palliative care. *Indian Journal of Palliative Care*, *31*(1), 21–28. DOI: 10.25259/IJPC_235_2024 PMID: 40027977

Koehler, F., Martin, Z.-S., Hertrampf, R.-S., Gäbel, C., Kessler, J., Ditzen, B., & Warth, M. (2021). Music therapy in the psychosocial treatment of adult cancer patients: A systematic review and meta-analysis. *Frontiers in Psychology, 11*, 651. DOI: 10.3389/fpsyg.2020.00651 PMID: 32373019

Köhler, F., Martin, Z.-S., Hertrampf, R.-S., Gäbel, C., Kessler, J., Ditzen, B., & Warth, M. (2020). Music therapy in the psychosocial treatment of adult cancer patients: A systematic review and meta-analysis. *Frontiers in Psychology, 11*, 651. DOI: 10.3389/fpsyg.2020.00651 PMID: 32373019

Li, Y., Zhang, L., Chen, X., Wang, J., & Zhou, H. (2025). The effect of music therapy on anxiety, depression, pain and sleep quality of lung cancer patients: A systematic review and meta-analysis. *Supportive Care in Cancer, 33*(3), 169. DOI: 10.1007/s00520-025-09213-2 PMID: 39928168

Mondanaro, J. F., Sara, G. A., Thoma, M. V., & Loewy, J. V. (2021). The effects of clinical music therapy on resiliency in adults undergoing infusion. *Journal of Pain and Symptom Management, 61*(6), 1099–1108. DOI: 10.1016/j.jpainsymman.2020.10.032 PMID: 33152443

Palmer, J. B., Lane, D., Mayo, D., Schluchter, M., & Leeming, R. (2015). Effects of music therapy on anesthesia requirements and anxiety in women undergoing ambulatory breast surgery for cancer diagnosis and treatment: A randomized controlled trial. *Journal of Clinical Oncology, 33*(28), 3162–3168. DOI: 10.1200/JCO.2014.59.6049 PMID: 26282640

Papanikolaou, E., Stratouli, E., Lianou, M., & Georgiadi, E. (2023). Guided imagery and music in the treatment for breast and gynecologic cancer: A randomized controlled trial. *Journal of Music Therapy, 60*(4), 410–434. DOI: 10.1093/jmt/thad011 PMID: 37503863

Rabinowitch, T.-C., Aberg, L., & Meltzer, L. J. (2023). Outcomes and experiences of an online Balance-Space music therapy intervention for cancer patients. *The Arts in Psychotherapy, 82*, 101998. DOI: 10.1016/j.aip.2023.101998 PMID: 36713463

Steinhardt, T. L., Mortvedt, S., & Trondalen, G. (2021). Music therapy in the hospital-at-home: A practice for children in palliative care. *British Journal of Music Therapy, 35*(2), 53–62. DOI: 10.1177/13594575211029109

Sumneangsanor, T., Thitipattanapong, S., & Thongruang, S. (2022). The effects of a biofeedback and music training programme in reducing stress in Thai patients living with cancer receiving palliative care. *International Journal of Palliative Nursing, 28*(10), 453–463. DOI: 10.12968/ijpn.2022.28.10.453 PMID: 36269291

Terzoni, S., De Vita, A., Ferrara, P., Sacchini, F., Cangelosi, G., Mancin, S., Petrelli, F., Lopane, D., Milani, A., Parozzi, M., & Lusignani, M. (2025). Biological effects of music therapy in end-of-life care: A narrative review. *Medicina, 61*(9), 1690. DOI: 10.3390/medicina61091690 PMID: 41011081

Vinayak, S., Dehkhoda, F., & Vinayak, R. (2017). The effect of music therapy on sleep quality of cancer patients undergoing chemotherapy or radiotherapy: A randomized control trial. *Journal of Social Sciences (COES&RJ-JSS), 6*(4), 734-743.

Warth, M., Keßler, J., Hillecke, T. K., & Bardenheuer, H. (2015). Music therapy in palliative care – A randomized controlled trial to evaluate effects on relaxation. *Deutsches Ärzteblatt International, 112*, 788–794. PMID: 26806566

World Health Organization. (2020). *Integrative health services: The role of music therapy in palliative and supportive care*. World Health Organization.

Chapter 9
Utilise Artmaking for Its Therapeutic-Like Effects in Integrative Care Settings:
The Non-Art Therapist's Guide

Vinh Quang Ly
https://orcid.org/0009-0001-8018-6532
School of Media and Applied Arts, University of Management and Technology Ho Chi Minh City, Vietnam

ABSTRACT

Whilst professional art therapy is a well-established discipline with proven clinical benefits, access to formal services is often limited, especially for individuals in long-term care. This chapter defines clear boundaries between clinician-led art therapy and carer-delivered creative activities and positions itself as a bridge between the two. It summarises the theoretical rationale, the quality of existing evidence of art therapy to establish a foundational understanding of the discipline. Building on this, it offers practical guidance for self-organising simple art activities that utilise these mechanisms. The aim is to enable low-risk, evidence-informed creative activities that support emotion regulation, meaning-making and social connection in domestic care environments.

Whilst interest in integrative approaches to health is growing, a practical challenge often faces by family caregivers (or carers or home carers) is accessing reliable, evidence-informed strategies and methods that can be safely and effectively adapted

DOI: 10.4018/979-8-3373-4094-4.ch009

for domestic settings. It is particularly important when formal therapeutic services are not consistently available.

Whilst this chapter does provide some information about formal art therapy and its clinical efficacy, its main objective is to serve as a bridge between the specialised domain of art therapy and the everyday realities of post-treatment or long-term home care. Recognising that the main audience of this chapter is family caregivers who normally do not possess intensive therapeutic training or accredited qualifications, the focus will be on translating the established principles and therapeutic mechanisms derived from formal art therapy into more accessible, easy-to-implement art-based activities. These activities are not only pastime hobbies but also have therapeutic nature, which may include promoting emotional expression, cognitive engagement, relaxation, or granting sense of accomplishment for the person-in-care (or client or patient or participant). Again, they are not formal art therapy sessions and are not meant to replace them. The intention here is to empower caregivers with practical knowledge about how to facilitate simple, safe, and meaningful creative experiences that draw upon the understanding of why art can be healing, without requiring the skills or knowledge of a clinical therapist.

In general, this chapter will first provide foundational context on the importance of integrative care, then offering an overview of formal art therapy to ground the adaptive practices, as well as exploring the science and mechanisms that explain how art engagement can foster well-being. Next, it dedicates significant attention to the practical application of these principles in home-setting, at a much lower level of clinical formality compared to institutional environments. This will include guidance on creating supportive environments, suggestions for specific activities, and considerations regarding potential challenges and limitations to ensure safe and beneficial use.

THE CALL FOR INTEGRATIVE SUPPORT

The shift from institutionalised to community-based models of care is increasingly presented. Institutionalisation occurs when certain assumptions about problems and their solutions become routinised and taken for granted (Weaver, 2000). The belief that care must be centralised in specialised hospitals or state-owned centres is one of the prime examples. Over time, this assumption was deeply embedded in policy, funding, professional training and public expectation, so that hospital-based care came to define legitimacy in health provision. However, when expectations shift or conflict, normative uncertainty may follow, and institutions' way of operation begins to drift away from everyday practice. In reality, persistent disagreement and changing political economies have weakened the dominance of the centralised model.

Most notable phenomena are the rise of neoliberal and managerialist ideologies, which concern more on cost, efficiency and market regulation than the quality of services itself. Several key societal shifts further spurred this development. Advances in medical science, for example, led to longer life expectancies and allowed more individuals with severe physical disabilities to live within community settings with appropriate support, rather than in often-isolated institutions (Rothman, 1991). Perhaps one of the most significant catalysts for exploring integrative approaches was the widespread decentralisation movement in mental health. Key decision-makers of various levels from government to institutional management have been persuading and relocating patients from large mental hospitals to less restrictive community environments (Rothman, 1991). Such forces contribute to a gradual deinstitutionalisation state. As the response, greater emphasis on family participation in care thrived (Hepworth et al., 2010; McDonald, 2006). However, this transition frequently occurred without commensurate funding or the establishment of robust, organised support systems within the community - leaving many vulnerable individuals without adequate care (Rothman, 1991).

Collaboration within a support system is therefore central for disempowered people in such context. It is believed that an extensive, unified and integrative network is what needed to increase the people's chances of accessing what they need (E. Moore, 2009; S. Moore, 1992; Moxley, 1997). Case management emerged as a practical response to this complexity (E. Moore, 2009; Rothman, 1991). Drawing on psychodynamic, critical, developmental and ecological ideas, it was introduced to provide extended, continuous support across fragmented service fields (Coady & Lehmann, 2008; Gronda, 2008; E. Moore, 2009; Tilbury, 1977). Unlike traditional one-to-one casework, contemporary case management emphasises resource coordination, care planning and capacity-building for autonomy and self-sustenance. The case manager acts as coordinator who locates and links clients to suitable services and tapping to underutilised supports such as family networks (Gladstone et al., 2014; E. Moore, 2009). The degree of service integration and the level of available resources shape a case manager's options. In low-resource or highly fragmented systems, care is often designed around the client and their immediate social ties (such as family, friends, or neighbours) (S. Moore, 1992). More importantly, this evolution opens space for more flexible, person-centred approaches: integrating formal services with community and home-based supports, and empowering home carers to deliver modest therapeutic activities - such as painting or drawing - within a supervised and accountable care plan. This approach has both strengths (i.e., maximising the personal knowledge about the person-in-care, having familiarity with the continuity of care) and limitations, since professional practice requires specific skills, values and knowledge that untrained caregivers may not possess (Chenoweth & McAuliffe, 2012). Domains such as mental health, aged care and homelessness are therefore especially suited to case-management models that combine professional oversight with mobilisation of informal supports (Gronda, 2008; Rothman, 1991).

THEORETICAL FRAMEWORKS FOR EFFECTIVE SUPPORT IN COMMUNITY SETTINGS

A wide variety of theoretical frameworks can be used to explain and support individuals or groups. These theories provide structured ways to conceptualise human experience, guide assessment, and inform interventions. They are proving invaluable in navigating the complexities of in-home and person-centred support.

Firstly, ecological systems theories can be used to understand the interrelations between people and their social environments, and to identify both risky and protective factors (Connolly & Harms, 2011a). As an instance, Bronfenbrenner's ecological model formulates that an individual is a part of an intricate system, and this structure has the tendency to stabilise itself against minor changes. The model is represented as a series of concentric circles, with the layers include (from the inner-most to the outermost) the person's self, their microsystem (i.e., family, friends, school, workplace), their mesosystem (the intermediate level demonstrates the interactions between different microsystemic groups), their exosystem (i.e., local government, mass media), their macrosystem (i.e., societal values, law, culture), and the chronosystem (time and history). Changes, according to this theory, can occur through interventions that target the interactions between the self with each component of said layers. However, it is emphasised that interventions must be initiated at many levels at the same time. Otherwise, the system will regulate itself and push everything back into the original state. This perspective is particularly vital in homecare setting, as it acknowledges the importance of supports from individual's family and the inner circles beside professional treatments in any comprehensive support plan.

In contrast, psychodynamic theories illuminate the profound influence of past experiences and unconscious processes on emotions, behaviours, and relational patterns (Chenoweth & McAuliffe, 2012). These approaches seek to peel back layers of experience to reach the undiscovered trauma by analysing one's relational systems and their internal psychological structures. They posit that the self, both conscious and unconscious, emerges through systems of relationship with others, with many patterns emerging from early childhood experiences within family structure – such as attachment theory. These theories provide useful frameworks for conceptualising complex dynamics within any relationship, as well as highlighting the importance of family members in mental development processes.

Growing from psychoanalytic traditions, the humanistic or person-centred approach redirected attention from unconscious drives to the experience of the individual and the relational field. Central to this perspective is the concept of intersubjectivity - the reciprocal connection between people within a helping relationship (Connolly & Harms, 2011c). Connolly & Harms (2011c) stated that the most significant contributor to positive changes is not the practitioner's mastery of techniques or their theoretical knowledge, but mostly the client's perception of the quality of the relationship and the genuineness of the encounter. As the response to this, person-centred practice emphasises on three basic conditions: empathy, unconditional positive regard and congruence as the pillars for professional interactions (Chenoweth & McAuliffe, 2012). Recognising clients' inherent capacity for self-direction, this practice resonates strongly with contemporary empowerment models and well aligns with the shift towards integrated and community-based support systems. Clients, in this instance, are recognised as active agents of changes rather than just passive patients.

At the other end of the spectrum, cognitive and behavioural theories in general and Cognitive Behavioural Therapies (CBT) examine the powerful interplay between thoughts, feelings, and actions (Connolly & Harms, 2011b). They tend to be more structured and directive than other theories, focusing on actively changing thoughts and behaviours. A core assumption is that psychological distress can often stem from "faulty" or unhelpful thinking patterns rather than simply from external events themselves. And thus, by changing a person's perception to a situation, it would help them to "fix" these undesirable behaviours (Chenoweth & McAuliffe, 2012). CBT - as an intervention method - provides practical, evidence-based tools that aid both individuals and caregivers with tangible strategies for managing distress, challenging unhelpful assumptions, and fostering coping skills within various life contexts.

Finally, aligning closely with humanistic and strength-based ethos that were increasingly represented in contemporary care, narrative theories focus on the power of the stories individuals and communities live by (Connolly & Harms, 2011d; Saleebey, 2006). These approaches propose that human beings make sense of their lives through narratives – heard, imposed and told by themselves. These stories, passed down or newly constructed, profoundly influence identity, well-being, and how people think, feel, and act. Thus, narrative therapists state that stories can be "re-authored" to enable more positive and rewarding life outcomes (Connolly & Harms, 2011d). They believe that by listening to the clients' stories, they can externalise the problems from the person, unearth the hidden meanings and discover factors that contributed to the establishment of the narrative. From the pieces, the stories can be re-organised or retold in a way that amplify strengths and resilience. This perspective is particularly relevant for reframing experiences of illness, disability, or caregiving. It can empower individuals to challenge problem-saturated narratives and collaboratively construct stories that reflect their strengths, agency, and preferred identities.

THE ORIGIN OF ART THERAPY AND ITS DEFINITION

The origins of creative arts therapies reach far back into human history. Since the early years, people have created marks, drawings, carved, or scratches as forms of visual communication and expression (Case et al., 2022). Indigenous healers and shamans across many cultures have used dance, song, drumming, storytelling, masks, costumes and ritual props as central elements in rites aimed at healing and illness prevention. These practices mobilised symbolic, bodily and communal resources to effect change (Feldwisch, 2022; Orkibi & Keisari, 2023). In ancient Greece, dramatic enactments combining dance, music and narrative sought to produce catharsis in audiences, a notion that directly links artistic enactment with emotional release. There are also accounts of artistic practices being embedded in medical and therapeutic settings through the Middle Ages and later during the Enlightenment. In nineteenth century, the rise of psychiatry resulted in further experiments in integrating the arts within institutional healthcare, laying groundwork for clinical approaches that followed (Orkibi & Keisari, 2023).

The modern profession of art therapy is traced back to the mid-twentieth century. Adrian Hill, an artist recuperating from tuberculosis at King Edward VII Sanatorium in England, is credited with the first explicit description of "art therapy" in the 1940s (Cheng et al., 2023; Nearney, 2006). Hill observed that making art occupied patients' attention, encouraged participation, and had both diversionary and expressive functions. Patients' artworks, the author stated, could be used as a medium through which anxiety, trauma and internal conflict could be revealed and worked through to support psychological recovery.

Practice and organisation of art therapy developed rapidly after these early clinical observations. In the 1950s art therapy frequently took the form of informal, open-studio groups in which patients could come and go and discussed their work with a therapist on an individual basis. By the late 1960s and into the 1970s, practice became more structured. Formal group formats with defined boundaries emerged and clinicians paid closer attention to group dynamics, therapeutic frame and the processes through which images carried meaning (Nearney, 2006).

In the modern day, art therapy sits within the wider family of creative arts therapies (CAT). It is an umbrella term that includes visual art therapy alongside dance-movement, drama, psychodrama, music therapy and bibliotherapy. All these professions apply creative processes within a therapeutic relationship, and their outcomes are to optimise health and wellbeing of the clients (Orkibi & Keisari, 2023). Art therapy, as a discipline, is defined as a form of psychotherapy that encourages expression and healing through artistic media (American Art Therapy Association, n.d.). According to Minhaj & Rauf (2023), its goals are to "improve cognitive and sensorimotor functions, foster self-esteem and self-awareness, cultivate emotional resilience, promote insight, enhance social skills, reduce conflict and distress, and support wider societal and ecological change". It privileges the meaning of the artworks and the act of creation over technical skill or aesthetic quality and focus on what these images, marks or materials communicate about the client's internal world and experience (Cheng et al., 2023; Emilia, 2021b; Nearney, 2006).

Art therapy, in most cases, is delivered by trained and licensed art therapists who can work safely with imagery that may reveal deep or distressing thoughts (Minhaj & Rauf, 2023). The art therapist's role is to facilitate their client's non-verbal and verbal self-expression and reflection through the making and discussion of images (Cheng et al., 2023; Orkibi & Keisari, 2023). As a therapeutic modality, art therapy can draw on a range of theoretical frameworks. Practitioners may integrate psychoanalytic, humanistic, cognitive–behavioural or Gestalt ideas to shape intervention strategies. Thus, a particular case can be approached differently depending on the therapist's conceptual orientation, knowledge and training (Demir et al., 2024; Rastogi, Paige Feldwisch, et al., 2022). Cathy Malchiodi's MSSS model, for example, organises creative modalities into Movement, Sound, Storytelling and Silence, highlighting how different media may be combined to access embodied, narrative and reflective processes (Minhaj & Rauf, 2023).

MECHANISMS OF ART THERAPY

Art therapy utilises the activity of making artworks in two ways. Firstly, there is the idea of "art as therapy". It means the creative process itself – such as making marks, shaping clay, etc. - can be intrinsically healing (Cheng et al., 2023; Rastogi, Paige Feldwisch, et al., 2022). This concept will be further discussed in a section below. Secondly, practitioners explicitly integrate psychological approaches (i.e. Psychoanalytic, humanist, CBT etc.) in specifically designed exercises to support their clients mentally (Case et al., 2022). To be more precise, the therapists identify and cultivate clients' creative potential, scaffold expression, and support social integration through shared artistic activities (Hosu, 2022). Some sensory and motor modes of expression cultivated from art therapy sessions enable clients to access perspectives beyond purely verbal reflection. Many clinicians combine artmaking with talk therapy, mindfulness, aromatherapy or other adjuncts to enhance regulation and insight (Emilia, 2021a; Minhaj & Rauf, 2023). For example, psychoanalytic art therapists explore transference and countertransference (both of them are concepts within the school of psychoanalytic/ psychodynamic) within the triadic relationship of artwork, client and therapist (Connolly & Harms, 2011c). Here the image becomes a projective surface through which unconscious thoughts within the client are surfaced and worked upon (Cheng et al., 2023). In reality, both strands coexist in contemporary practice. Depends on the situation, the therapists may want to place the emphasis on facilitating a non-verbal, sensory route to feeling and regulation or focus on using the picture or product as a catalyst for dialogic exploration.

Duncan & Miller (2001)'s "client-centred theory of change" underscores that the resources clients bring into the therapy room - such as persistence, openness, faith and external supports - are often the primary contributors to outcome. Hence, the most effective interventions are those that fit a particular client's self-understanding and meaning-making ability rather than those that statistically boast the highest average success rates in general. In practice, this means that the art process becomes therapeutic when it resonates with the client's own interpretations, goals and personal narrative. Therapy is therefore a co-constructed enterprise in which the client controls content whilst the therapist guides the unfolding of that content toward changes. In most cases, the therapeutic quality may not be affected even when the clients refuse to share their artworks because the process of "making art" is deemed more important than the final products themselves. (Case et al., 2022). The reason for this, according to Case et al. (2022), is that the state of a client when they go back to paint an unfinished piece maybe vastly different from when they started, or the "concrete form outlasts the actual experience of making it".

The therapeutic partnership is central to effective co-construction of meaning in any intervention. It consists of four interrelated elements: the client's affective bond with the therapist; the client's capacity to work with purpose; the therapist's empathic involvement; and mutual agreement on goals and tasks (Duncan & Miller, 2001). In talk therapies, however, the interaction between stakeholders can easily be strained and changes are usually hindered by resistance, even in voluntary cases (Westra & Aviram, 2013). In general, clients' resistance usually is the result of their internal conflicts, that may be either about competing motivations or opposition to the therapist/treatments. By contrast, if middle ground mediums are used (like using artworks), they can potentially help mitigating this issue. In this instance, art therapy is comparable to motivational interviewing (MI) in resistance management. In both methods, clients are positioned as the experts of their own lives and the therapist acknowledges the clients' authority within the therapeutic relationship (Hohman, 2012; Westra & Aviram, 2013). In MI, resistance is regarded as a valuable source of information. The therapists are encouraged to "roll" with the clients' stories by elaborating the conversations in a way that make the clients discussed about "changes" themselves, not by forcing them to (Hohman, 2012). Art therapy achieves a similar outcome through non-threatening, indirect channels. By externalising emotions into images, artmaking often reduces perceived threats and creates openings for undiscovered expression. This allows subconscious material to surface, deepening self-understanding and enhancing communication in ways that exceed purely rational or verbal processes (Orkibi & Keisari, 2023). Emerging neuroscientific models suggest that artmaking recruits non-verbal processing networks and may influence stress-response systems in ways that aid the linking of sensory-emotional memory with narrative representations (Wang et al., 2025). In the other words, the person-in-care naturally paints the stories in their own view without fear of facing judgements from the therapists. Therapists can still ask questions, but those inquiries in this context are deliberately open and minimally directive so that the client's associations, emotions and bodily responses have maximal space to surface. Such an invitational stance allows new connections and distinctions to be discovered rather than imposed, enabling the client to re-authorise aspects of their life story. This indirect pathway fosters psychological safety, reduces defensive interactions, and sustains engagement (Westra & Aviram, 2013). Trauma-informed practice, for instance, commonly position creative arts as adjunctive to talk-based therapies because they open non-verbal, embodied routes to sensory and affective memory traces that can be resistant to verbal processing.

In additional, creativity itself is recognised as a core human capacity for adapting to life's challenges. Some theorists even suggested that creativity is essential for psychological survival (Orkibi & Keisari, 2023). The construct of creative adaptability refers to the integration of cognitive, behavioural, and emotional resources that enable people to respond flexibly to issues, or stress. Artistic practice helps transforming the often complex and subtle range of feelings into symbolic, tangible forms. As clients tell their stories through images, they reveal plotlines, characters, conflicts and desires, which are the refection of their perception to situations in life (Connolly & Harms, 2011d). The therapist's attunement to a client's symbolic language (understanding their choices of colour, forms, space, and material represented in the artpieces) may exemplify empathic involvement. Artworks thus function simultaneously as both record/product and process/experiment (Rastogi, Paige Feldwisch, et al., 2022). Through symbols, metaphors, and evocative images, art conveys implicit messages about inner experiences that might otherwise remain unspoken (Orkibi & Keisari, 2023). Because such communication can operate with little or no reliance on words, it often bypasses conventional barriers to expression. These visual forms also serve as focus for reflection and revision whilst collaboratively negotiated art tasks provide concrete goals and shared agreement about next steps.

From a psychodynamic perspective, object relations theory helps explain why art-based works can be therapeutic and promote psychological changes in non-clinical or home contexts (Brandell & George, 2015). It emphasises how people internalise their early relationships by referring both to actual interactions with important figures and to the inner mental images (objects) that represent those people and the self (Brandell & George, 2015). In this view, human beings are not simply driven by instinct but are fundamentally motivated to relate. A key concept here is "transference", which is defined as the tendency to unconsciously repeat old patterns of feelings, attitudes and behaviours from early relationships in new connections. In most therapy sessions, these patterns emerge during the engagements with the therapist, where they can be recognised, worked through, and changed (Brandell & George, 2015). In art therapy, artworks and materials act as symbolic objects that invite projection and transference. Clients may project disavowed parts of relational experience onto materials, re-experience familiar relational scripts through the art process, and may be able to reorganise maladaptive internal objects. More importantly, this psychodynamic process is not confined to formal clinical settings as encounters with artworks outside therapy can elicit similar movements. In case of an exhibition, a created image may afford projection and symbolic re-enactment, whilst an audience's reflective response can offer mirroring functions that parallel the therapist's role. Where no external force is present, an internalised or imagined audience may suffice to sustain therapeutic effects.

Beyond relational and intrapsychic mechanisms, creative activity is also multidimensional. From biopsychosocial–spiritual perspective, artmaking engages the body through sensorimotor activity, affects physiological arousal, supports emotional regulation, and fosters social connection when shared. It can also generate existential or spiritual meaning for the individual (Harms, 2010). Since these subjective perceptions of wellbeing often have greater affection on resilience, an activity that changes perceptive experience, meaning and social belonging can have remarkable effects on overall functioning. The effects of creativity can also be understood within an ecological framework. The mesosystem is where shared creative activity can strengthen relationships (i.e., family and the home environment), such as collaborative tasks or group viewing activities foster belonging, mutual recognitions (Connolly & Harms, 2011a). It is important to understand that at broader levels, the exosystem (i.e., government, mass media, funding) and macrosystem (i.e., cultural norms, professional ideologies) may affect the state of art-based practices. They decide whether art in general or art-based interventions is supported or sanctioned. This reflect through the level of material accessibility, validation from community groups, commissioning priorities, cultural attitudes toward creativity and whether home-based art activity is treated as legitimate care or informal pastime.

Visual art therapy has been shown to also foster emotion regulation capability. Firstly, it can enhance participants' ability to modulate their emotions directly through the art-making process. This engagement often involves a pleasurable sensory experience with the art materials and can provide a profound sense of relief or release (Orkibi & Keisari, 2023). Secondly, art therapy can significantly increase participants' capacity to reflect upon their own emotions, to express and communicate these feelings effectively to others, and, more importantly, to discover new meanings and insights related to their emotional states and experiences. This enhanced capacity for emotional processing is widely considered a primary mechanism through which art therapy leads to demonstrable reductions in both psychological and physical symptoms. These characteristics have been shown, for instance, in some studies involving patients with breast cancer, according to Orkibi & Keisari (2023).

APPLICATION OF ART THERAPY

Art therapy itself and techniques of choices are defined by the alignment of purpose, medium and context. When choices are intentionally mapped – including selecting materials and tasks that afford the desired psychological process, accounting for cultural and practical constraints, and honouring the person's autonomy and preference - art-based interventions become adaptable tools for regulation, expression, narrative integration and social belonging in a wide variety of real-world settings (Demir et al., 2024; Orkibi & Keisari, 2023).

Art therapy can be applied across the lifespan and in a remarkably wide range of clinical and community contexts, tailoring approaches to developmental stage and presenting needs. Practitioners can work with children, adolescents, adults and older people. The literatures also reported benefits of art therapy in mood disorders, schizophrenia-spectrum conditions, trauma-related problems and broader indices of wellbeing and coping (Cheng et al., 2023; Putri et al., 2025). For children, art provides a developmentally appropriate, non-verbal means to process and integrate experiences that are hard to put into words. For older adults, short-course creative programmes have demonstrated reductions in anxiety, diminished loneliness and improvements in confidence and agency (Putri et al., 2025). These diverse age groups and clinical presentations call for an equally diverse repertoire of techniques, each selected for the affordances it provides. The repertoire may range from low-threshold activities (i.e. free drawing, mandala colouring and collage) to kinaesthetic and tactile work such as clay modelling and assemblage, to narrative devices like timelines and storyboards. Integrated models such as Mindfulness-Based Art Therapy can combine attentional training with creative practice (Demir et al., 2024; Orkibi & Keisari, 2023). Each method affords different psychological functions. For examples, patterned or repetitive mark-making often supports attentional regulation and calming whilst heavy, manipulative media provide strong proprioceptive feedback useful for embodied release. Guided imagery and narrative formats, on the other hand, encourage memory integration and identity work and collaborative or object-based projects foster social recognition and shared meaning.

Due to its versality, contexts of delivery are quite varied. In some Western countries, social prescribing schemes in some jurisdictions formalise clinical referrals to local creative activities and integrate arts engagement within a broader model of community care (Stevenson & Alzyood, 2025). Art-based practice is embedded in hospitals and palliative-care services, mental-health clinics and schools. Correctional institutions and community centres usually offer creative programmes aimed at rehabilitation and social reintegration. Cultural institutions, notably museums and galleries, increasingly partner with health and community services to deliver object-based and participatory programmes that foreground public validation and communal meaning-making. Digital and hybrid modalities - such as tele-art therapy, guided online workshops, creative apps and moderated online communities - have rapidly expanded access, reducing barriers of distance, mobility and stigma. This was especially evident during the pandemic and lockdown periods, according to Stevenson & Alzyood (2025).

Implementation decisions are thus shaped by both therapeutic purpose and pragmatic constraints. Important practical considerations include the available space, the cost and portability of materials, cultural meanings attached to media or images, and the level of relational containment required by the material being worked with. These factors determine whether an activity is most appropriately delivered one-to-one, in a small, structured group, through community partnerships, or via digital platforms. Equally, facilitator skills and the degree of clinical oversight available influence decisions about technique and setting. Some contexts require trained art therapists whilst others can safely use low-threshold, facilitator-led activities that emphasise process over product.

COMPILATION OF EMPIRICAL STUDIES

A growing body of empirical evidence has examined these applications, providing evidence for their effectiveness, though methods and samples vary widely.

Table 1.

Study	Design, method & sample	Key outcomes/ statistic
Korostiy & Hmain (2013)	Design: Clinical sample of 40 patients with depressive disorder (ages 18–30, both genders), form into 2 groups that had Art therapy sessions and group that did not (control group). Method: Contents of their pictures analysed and compared with subjective experience to evaluate the effect of treatments	Outcome: - 90% linked picture content to experience - 70% reduced anxiety - 75% mood improvement - 77% increased self-esteem - 80% sustained remission reported - 68% positive outlook.
Kozhyna et al. (2017)	Design: 135 patients aged 18-30 with major depressive disorder. Method: Comparison between combined treatment group (with group art therapy) and standard care.	Outcome: ~60% reported decreased melancholic symptoms early in treatment when group art therapy added Improved Quality of life during remission.
Cheng et al. (2023)	Referred to trial from Beebe et al. (2010). Design: Randomised controlled trial with children with asthma. Methods: Pre-post comparison after 7 weekly sessions of art therapy.	Outcome: Post-treatment result: reduced anxiety and improved self-concept (reported RCT outcome).
Lin & Yang (2023)	Design: Divided 100 university students with autism into 2 groups (experimental and control). Method: Both groups were evaluated pre/post experiment using Kirschner Autism Behaviour Scale. Controlled trial last for 1 month.	Outcome: In experimental group severe emotional-understanding cases fell from 12 to 3. Overall improvement in emotional comprehension vs no-treatment control.
Demir et al. (2024)	Mindfulness-based Art Therapy (MBAT) quasi-experimental study. Design: Study group consist of 10 patients (80% female, between 26 and 41 years of age) in outpatient clinic who were diagnosed with migraine. Method: Depression-Anxiety-Stress Scale and Oxford Happiness Scale Short Form were used pre and post treatment to evaluate the effectiveness of intervention (8 sessions).	Outcome: Pre/post changes: happiness $z = -2.314$ ($p < 0.05$); depression $z = -2.150$ ($p < 0.05$); stress $z = -1.995$ ($p < 0.05$); anxiety nonsignificant ($z = -1.541$, $p > 0.05$).

continued on following page

Table 1. Continued

Study	Design, method & sample	Key outcomes/ statistic
Putri et al. (2025)	Design: 35 community older adults (age 60-74, ~85% were female) in Posyandu Mugi Sehat Ledug, Indonesia with signs of anxiety. Method: Single group pre/post-test model, last one month. The intervention method is colouring therapy. Data was gathered by administering interviews with Geriatric Anxiety Scale questionnaire.	Outcome: Wilcoxon $Z = 20.19$, $p < 0.001$; mean anxiety 22.4 → 12.1 (difference 10.3) after programme. Proportion of people who had moderate and severe anxiety at 65.7% and 8.6% dropped to 40% and 2.9%, respectively.
Toroghi (2015)	Design: 21 housewives in West of Tehran. Method: Data was gathered from taking general health, Sherer general self-efficacy and Beck anxiety tests before and after intervention (12 art therapy sessions)	Outcome: Statistically significant improvements in general health, anxiety and self-efficacy after intervention. - Physical modelling: pre/post means: 1.56/1.55, t-test: 3.13 - Anxiety: pre/post means: 1.92/1.97, t-test: 4.02 - Karkrdajtmay (translation: Social functioning): pre/post means: 1.17/1.09, t-test: -5.50 - Depression: pre/post means: 0.97/1.02, t-test: 4.69 - Overall public health: pre/post means: 2.69/2.69 (Standard deviation dropped), t-test: -5.54
Minhaj & Rauf (2023)	Design 15 participants (psychologists, neurologists and a special educator) in Karachi (Pakistan) Method: Used qualitative survey to gather information from their clients. Purpose is to explore the perspectives of mental health providers on the effectiveness of art therapy)	Outcome: Clinician reports of symptomatic reduction up to ~80% across various disorders (practitioner-reported).

Note. This table is a compilation of controlled trials, from cited sources.

It is noticeable that the above empirical reports display heterogeneity in sample size, outcome measures and intervention types. Some studies are small or non-randomised, others use clinician-rated outcomes or practitioner surveys. Nonetheless, the statistical findings above, including records of pre/post score changes and test statistics, still provide quantifiable evidence that art-based interventions produce measurable improvements across a variety of populations and settings (Korostiy & Hmain, 2013; Kozhyna et al., 2017; Lin & Yang, 2023; Putri et al., 2025).

CHALLENGES

Despite promising indications, the translation of art therapy into widely endorsed, first-line practice faces several clear challenges.

Methodologically, the evidence base remains uneven. Many reports are case studies, expert opinions or small quasi-experimental trials rather than large, well-designed randomised controlled trials. As Wang et al. (2025) noted, systematic reviews of creative arts therapy in trauma lack quantitative meta-analyses capable of consolidating disparate findings, and this limited empirical robustness constrains formal endorsement and commissioning of services. Responsible application therefore requires skilled facilitation, cultural sensitivity, clear safety boundaries and pathways for referral where deeper clinical intervention is needed.

Practical and clinical obstacles further complicate implementation. Art therapy is not for everyone, and certain approaches are more suitable for specific cases than others (Viganò et al., 2019). In general, outcomes of therapy vary according to client preference, the fit between method and individual worldview, therapist skill, and the quality of the therapeutic frame. As an example, CBT approaches are widely considered suitable for people with phobias, though this is not always accurate, as stated by Case et al. (2022). So, unless clients are matched with an appropriate therapist and approach early in treatment, they may disengage before finding a method that fits their needs.

Group work can also suffer strong resistance and boundary-related problems. Nearney (2006) concerns that quiet, reflective art tasks may leave participants confronting distressing material, sometimes provoking avoidance. These tasks can also make the person exits intervention plan prematurely, destroys their works, or mould them into defensive styles of production. Moreover, individual differences further limit applicability when working in a group. Some clients initially resist art activities and consider them as childish or irrelevant and it may affect the dynamism in the group. The therapists must then spend more effort to build rapport to each individual (Minhaj & Rauf, 2023). In worse cases, group sessions can also become a forum for protest or a vehicle for collective processing. Thus, managing these variable dynamics requires experienced facilitation, clear boundaries and structured procedures for after-group supervision and follow-up.

Implementation is additionally constrained by resource and workforce factors. Trained, licensed art therapists are not universally available and clinical settings often lack material resources or dedicated spaces (Demir et al., 2024; Minhaj & Rauf, 2023). It is a vital issue since ethical and safety considerations (may consist of dealing with distressing imagery, ensuring appropriate consent, and knowing when to escalate to specialist mental-health care) require clear protocols and supervision that many community or home contexts do not yet provide.

ART AS A THERAPEUTIC ACTIVITY FOR HUMAN BETTERMENT

Whilst it is beyond doubt that trained art therapists have an important place in formal therapeutic settings, according to Trevithick (2003) and Westra & Aviram (2013), the overemphasise on psychological techniques and mechanisms can provoke resistance or unintended behaviours in some care contexts. As argued from the earlier section, it is important to consider the strengths of community models and empowerment perspectives. Furthermore, even without the intervention of professional therapists, artworks and the process of making them are said to already have healing effects (Cheng et al., 2023; Rastogi, Paige Feldwisch, et al., 2022). Thus, everyday art-related activities, when designed with an understanding of art-therapy mechanisms or directly retrieved from established branches of art therapy, can be a valuable component of a person's recovery regimen and of broader integrative support system. It would be even more beneficial if that are deliverable by lesser trained carers and family members.

From an evolutionary and neuroscientific perspective, artmaking is a deeply embedded hominin practice that co-evolved with our capacity to shape the material world (Rastogi, Strang, et al., 2022). Human's nervous system receives multimodal sensory inputs (including sight, touch, sound, smell, taste), transforms them into electrical and chemical signals, and produces coordinated motor and affective responses. For everyday creative practice, these processes operate at both automatic (subcortical, sensorimotor) and controlled (cortical, executive) levels. Art materials therefore serve as affordances that can either activate a sympathetic, energising response (for example, vigorous clay work) or a parasympathetic, calming response (for example, slow smoothing of clay), allowing simple, low-risk modulation of arousal through material selection and guidance (Rastogi, Strang, et al., 2022).

According to Rastogi, Strang, et al. (2022), the idea of neuroplasticity provides a physiological explanation for the longer-term benefits of repeated creative engagement. Synaptic plasticity - or the strengthening and weakening of synapses in response to activity - underpins learning, habit formation and the gradual reorganisation of cognitive-affective networks by physically alter the brain's cerebellum and motor cortex. As an instance, repeated intentional artful behaviours (from brief daily doodling to collaborative collage) can reinforce adaptive neural pathways and attenuate maladaptive associations. Thus, contemporary therapeutic frameworks explicitly aim to wire new relational and regulatory patterns by harnessing such practice-dependent plasticity.

Next, contemporary neurocognitive models of creativity emphasise the coordinated action of large-scale brain networks rather than isolated loci. Creative activity typically involves dynamic interaction among the default mode network

(DMN - implicated in internally directed thought and imagery), the executive control network (ECN - supports focused attention, evaluation and planning), and the salience network (SN - mediates switching between internal exploration and externally guided appraisal) (Rastogi, Strang, et al., 2022). Artmaking reliably engages these networks in complementary ways: spontaneous ideation and imagery recruit DMN processes, evaluative refinement draws on ECN functions, and the SN enables transitions between exploratory and critical modes of processing. The flexible coupling of these networks may produce "flow" - an absorbed, time-dilated state that can reduce anxiety and enhanced engagement - which can be fostered by tasks that appropriately balance challenge and skill.

It is also argued that art can greatly influence one's vision and thus their perception (Rastogi, Strang, et al., 2022). The visual system is tightly linked with memory and emotion, making visual expression a powerful route to autobiographical material and affective states. At the same time, the sensorimotor and kinaesthetic aspects of artmaking (gesture, texture, movement) provide preverbal channels for expression and regulation, especially where verbal processing is limited or distressing.

More importantly, the neuroscientific processes outlined above do not exist in isolation from the richer psychological phenomena that therapists and carers observe in practice. Rather, they provide the physiological and functional substrate that makes those phenomena possible and tractable. The fundamental role of art extends far beyond the mere application of previously acquired artistic skills or knowledge. It is, more profoundly, a journey into the discovery of the yet-known and unarticulated aspects of the self (Emilia, 2021b).

Firstly, creative engagement can help establishing a psychological "distance" from the often-overwhelming immediacy of perceived reality. This dynamic interplay between identification with and separation from subjective experiences is a core mechanism shared with other therapeutic modalities, such as solution-focused brief therapy (SFBT). For example, the miracle question in SFBT functions in a similar way by prompting the individual to verbally "paint" an alternative reality where their problems have been resolved. This technique requires the person to both internally and externally recognises their strengths and the agents for change in relation to their problems, which promotes a similar process of psychological distancing and cognitive clarity (Connolly & Harms, 2011d; Orkibi & Keisari, 2023). Another central operational mechanism is "concretisation," a term that describes the transformative process whereby abstract and often formless internal psychological content - such as diffuse emotions, fleeting thoughts, or fragmented memories - is actively changed into an externalised, tangible, and observable artistic presentation through the deliberate use of artistic elements like colour, shape, line, or composition (Orkibi & Keisari, 2023). It makes otherwise elusive material observable and discussable, enabling new meanings to be generated and integrated. By externalising an internal experience through the physical act of creation, the individual can engage with and reflect on difficult emotions from a safer, more objective perspective.

Within this framework, a secure and supportive therapeutic environment is designed to actively encourage "playfulness." In this specialised context, playfulness is understood as an intrinsically motivating state characterised by psychological flexibility, an openness to arts-based experiences, and a willingness to engage in authentic self-exploration and expression - all of which are foundational to fostering creativity and facilitating profound therapeutic change. This form of therapeutic playfulness empowers clients to spontaneously and safely interact with, and gain mastery over, emotionally challenging experiences (Orkibi & Keisari, 2023). This cultivated detachment that can render the exploration of self through various artistic forms a more manageable and insightful endeavour.

Creative engagement also promotes emotion regulation via two principal pathways. First, the sensory-motor experience of artmaking can directly modulate affective arousal, offering relief or catharsis through pleasurable interaction with materials. Second, the reflective aspect of art - interpretation of images and metaphors - enhances meta-emotional awareness, verbalisation and interpersonal communication about feelings. This dual pathway is implicated in documented symptom reduction across a range of conditions (for example, in oncology settings where visual arts interventions have been associated with reduced distress) (Orkibi & Keisari, 2023).

Finally, the benefits of art extend beyond individual change to communal and collective wellbeing. During the COVID-19 pandemic, for instance, art-based activities and digital creative platforms were mobilised to mitigate distress, sustain social ties and enable collective meaning-making. Collaborative creative practices can foster resilience by reframing shared adversity into narratives of endurance and growth (Stevenson & Alzyood, 2025). Such applications highlight the arts' capacity to restore agency, facilitate post-traumatic growth and reinforce social belonging.

THE APPLICATION TO HOME SETTINGS

The theoretical and neuroscientific accounts explained earlier provide not only a rationale but also clear parameters for translating art-based mechanisms into low-risk, home-deliverable interventions. Carers who work outside clinical settings can facilitate deliberately designed creative activities that leverage sensory affordances, network-level engagement and practice-dependent neuroplasticity to support emotion regulation, attentional control, identity work and social connection (Orkibi & Keisari, 2023; Rastogi, Paige Feldwisch, et al., 2022). Importantly, it must be clearly defined that the aims of such applications are more supportive and adjunctive rather than therapeutic in specialist sense. Everyday art practices can be offered as potential opportunities, but caregivers should remain alert to the limits of their role and to indicators that require professional referral (Trevithick, 2003).

First and foremost, successful translation into home contexts begins with pragmatic attention to setting and safety. At the outset, carers may need some guidance since some procedures that are a crucial part of professional therapy, regardless talk or art-based, must be completed. Ideally, certified art therapist or psychologist or social workers can give some instruction at the end of the formal treatment and/or at the beginning of home-based support. This is plausible as the family caregivers should have always been a pillar of support and an integrated part of the therapeutic process in contemporary settings. In many instances, the caregivers are considered as co-therapists in dyadic art therapy systems (Case et al., 2022). Regarding the environment, a predictable, well-ventilated work area, basic protective coverings for surfaces, and the exclusive use of non-toxic, washable materials reduce physical risk and lower barriers to participation. They should also be easy to clean because messes during the activities are unavoidable (Case et al., 2022). Furthermore, if the situation allows, practicing activities involving environmental manipulation, such as art installations or costume making, are found to have great effects in improving one's self-esteem and other skills (Hosu, 2023).

Before starting any activity, caregivers must gain consents, offer clear choices and acquire agreement on time limits and rules. These steps protect dignity and autonomy of the person-in-care and minimise the likelihood of coercion. A short pre-activity plan that includes when and where to pause the session, as well as emergency contact should also be prepared as an essential part of ethically responsible practice. In cases when there is risk of self-harm, intense trauma recalls or medical issues, the caregivers must contact appropriate people on the plan and never attempt to manage the crises alone.

Although the family caregivers might have no formal training in psychology or therapy, it is possible to learn some fundamental principles that can be easily applied by non-specialists. Firstly, they can be taught to use appropriate language when working with the person-in-care since discourses have the power to either empower or oppressed the person-in-care (Ellermann, 1998). Caregivers should use open-ended prompts and non-evaluative language to reduce the person-in-care's performance anxiety and let them know that it is more important to focus on the process than the final product. Secondly, it is important for caregivers to observe and reflect but not interpret the work or the person-in-care's actions. Case et al. (2022) admitted that even professional analytical art therapist can misinterpret the works. By prematurely interfering or interpreting, it robs the person the opportunity to learn and reflect about themselves. Caregivers can also support meaning-making by mirroring observed actions (For example, using sentences like "I notice you used a lot of [colour name]. What does that feel like?") but must avoid imposing psychological explanations. Finally, if there is no specific requests from the person, the caregivers should select materials and tasks to match the goals, thus aligning activity design with the neuro-psychological pathways described previously.

To expand on this, art materials should be chosen deliberately with an eye to their predictable psychological affordances rather than by aesthetics or availability alone. Caregivers can refer to Expressive Therapies Continuum (ETC) and the media-dimension variables (MDV) models to understand simple, practical taxonomy (Rastogi, Paige Feldwisch, et al., 2022). They can provide evidence-informed way to match a medium to a mechanism rather than leaving selection to chance. In general, the ETC classifies art materials accordingly to three continua: The physical qualities of the medium (from fluid to resistive), the levels of complexity (from low to high) and the amount of liberty that the participants have (from unstructured to structured). These properties reliably influence whether an activity invites affective release, sensorimotor engagement, perceptual containment or cognitive sequencing (O'Neill Haaga & Schwartz, 2022). As an instance, when the aim is emotional release or mood exploration, fluid, colourful media such as tempera, watercolour pans or soft chalk pastels can be used. It is discovered that painting with oil pastels show increases in brain activity link with the Alpha frequency band, which is typically associated with the state of relaxed alertness. On the other hand, resistive, tactile materials such as clay or firmer modelling dough give strong proprioceptive feedback and suit grounding or discharge work, help enhancing memory and motor control (Rastogi, Paige Feldwisch, et al., 2022). In additional, other low-tech structured media – for examples, pre-cut collage kits, simple print stamps or timeline templates - support narrative organisation and cognitive sequencing when reflection or memory work is the objective.

Another advantage that caregivers have when organising art activities in home settings is that they can find materials and resources quite easily and less restrictive than in institutional settings. A few short facilitation rules help ensuring materials achieve their intended effect and aiding fresh starters to learn how a given paint, clay or collage glue behaves. Caregivers may offer a modest range of culturally relevant options so the person can choose what feels comfortable to work with. For inexpensive options, they can utilise cheap crayons, coloured pencils water-soluble markers, tempera cakes, or student-graded acrylics for drawing exercises. For collage and mixed media works, newspapers, magazines, old calendars, fabric scraps, ticket stubs and packaging can be obtained from many sources and even free. Whilst clay and other sculpting materials can be expensive, kitchen-made items (such as salt-dough, sponge brushes, cork stamps) can be fine substitutes and still preserving the therapeutic affordances of the medium. These media-informed administrative choices turn everyday household supplies into reliably therapeutic tools when mapped to the ETC-based mechanisms described earlier.

Adapting materials and delivery to individual needs is central to accessibility. For children, activities should be playful, brief and game-based, with concrete prompts and immediate rewards. Adolescents typically require autonomy and anonymity options so digital drawing tools or private sketchbooks can be effective. With older adults and those living with cognitive impairment, tasks that foreground large shapes, high-contrast colours, and short predictable steps are preferable; sensory materials and reminiscence prompts enhance engagement and may support preserved procedural and episodic memory (Rastogi, Paige Feldwisch, et al., 2022). For individuals with mild mental disability and other neurodivergent issues, a prior discussion of sensory preferences and tolerances will guide material choice whilst providing precise, stepwise instructions and visual examples can reduce anxiety.

The caregivers also must keep track of the progress to detect unusual patterns in behaviours. The notes recording session length, materials used, and any distressing content provides continuity and assists other care workers or clinicians who may later review the person's progress. Brief observation/case notes are usually adequate in this context (Chenoweth & McAuliffe, 2012). If an activity consistently produces unmanageable distress, intrusive memories, or sustained dysregulation, the carer should cease the activity and seek professional assessment. Similarly, when interpersonal conflict arises during collaborative work, the option of a planned pause can help to contain escalation.

In home-based applications, ethical responsibility centres on respecting autonomy, privacy and authorship. Artworks belong to their makers. Caregivers should not photograph, exhibit or distribute work without explicit permission and should always be attentive to the privacy and dignity of the person (Rastogi, Paige Feldwisch, et al., 2022). Colour symbolism, material taboos and different cultural modes of expression must be elicited respectfully rather than assumed.

A set of activities, each chosen for specific affordances, can serve as a core repertoire for caregivers. Simple free-drawing or doodling exercise is often the least demanding entry point. It supports rapid expression and requires minimal instruction or specialist materials. Sensory collage - a tactile assemblage of fabric, paper and found objects - capitalises on kinaesthetic and haptic input to ground attention and provide a non-verbal mode of expression that is accessible to people with limited verbal capacity. It is also highly accessible an ideal low-threshold option for many carers. The manoeuvres, such as selecting, cutting and placing found imagery engage sensory, perceptual and symbolic processes without demanding advanced fine-motor skills. In cases where cognitive load is a concern, using pre-cut elements or offering templates are also options to simplify the multi-step processes so that tasks neither bore nor overwhelm (Rastogi, Paige Feldwisch, et al., 2022). Clay manipulation and playdough activities afford strong proprioceptive feedback and can be particularly useful when the objective is physical release, reduction of tension or the restoration of bodily agency. Guided drawing practice, where a brief verbal visualisation precedes image-making, recruits the DMN and supports the externalisation of inner images for reflection and can be useful for mood exploration and memory activation. Longer, paced interventions such as life-story storyboards or timelines allow autobiographical organisation and identity repair through narrative externalisation, whilst collaborative projects (dyadic or family) facilitate co-regulation, repair of relational ruptures and shared achievement. Taken together, such processes help translate complex feelings into tangible, expressive, and often illuminating forms (Hosu, 2022; Minhaj & Rauf, 2023). The person-in-care, thus not only has opportunities to express themselves but also is able to divert their attention from pervasive negative thoughts, improve their stress-coping mechanisms and strengthen self-confidence (Putri et al., 2025). The engagement with colours and art materials within a supportive and non-judgmental environment is also stated to allow breathing-room and providing a valuable retreat from daily frustrations and stressors (Minhaj & Rauf, 2023).

Within art therapy practice that can be directly adapted to home setting, activities such as drawing and colouring mandalas are often suggested as stress-relieving tools. The mandala can be perceived as a symbol of "the self" in Jungian's archetypes concept. Thus, it can be a symbolic pathway to inner balance and relaxation (Orkibi & Keisari, 2023). In another word, people may be able to re-centre their sense of identity by creating and colouring mandalas. The mechanism is explained by studies, such as works by Curry & Kasser (2005) and Babouchkina & Robbins (2015). They indicate that working with repetitive geometric patterns may encourage a calm, almost meditative focus, which can improve mood and reduce anxiety (Orkibi & Keisari, 2023). However, these exercises' comparative efficacy against other free-drawing activities can vary depending on the individual and context.

CONCLUSION

This chapter has argued that everyday home-delivered creative activities can serve as a pragmatic and evidence-informed adjunct to formal therapeutic provision. Drawing on biopsychosocial frameworks, and supported by contemporary neuro-scientific accounts, the chapter showed why artmaking is not merely recreational but has specific affordances for regulation, expression, habit formation and social connection. By choosing and matching the appropriate art-based activity to the suitable treatment goals, caregivers can create low-risk opportunities that promote emotional relief, reflective meaning-making and relational repair within ordinary domestic routines.

For family caregivers who plan to implement creative exercise into practice, the chapter offers explanation on the basic principles of art-based exercises and how they connected to a more developed discipline of art therapy. It also provides suggestions on simple activities, as well as basic safety procedures before organising them at home and without professional supervision. These measures allow the practice to be integrated into an individual's everyday life in ways that honour autonomy and dignity whilst enabling incremental, practice-dependent benefits.

At the same time, the chapter acknowledges limitations of this method. Home-based exercise is supportive rather than substitutive. It is not a replacement for proper art therapy in situations of severe distress, active self-harm, suicide risk, or complex trauma. Thus, carers and service providers should apply these methods with caution and with well-defined escalation pathways to clinical care where needed. Ethical considerations - such as getting consent, negotiating about ownership of artwork, protecting cultural meanings and privacy - must remain central to practice.

There are two priorities that should be considered for future implementation. Firstly, the issue of lacking evidence on the efficacy of deinstitutionalised art-based exercises must be addressed. This may require pragmatic trials, clearer parameters and evaluation of fidelity when interventions are delivered by non-specialists. Secondly, trained professionals can aid this practice by creating and disseminating relevant resources (one-page guides, session templates, escalation flowcharts and brief training modules) and make them available to public. These guide and templates will help easing the entry of new family caregivers and reduce the risk of malpractice. Until such evidence and resources are widely available, the safest and most ethical approach is cautious, intentional use is adopting well-defined activities that map onto known mechanisms, monitor effects, respect cultural and personal meaning, and escalate to professionals whenever responses exceed the carer's competence.

In sum, everyday art practices - when delivered with care, sensitivity and a clear understanding of their mechanisms - offer an accessible, low-cost and humanising means of supporting well-being in home care environments. They extend the reach of therapeutic intent into daily life, strengthening the relational and regulatory scaffolding that so often determines recovery and quality of life.

ACKNOWLEDGEMENTS

This paper is supported by University of Management and Technology Ho Chi Minh City, Ho Chi Minh City, Vietnam.

The author did use AI to review, check and fix sentences thorough the chapter.

REFERENCES

American Art Therapy Association. (n.d.). *What is Art Therapy? Fact Sheet.* Retrieved 3 September 2025, from https://arttherapy.org/what-is-art-therapy/

Brandell, J. R., & George, L. J. (2015). Social Work and Psychodynamic Thought. In *International Encyclopedia of the Social & Behavioral Sciences* (2nd ed., pp. 761–768). Elsevier Inc., DOI: 10.1016/B978-0-08-097086-8.28117-8

Case, C., Dalley, T., & Reddick, D. (2022). The handbook of art therapy. In *The Handbook of Art Therapy* (4th ed.). Taylor and Francis., DOI: 10.4324/9781003197850

Cheng, C., Elamin, M. E., May, H., & Kennedy, M. (2023). Drawing on emotions: The evolving role of art therapy. *Irish Journal of Psychological Medicine, 40*(3), 500–502. DOI: 10.1017/ipm.2021.20 PMID: 33870885

Chenoweth, L., & McAuliffe, D. (2012). *Road to Social Work and Human Service Practice.* Cengage Learning Australia.

Coady, N., & Lehmann, P. (2008). *Theoretical Perspectives for Direct social Work practice: A generalist-eclectic Approach* (2nd ed.). Springer.

Connolly, M., & Harms, L. (2011a). Ecosystems theories. In *Social Work: From Theory to Practice* (pp. 47–72). Cambridge University Press. DOI: 10.1017/CBO9781139192521

Connolly, M., & Harms, L. (2011b). Faulty-engine theories. In *Social Work: From Theory to Practice* (pp. 101–123). Cambridge University Press. DOI: 10.1017/CBO9781139192521

Connolly, M., & Harms, L. (2011c). Onion-peeling theories. In *Social Work: From Theory to Practice* (pp. 73–100). Cambridge University Press. DOI: 10.1017/CBO9781139192521

Connolly, M., & Harms, L. (2011d). Story-Telling Theories. In *Social Work: From Theory to Practice* (pp. 124–144). Cambridge University Press. DOI: 10.1017/CBO9781139192521

Demir, V., Eryürek, S., & Savaş, E. (2024). The effect of mindfulness-based art therapy on psychological symptoms and happiness levels in patients with migraine: A pilot study. *Current Psychology (New Brunswick, N.J.)*, *43*(19), 17664–17672. DOI: 10.1007/s12144-024-05634-0

Duncan, B., & Miller, S. (2001). Using the Client's Theory of Change: Research and practice. *Psychotherapy in Australia*, *8*, 16–23.

Ellermann, A. (1998). Can discourse analysis enable reflective social work practice? *Social Work Education*, *17*(1), 35–44. DOI: 10.1080/02615479811220041

Emilia, C. (2021a). Art therapy with children surviving cancer used to relieve symptoms associated with death, loss and pain. *European Psychiatry : the Journal of the Association of European Psychiatrists*, *64*(S1), S682–S683. DOI: 10.1192/j.eurpsy.2021.1809

Emilia, C. (2021b). Implementing new digital options in education/ occupational/ play/ art therapy as tools for self- knowledge, self-managements, self-esteem. *European Psychiatry : the Journal of the Association of European Psychiatrists*, *64*(S1), S681–S682. DOI: 10.1192/j.eurpsy.2021.1808

Feldwisch, R. P. (2022). History, profession, and ethics of art therapy. In *Foundations of Art Therapy* (pp. 3–30). Elsevier., DOI: 10.1016/B978-0-12-824308-4.00007-7

Gladstone, J., Dumbrill, G., Leslie, B., Koster, A., Young, M., & Ismaila, A. (2014). Understanding worker-parent engagement in child protection casework. *Children and Youth Services Review*, *44*, 56–64. DOI: 10.1016/j.childyouth.2014.06.002

Gronda, H. (2008). Case Management for People Experiencing Homelessness: What Makes It Work? Evidence for Practice. *Parity*, *21*(10). http://www.yp4.org.au/

Harms, L. (2010). A multidimensional approach. In Harms, L. (Ed.), *Understanding human development* (2nd ed., pp. 3–35). Oxford University Press.

Hepworth, D. H., Rooney, R. H., Rooney, G. D., Strom-Gottfried, K., & Larsen, J. (2010). *Direct Social Work Practice: Theory and Skills* (8th ed.). Cengage Learning.

Hohman, M. (2012). *Motivational interviewing in Social work Practice*. The Guilford Press.

Hosu, L.-M. (2022). Art therapy focused on stimulating the emotional and expressive skills of the atypical children. *European Psychiatry : the Journal of the Association of European Psychiatrists*, *65*(S1), S236–S237. DOI: 10.1192/j.eurpsy.2022.612

Hosu, L.-M. (2023). Environmental manipulation and stimulation of atypical children through art therapy. *European Psychiatry : the Journal of the Association of European Psychiatrists, 66*(S1), S820–S821. DOI: 10.1192/j.eurpsy.2023.1738

Korostiy, V., & Hmain, S. (2013). Art Therapy In The Treatment Of Patients With Depressive Disorder. *European Psychiatry : the Journal of the Association of European Psychiatrists, 28*(S1), 1. DOI: 10.1016/S0924-9338(13)77177-3

Kozhyna, H., Korostiy, V., Hmain, S., & Mykhaylov, V. (2017). The use of art therapy in complex treatment on the quality of remission in patients with melancholy in major depressive disorder. *European Psychiatry : the Journal of the Association of European Psychiatrists, 41*(S1), s777–s777. DOI: 10.1016/j.eurpsy.2017.01.1473

Lin, Y., & Yang, F. (2023). Intervention of emotional interaction in college art and design courses for autism patients' emotions. *CNS Spectrums, 28*(S2), S124. DOI: 10.1017/S1092852923005667

McDonald, C. (2006). Challenging social work, the politics of change. In *Challenging social work: The context of practice* (1st ed., pp. 61–75). DOI: 10.1007/978-0-230-50549-0_4

Minhaj, U., & Rauf, K. (2023). The psychology of art therapy: An effective approach for mental disorders. *Pakistan Journal of Psychology, 54*(1), 47–63.

Moore, E. (2009). *Case Management for Community Practice*. Oxford University Press., www.touchingthecorners.com/index.htm

Moore, S. (1992). Case Management and the Integration of Services: How Service Delivery Systems Shape Case Management. *Social Work, 37*(5), 418. DOI: 10.1093/sw/37.5.418

Moxley, D. (1997). Sorting out the purpose of case management. In *Case management by design: Reflections on principles and Practices*. Nelson-Hall.

Nearney, H. (2006). Art therapy: A senior house officer's perspective. *Psychiatric Bulletin, 30*(3), 109–110. DOI: 10.1192/pb.30.3.109

O'Neill Haaga, M., & Schwartz, J. B. (2022). Understanding media: Laying the groundwork for art-making. In Rastogi, M., Paige Feldwisch, R., Pate, M., & Scarce, J. (Eds.), *Foundations of Art Therapy* (pp. 31–80). Elsevier., DOI: 10.1016/B978-0-12-824308-4.00013-2

Orkibi, H., & Keisari, S. (2023). Creative Arts Therapies - Processes and Outcomes for Emotional Well-Being. In Ivcevic, Z., Hoffmann, J. D., & Kaufman, J. C. (Eds.), *The Cambridge Handbook of Creativity and Emotions* (pp. 411–433). Cambridge University Press., DOI: 10.1017/9781009031240.027

Putri, N. R. I. A. T., Cahyaningrum, E. D., Wurdaningsih, T. K., Syangadah, Z., & Mesayu, S. F. (2025). Evaluation of coloring therapy as an anxiety reduction strategy in the older adults in the community area. *BIO Web of Conferences, 152*. DOI: 10.1051/bioconf/202515201032

Rastogi, M., Paige Feldwisch, R., Pate, M., & Scarce, J. (2022). Foundations of Art Therapy: Theory and Applications. In *Foundations of Art Therapy: Theory and Applications*. Academic Press.

Rastogi, M., Strang, C., Vilinsky, I., & Holland, K. (2022). Intersections of neuroscience and art therapy. In *Foundations of Art Therapy* (pp. 123–158). Elsevier., DOI: 10.1016/B978-0-12-824308-4.00014-4

Rothman, J. (1991). A Model of Case Management: Toward Empirically Based Practice. *Social Work, 36*(6), 520–528. DOI: 10.1093/sw/36.6.520 PMID: 1754929

Saleebey, D. (2006). Power in the People. In *The strengths perspective in social work practice* (4th ed., pp. 1–24). Pearson/Allyn & Bacon.

Stevenson, H., & Alzyood, M. (2025). Healing through art: A thematic synthesis within a quasi-systematic review of art's impact on adult mental well-being during the COVID-19 pandemic. *BMC Public Health, 25*(1), 1641. Advance online publication. DOI: 10.1186/s12889-025-22741-0 PMID: 40319249

Tilbury, D. E. F. (1977). *Casework in Context*. Elsevier., DOI: 10.1016/C2013-0-05717-9

Toroghi, L. M. (2015). The Effectiveness of Art Therapy On Housewives General Health, Anxiety and Self-efficacy in Tehran. *European Psychiatry : the Journal of the Association of European Psychiatrists, 30*, 852. Advance online publication. DOI: 10.1016/S0924-9338(15)30665-9

Trevithick, P. (2003). Effective relationship-based practice: A theoretical exploration. *Journal of Social Work Practice, 17*(2), 163–176. DOI: 10.1080/026505302000145699

Viganò, C., Wenk, M., Ferrara, L., Magnotti, R., & Borsani, S. (2019). The "State of The Art" of Art Therapy in Psychiatry: Reflections on International Evidences and Italian Experiences. *Journal of Complementary Medicine & Alternative Healthcare, 10*(5). Advance online publication. DOI: 10.19080/JCMAH.2019.10.555796

Wang, J., Zhang, B., Yahaya, R., & Abdullah, A. (2025). Colors of the mind: A meta-analysis of creative arts therapy as an approach for post-traumatic stress disorder intervention. *BMC Psychology*, *13*(32), 32. Advance online publication. DOI: 10.1186/s40359-025-02361-4 PMID: 39799380

Weaver, D. (2000). Organizational Technology as Institutionalized Ideology: Case Management Practices in Welfare-to-Work Programs. *Administration in Social Work*, *24*(1), 1–19. DOI: 10.1300/J147v24n01_01

Westra, H. A., & Aviram, A. (2013). Core skills in motivational interviewing. *Psychotherapy (Chicago, Ill.)*, *50*(3), 273–278. DOI: 10.1037/a0032409 PMID: 24000834

Chapter 10
Safe and Effective Application of Aromatherapy in Home Care

Tuong-Minh Ly-Le
https://orcid.org/0000-0001-8203-7357
School of Media and Applied Arts, University of Management and Technology Ho Chi Minh City, Vietnam

ABSTRACT

The shift toward home-based care has increased demand for efficient and safe non-pharmacological interventions. Aromatherapy, a well-known integrative therapy, offers symptom relief through essential oils but is often applied without evidence-based guidance. This chapter presents a review of 49 randomized controlled trials (2021–2025) to examine the operational effectiveness of aromatherapy in home or caregiver-assisted settings. Going beyond mere oil selection, the chapter explores usage variables of relevance – route of delivery, dosage, frequency, and duration – and refers to typical mistakes and contraindications. The objective is to offer care-givers accurate, evidence-based recommendations for symptom-specific applications, including anxiety, pain, sleep disturbance, and fatigue. Blending clinical evidence with the realities of day-to-day caregiving, this chapter presents a practical guide to informing safe and effective aromatherapy use in home care practice.

DOI: 10.4018/979-8-3373-4094-4.ch010

1. INTRODUCTION

The global health care system is undergoing profound transformations, which are characterized by aging populations, the increasing prevalence of chronic illnesses, and a gradual shift toward deinstitutionalized models of care. As health systems around the world face the increasing pressure on institutional resources, an equal demand is rising for high-quality, patient-centered care to be provided at home, where the patient has utmost comfort and familiarity. This shift has considerably increased the emphasis on the support that family members and informal caregivers provide in managing physical and emotional symptoms across an array of health conditions (World Health Organization, 2022).

In this evolving paradigm, aromatherapy has emerged as one of the most common and accessible integrative therapies in home care environments. Aromatherapy is the therapeutic use of plant-derived essential oils by inhalation, topical application, or, in certain cases, oral consumption, to enhance health and well-being (National Association for Holistic Aromatherapy, n.d.).

Historical precedent exists for the use of essential oils. Ancient Egyptian, traditional Chinese, and Ayurvedic systems all reference aromatic healing thousands of years ago. Nevertheless, their resurgence in contemporary care settings involving family caregivers, hospice workers, and community health aides reflect larger structural changes within integrative and complementary medicine. The big draw for aromatherapy is that it is cheap, non-invasive, and flexible across cultures; this is attractive for practitioners in settings from the third world to the first (Kang et al., 2023).

The purpose of aromatherapy is not to substitute conventional medication within chronic illness, mental health treatment, and palliative care but to work alongside it and be equally effective in bringing comfort, emotional well-being, and quality life. According to Herz (2009), the sense of smell is uniquely linked with brain regions involved in memory, emotion, and autonomic regulation. This is the reason aromatherapy can manage challenging symptoms such as emotional distress, grief, or existential suffering which appear to be difficult to quantify or pharmacologically manage.

For these reasons, aromatherapy has been recommended by many clinicians as an adjunctive technique in integrative care models. Yet, professional standards are not always translated into readily accessible information for caregivers. Despite its extensive use and apparent benefits, aromatherapy in homecare remains largely anecdotal, with users very frequently relying on websites, networks, or personal experience for patterns of use. In practice, the use of essential oils is always rather likely to be concerned with questions like, "What oil do you use for pain?" or "What scent do you use for sleep?" Such use, although well-intended, has the track record of ignoring some of the finer operational details that are essential to therapeutic outcomes-such as methods of application, doses, duration, and frequency. Furthermore, inconsistent information, mislabelling of products, and the absence of caregiver training frequently led to inappropriate use, diminishing potential benefits and introducing risks of skin irritation, respiratory issues, or ineffective symptom control (Haramshahi et al., 2024; Başdaş et al., 2024).

Instead of merely listing essential oils for specific conditions, this chapter explores the operational variables that mediate efficacy in caregiver-applied aromatherapy. It shifts the focus from "what oil should be used" to "how aromatherapy should be properly applied." The chapter seeks to provide guidance to caregivers so that they no longer rely on trial and error, but instead on balanced evidence-based practice through high-quality research synthesis. This is in line with other efforts in health care to nurture dignity, autonomy, and patient-centered care throughout the caregiving process.

The review is guided by the following research questions:

- RQ1: What are the most common and effective aromatherapy delivery methods (e.g., inhalation, massage, oral use) used for specific symptoms in home care contexts?
- RQ2: What effect does dosage, frequency, and duration of aromatherapy have on therapeutic effects?
- RQ3: What types of mistakes, adverse effects, or contraindications are documented in caregiver-relevant aromatherapy applications?

2. CONCEPTUAL FRAMEWORK

Aromatherapy is an integrative therapy using plant-based essential oils to improve physical, mental, and spiritual well-being. People are increasingly using aromatherapy in hospital and home settings. However, the mechanisms that determine its effectiveness are usually not known or are oversimplified. This research explores the foundations upon which safe and effective aromatherapy delivery can occur within home care in three dimensions: (1) delivery methods, (2) dosage, frequency and duration, and (3) common mistakes and contraindications.

2.1. Therapeutic Mechanisms of Aromatherapy

The therapeutic action of essential oils is regulated through two main physiological pathways: olfactory stimulation and percutaneous absorption.

The olfactory pathway refers to when inhaled essential oil molecules stimulate olfactory receptors in the nasal cavity, transmit signals to the limbic system, including amygdala and hippocampus (Herz, 2009). This reaction initiates emotional and memory responses (Ahn et al., 2024; Pourshaikhian et al., 2024) as well as autonomic control through which activation of emotions occurs regarding anxiety, stress, and mood disorders (Lu et al., 2023; Dehghan et al., 2022).

In the percutaneous pathway, the basic oils are administered topically and penetrate via the dermis and enter systemic circulation via the capillaries within approximately 20-40 minutes (Riedler et al., 2023). The delivery route is suited for local analgesic, anti-inflammatory, or antispasmodic action, as desired for musculoskeletal pain, joint stiffness, or fatigue (Lu et al., 2023). The use of massage and deep pressure massage allows absorption through the skin as well as some therapeutic benefit from the stimulation and vasodilatory action.

2.2. Delivery Methods and Symptom Matching

Understanding the routes of application is critical for caregivers aiming to use aromatherapy effectively at home. The three main methods used in reviewed RCTs are: (1) inhalation (via diffusers, cotton balls, or personal inhalers), (2) topical application (via massage, compresses, or baths), and (3) oral use (rare and typically under clinical supervision)

Each route influences not only the speed and intensity of the therapeutic response but also determines which symptoms are best addressed. Inhalation is particularly suited for anxiety, nausea, and respiratory symptoms, whereas topical application is more effective for localized pain and musculoskeletal tension (Ahn et al., 2024; Tohidi et al., 2022). And as Herz (2009) notes, contextual factors, including the patient's psychological state, setting, and previous experiences with scent, also modulate effectiveness. This emphasizes the need for individualized intervention planning within caregiving contexts.

2.3. Dosage, Frequency, and Duration as Operational Determinants

Operational parameters of frequency, duration, and dosage represent a second pillar of the conceptual framework. Since essential oils are not standardized like pharmaceuticals, safe and effective application demands employing generalizable but flexible dosing concepts.

Dosage refers to the quantity or proportion of drops used with each application. Topical use is safe in adults with a 2–5% dilution (Başdaş et al., 2024).

Frequency refers to how often the oil is applied. Daily use may be extended for chronic issues, while acute or situational needs may justify use of 1 day or up to 2 days per week. Again, acuity of the situation should be considered.

Duration measures how long aromatherapy applications will last (for example, 5 days versus 8 weeks). Most RCTs report effective symptom management 2-4 weeks in with steady use (Aslan & Altın, 2022).

Together, these variables are the "posology" model in pharmacology, where dosage, interval, and course duration determine therapeutic impact. Applied to aromatherapy, they provide tangible anchors that caregivers could use to maintain their own application.

2.4. Caregiver as Therapeutic Agent

In the home context, the caregiver is said to be an alternative a co-therapist, and their role is instrumental to the successful outcome of an aromatherapy program. The conceptual framework draws from Bandura's self-efficacy theory, which states that a person's belief in his or her ability to carry out actions will determine behavior and outcomes (Bandura, 1997). This includes the caregivers themselves, that is, they that would have good access to protocols, safety training, and positive reinforcement are more likely to apply aromatherapy product use in a consistent and effective manner.

In trials where caregivers received structured guidance, such as checklists or dosing charts, outcomes were superior compared to studies where aromatherapy was introduced without structured support (Yildirim et al., 2025; Lu et al., 2023). This underscores the need for a user-centered design in protocol development, ensuring that interventions are not only clinically sound but also practically executable in diverse caregiving environments.

This conceptual framework reconceptualizes aromatherapy as a structured, operationally guided, and evidence-aligned modality within home care. It emphasizes the physiological mechanisms of action, the need for delivery-method alignment with symptoms, the importance of dosing precision, and the central role of caregivers.

3. METHODOLOGY

This chapter is a systematic narrative review looking through randomized controlled trials (RCTs) to observe the use of aromatherapy within home-based or caregiver-assisted contexts. The aim was to synthesize existing evidence, not only regarding the efficacy of aromatherapy but more importantly, to operationalize best practices – so that they can be directly applicable to informal caregivers and professional caregivers alike – including delivery methods, dosage, frequency, duration, and safety considerations.

Unlike meta-analysis, which relies on statistical aggregation, this review focuses on practical implementation insight. It provides an overview of real-world applications of aromatherapy intended for use by caregivers, especially during this post-pandemic period of increased emphasis on home care as a central tenet of global healthcare strategies.

To ensure the results would be useful and actionable for home-based care, strict inclusion and exclusion criteria were applied.

Inclusion criteria:

- Study type: Randomized controlled trials (RCTs)
- Language: English
- Publication period: January 1, 2021 – March 30, 2025
- Intervention: Aromatherapy (use of essential oils) as a primary treatment, using inhalation, topical application (massage or compress), or oral administration

Exclusion criteria:

- Aromatherapy was used only as one of several components in a multimodal intervention (e.g., aromatherapy + acupuncture + yoga)
- Studies that took place exclusively in highly medicalized settings (e.g., surgical ICUs, emergency rooms) with no home care relevance
- Non-randomized trials, observational studies, or qualitative research

The search strategy employed combinations of the following terms: ("aromatherapy" OR "essential oil") AND ("home care" OR "caregiver" OR "self-care" OR "family care") AND ("randomized controlled trial" OR "RCT") AND ("anxiety" OR "pain" OR "sleep" OR "fatigue" OR "mood" OR "nausea").

All results were sorted by relevance, using the database's default ranking algorithm. The first 49 studies that met all inclusion criteria and that appeared in this sorted list were selected for inclusion in the review. This approach was taken to put studies most relevant to practical, home-based applications of aromatherapy first. Duplicate studies were removed manually. Backward citation tracking or snowball sampling was not used beyond this top 49 to allow for consistency and feasibility.

Given the heterogeneity of interventions, populations, and outcome measures, a narrative synthesis method was used. Key themes were grouped according to:

- Delivery method: Most commonly used applications and their clinical targets
- Operational factors: Dosage, frequency, and intervention length
- Symptom categories: Anxiety, sleep, pain, fatigue, mood disturbance, and nausea
- Safety and contraindications: Common mistakes, risk populations, and recommendations for safe use

Rather than pooling statistical effect sizes, findings were presented using descriptive frequencies, pattern recognition, and illustrative comparisons across studies. Tables were developed to highlight recommended practices for caregivers and summarize symptom–method–oil pairings.

This research was based entirely on publicly available published studies. As such, it involved no direct participation of human subjects and did not require ethics committee approval.

4. RESULTS

This chapter synthesizes the findings of 49 randomized controlled trials (RCTs) published between 2021 and 2025 that studied the effects of aromatherapy interventions in home settings or with caregiver assistance. It presents a general profile of the studies under consideration with respect to target populations, therapeutic goals, types of essential oils used, modes of application, duration of interventions, and clinical outcomes.

The 49 included studies involved a total of approximately 5,230 participants, with sample sizes ranging from 30 to 200. Most of the studies were conducted within hospital-affiliated settings (e.g., outpatient clinics, rehabilitation units), but the interventions themselves were designed to be used in home or home-like settings (e.g., massage by a caregiver, self-inhalation by a patient, or evening diffuser use). Studies recruited participants across the lifespan, from neonates to older adults, though the majority recruited women (72%), particularly postmenopausal women, surgical patients, and those with chronic diseases.

In a geographical context, the studies put places across a variety of countries, including South Korea, Turkey, Iran, and Taiwan, along with several European countries, which directly impacts regionally contextualized evidence through several multicenter studies. This diversity helped the review in recognizing cultural differences in aromatherapy use, mainly in terms of dosing and oil selection.

The clinical objectives of the studies were highly diverse but converged on the following core symptom domains:

- Anxiety and stress were studied in 28 trials with subjects ranging from surgical patients (e.g., cesarean section, cholecystectomies) to intensive care nurses, hemodialysis patients, and cancer patients or those with menopausal symptoms.
- Pain management was studied in 24 trials, which largely included pain during labor, migraine, postoperative pain, procedural pain, and joint pain (e.g., in arthritis).
- Sleep quality and fatigue features were studied in 22 trials mostly involving chemotherapy patients, menopausal women, and those with chronic fatigue syndrome or rheumatoid arthritis;
- Other 11 studies looked at mood and depression, targeting mostly postpartum women, stroke patients, and patients with neuropsychiatric comorbidities;
- Other functional outcomes include the improvement of memory in the elderly or electroconvulsive therapy patients, quality of life for terminal patients, and sexual function among postmenopausal women.

The interventions utilized a variety of different delivery methods:

- Inhalation (33 studies): Essential oils were inhaled by the participants using cotton balls, diffusers, aroma necklaces, or masks. Duration was 5–60 minutes and frequency was once to twice daily.
- Massage (15 studies): Oils were applied via full-body or localized massage (e.g., hand, feet, abdomen), typically diluted to 2–5% in carrier oils like sweet almond.
- Oral ingestion (2 studies): Standardized lavender softgel capsules, 80 mg/day, for 60 days.
- Bath or self-application (4 studies): Oils were applied by patients or caregivers via bathing or compresses, especially in the pediatric or neonatal environment.
- A few studies used multimodal interventions, combining aromatherapy with music therapy, foot massage, or guided breathing to enhance therapeutic effect.

The lengths of intervention of these studies included:

- Short: up to 1 week, usually in association with acute symptom management such as recovery from surgery or a labor type.

- Mid-term: 2 to 4 weeks; mostly targeting fatigue, sleep, and anxiety included 21 studies.
- Long term (>4 weeks): 10 studies target chronic pain, menopausal symptoms, or dermatological healing.
- Frequency from once daily (most are standard in inhalation trials) to 3-5 times per week (typical for massaged or self-administered sessions). Some of the studies designed flexible timing for caregivers that more closely represent real-life home care situations.

The key findings included:

- Improvement in quality of sleep was seen in 19 of the 22 studies, with distinctive lavender and citrus-based inhalation just before bed.
- Pain reduction was significantly present in 20 out of the 24 studies, including those that have migraine, procedural, labor, and arthritis-related pain.
- Levels of anxiety that were reduced by a significant margin were observed in 25 of 28 studies, particularly in perioperative and chronic disease populations.
- Fifteen out of 17 studies indicated increased improvement in terms of fatigue and yielded regular positive effects for cancer, MS, and RA patients.
- No serious adverse events were associated with the use of essential oils; however, some studies were given a precautionary note against such application in neonates or oral ingestion.

Overall, most studies depicted methodological rigor, but there were some issues that emerged:

- Heterogeneity of sample sizes: The majority of trials used small numbers ($n < 60$), limiting generalizability.
- Heterogeneity of outcome measures: While shared symptom targets, tools varied, complicating meta-analysis.
- Lack of sufficient blinding of massage or inhalation research, particularly where the odor was unequivocal.
- Short follow-up periods: Most only reported immediate or short-term effects, with only 8 having post-intervention follow-up over one month post-intervention.

Despite this, the dataset as a whole offers rich operational information, particularly regarding real-world utility, safety, and flexible formats of delivery applicable to caregiver-administered environments.

4.1. Delivery Methods and Symptom Matching

Evidence gathered from all studies giving the delivery methods and oil combinations most effective for each major symptom cluster is presented in Table 1 below.

Table 1. Symptom-Method-Oil Matching Matrix

Symptom	Best delivery method(s)	Effective essential oil(s)	# of supporting RCTs	Effectiveness
Anxiety	Inhalation	Lavender, Citrus aurantium, Damask rose	25+	Rapid, significant reduction
Sleep disturbance	Inhalation, massage	Lavender, Chamomile, Geranium	22	Sustained improvement
Pain (e.g., migraine)	Massage, inhalation	Peppermint, Lavender, Ginger	20+	Moderate to strong relief
Fatigue	Massage, inhalation	Lavender, Marjoram, Melissa officinalis	15	Gradual improvement
Menopausal symptoms	Oral, inhalation	Lavender (oral), Citrus aurantium, Geranium	10	Targeted symptom relief
Cognitive/memory issues	Inhalation	Rosemary, Clove, Orange	6	Mild to moderate benefit
Pediatric distress	Massage, mask inhalation	Lavender (diluted), Chamomile	5	Gentle symptom control

Inhalation is the most widely used and evidence-based method of essential oil administration, especially for symptoms associated with anxiety, sleep disorders, and nausea. Inhalation takes volatile compounds to the olfactory bulb, which is linked to the limbic system, the region of the brain that regulates emotions and autonomic functions (Herz, 2009). Out of the 49 studies, 33 used inhalation via devices like aroma necklaces, diffusers, cotton balls, or masks.

Lavender (Lavandula angustifolia) inhalation was particularly effective in the management of preoperative anxiety as well as improving sleep. For example, Yildirim et al. (2025) demonstrated that nocturnal inhalation of lavender over five days improved the quality of sleep as well as reduced fatigue in hematology patients undergoing chemotherapy. Similarly, Kang et al. (2023) showed that a combination of eucalyptus, lemon, chamomile, and peppermint oils inhaled using a mask considerably improved symptoms of rhinitis and fatigue during COVID-19 isolation. In addition, the use of peppermint-lemon oil mixture through inhalation was shown to have significant improvements in terms of decreasing nausea and increasing

appetite among the pediatric leukemia patients (Şancı et al., 2023), suggesting its use in gastrointestinal disturbances induced by chemotherapy.

The use of massage as a method of topical aromatherapy is strongly advocated in relieving pain, physical fatigue, and muscle relaxation. The importance of this method is that it helps for transdermal absorption of essential oils with the mechanical benefits provided by massage. From the total of 49 studies, 15 utilized massage or direct application, while intervention duration was cited as 10 to 30 min.

In a randomized trial of stroke, Aslan and Altın (2022) found lavender oil foot massage, three times a week over four weeks, to significantly improve fatigue and sleep. Massage and bath with diluted lavender oil had also been found to reduce pain behaviors and stress in neonatal subjects, hence serving as a model for the safe use in pediatrics (Başdaş et al., 2024).

Pain-related applications were extremely efficient under trained caregivers. Lu et al. (2023) revealed that in patients with rheumatoid arthritis, self-administration of hand massage using a compounded essential oil (cedarwood, sweet orange, and marjoram) significantly improved sleep, but had almost no treatment effect on joint pain. Alternatively, in a clinical trial for migraine patients, a significant decrease in pain intensity and a better quality of life were reported after massage with a peppermint-lavender blend (Akyüz et al., 2024). Most importantly, the concentration of the essential oil was of utmost importance: most massage oils were diluted 2%-5% in carrier oils such as almond or jojoba to prevent dermal irritation.

Oral dispensing of essential oils, for reasons of safety concerns and regulatory constraints, is only rarely indicated. Nevertheless, under the direction of an authorized practitioner, it has a favorable chance of alleviating hormonal symptoms, sexual disorders, as well as other mood disorder systems. In the setting of two trials encompassed within the review, oral dosing began during lavender capsules (standardized) (80 mg per day for 60 days).

Haramshahi et al. (2024) conducted a triple-blind RCT investigating oral lavender among postmenopausal women and found the effectiveness of notable sexual function and symptom-related anxiety improvements. No relevant alteration in lipid profile or cortisol level was shown, but menopausal symptoms and subjective mood improvement were remarkable. Likewise, Abbaspoor et al. (2022) showed Citrus aurantium, taken orally, had an encouraging effect on the quality of sleep among postmenopausal women, whose investigation did not include a drug formulation in comparison.

Few studies (n = 5) used combination methods or unorthodox approaches such as aromatherapy bath, inhalation with massage, or aroma mask. The combined methods were promising, particularly in COVID-19 recovery, burn rehabilitation, and postpartum.

4.2. Dosage, Frequency, and Duration

Dosage in aromatherapy varied according to route of administration, type of essential oil, patient's condition, and the symptom targeted. In the reviewed studies, dosage was typically quantified in drops (bath or inhalation), milliliters or percent dilution (massage), or per capsule milligrams (oral).

Two to five drops of essential oil per treatment were applied in most studies. Research (e.g., Yildirim et al., 2025; Nouira et al., 2024) presented that inhalation through cotton ball or aroma necklace always employed 3 drops of lavender could yield significant effects on anxiety and sleep following 15-30 minutes of exposure. The dose was decreased to 1-2 drops in child studies so that the child was not exposed too much (Başdaş et al., 2024).

For massage, essential oils were mixed with carrier oils (almond, coconut) 2–5%. The mix used for studies was 10 drops of essential oil and 10 ml carrier oil (3%), to local regions such as the neck, feet, or belly for 15-30 minutes (Aslan & Altın, 2022). Doses above this were given only under doctor's observation (Akyüz et al., 2024).

Oral ingestion often used standardized doses. The most common dose is 80 mg/day of Lavandula angustifolia softgels, as noted by Haramshahi et al. (2024), with positive results in mood and menopausal signs. The oil preparation was correctly formulated and consumed for 60 consecutive days without serious side effects.

Table 2 provides an overview of the operational characteristics for each delivery method based on the studies reviewed. These represent a starting point only, and titration to the patient based upon age, condition, and strength of the oil remains a necessity.

Table 2. Dosage Ranges by Method and Oil Type

Application method	Essential oil(s)	Dosage range	Delivery details
Inhalation	Lavender, Citrus, Peppermint	2-5 drops/session	Cotton ball, diffuser, mask (10-30 mins)
Massage	Lavender, Geranium, Ginger	2-5% dilution (10-15 drops/30ml)	1-2 ml per session, localized or full-body use
Oral (capsule)	Lavender (LEO)	80 mg/day	Standardized softgel, once daily for 60 days
Bath/Compress	Chamomile, Damask rose	5-10 drops per bath (2-3 L water)	15–20-minute soak

Each type of intervention would lead to a different application frequency. The standard frequency for inhalation was once or twice a day, or at night, or prior to an anxiety-inducing activity (Kang et al., 2023; Mahdood et al., 2022). Daily application of inhalation repeated for 5-7 days in cancer treatment could result in the alleviation of nausea and sleep support (Ahn et al., 2024). Massage therapy interventions were administered 2-5 times per week, while softgel capsules taken orally were administered once daily, with full compliance tracked on checklists and weekly telephone follow-up (Haramshahi et al., 2024). Most studies used a continuous dosing regimen with no missed days to maintain systemic activity.

Overall, daily usage was more common for sleep, anxiety, and hormonal symptoms, and every-other-day or alternate-day usage was acceptable for physical pain and fatigue, for which overstimulation may be countertherapeutic.

Aside from the frequency, the duration of intervention is also significant. It ranged from a single session to eight weeks, depending on the nature of the symptom and the mode of delivery of oil, as presented in Table 3.

Table 3. Intervention Summary by Duration

Duration	Common targets	Typical methods	Examples
1-7 days	Procedural anxiety, nausea	Inhalation	Pre-surgery (Nouira et al., 2024)
2-4 weeks	Sleep, mild fatigue, mood	Inhalation, massage	COVID recovery (Kang et al., 2023)
5-8 weeks	Menopause, chronic pain/ fatigue	Oral, massage	Menopause relief (Haramshahi et al., 2024)

Short interventions (1-7 days) were primarily used for relieving acute symptoms, such as procedural anxiety, labor pain, and postoperative discomfort. On the other hand, in a homecare setting, medium-term (2–4 weeks) was the most common intervention window, targeting fatigue, sleep, and mood. Longer durations (5-8 weeks) were routinely used in relation to other chronic or systemic issues such as menopausal symptoms, rheumatoid arthritis, or chemotherapy fatigue.

Longer durations were needed for chronic symptoms, while acute or episodic symptoms could be helped with short-term administrations that required immediate onset of delivery such as inhalation.

Safety concerns and dosing mistakes are another factor to take into consideration. Caregivers should be provided with simple-to-follow, visual charts of dosages and checklists to monitor frequency and symptom shift. Several studies (e.g., Başdaş et al., 2024; Lu et al., 2023) incorporated caregiver diaries or biweekly contact for monitoring compliance and detecting early signs of adverse effects. Although there were no severe side effects in most studies, but dosing and frequency mistakes could lead to irritation, allergic response, or desensitization.

4.3. Common Mistakes and Contraindications

Table 4 described the major categories of misuse of aromatherapy, as reviewed from the 49 studies.

Table 4. Common Aromatherapy Mistakes and Preventions

Mistake	Description	Potential consequences	Recommended solution
Overconcentration in topical use	Using oils undiluted or above 5% dilution	Skin irritation, burns, allergic reactions	Always dilute to 2–5% in carrier oil (almond, jojoba, etc.)
Excessive frequency (e.g., >3x/day)	Using inhalation or massage too often	Headaches, reduced efficacy, respiratory symptoms	Limit to 1–2x/day; ensure rest periods
Wrong method for symptom	E.g., using massage for anxiety or inhalation for joint pain	Reduced effectiveness	Match method to symptom: inhalation for mood; massage for pain
Use in infants or high-risk adults	Peppermint/eucalyptus used in children <2 or elderly with respiratory disease	Bronchospasm, aspiration risk	Avoid strong oils in vulnerable groups; consult provider
Improper storage	Oils stored in plastic or exposed to light and air	Loss of potency, chemical degradation	Use dark glass bottles; store in cool, dry places
Oral ingestion without supervision	Taking oils internally with no medical oversight	GI distress, liver burden, drug interactions	Only use oral forms if standardized and prescribed

The most common error is the application of undiluted essential oils in topical uses, causing skin irritation or sensitization. Various studies (e.g., Başdaş et al., 2024; Akyüz et al., 2024) reported adverse effects when caregivers used higher dilution concentrations (generally 2-5%) for massage or compresses. Moreover, frequent inhalation or massage may lead to desensitization, reduced efficacy, or increased respiratory irritation. Kang et al. (2023) described that patients who were treated with continuous inhalation of different oils complained of headaches or dizziness, especially in unventilated rooms.

The improper delivery mechanism for a particular symptom also reduces efficacy. For instance, the use of topical massage for acute anxiety has less benefit than inhalation (Nouira et al., 2024). Alternatively, giving intense oils like peppermint or eucalyptus to children below the age of two may result in respiratory distress (Başdaş et al., 2024). Likewise, the oral consumption of essential oils without clinical supervision is dangerous in patients with gastrointestinal or hepatic pathologies (Haramshahi et al., 2024).

Regarding the storage of essential oils, contact with light, heat, and air can diminish oil quality and strength. Researchers recommended caregivers use dark glass bottles, store opened oils in refrigerators and not use plastic containers to reduce chemical leaching (Lu et al., 2023).

Not only misuse, caregivers should also pay attention to contraindication (i.e., who should avoid aromatherapy). Aromatherapy is safe when given in proper doses, but there are patient populations for whom caution is necessary.

Another consideration is quality control. Not all essential oils are created equal. Some studies used pharmaceutical-grade or ISO-standardized oils, while others utilized either products of pharmacy shops or from local dealers without any chemical analysis. This discrepancy may introduce variability in the results, particularly in home settings where it is difficult to establish quality. It could be implied that, when possible, caregivers should be instructed to use oils approved by regulatory bodies or recommended by clinical research to ensure reproducibility and safety.

5. DISCUSSION

The growing shift toward decentralized, home-based health care has prompted increased interest in integrative therapies such as aromatherapy. This chapter has strived to narrow the gap between science and practice at home by systematically examining 49 RCTs from 2021 to 2025. To remind, the discussion examines three research questions: (1) What are the most common and effective aromatherapy delivery methods used for specific symptoms in home care contexts? (2) What effect do dosage, frequency, and duration have on therapeutic outcomes? (3) What types of mistakes, adverse effects, or contraindications are commonly documented in caregiver-relevant aromatherapy applications?

To answer the first research question, the review confirms that certain routes of administration are more likely to be effective for certain symptom categories. Inhalation is best for psychological symptoms including anxiety, emotional distress, and insomnia; and topical massage works best for physical pain and fatigue.

In response to RQ2, the review presents that one of the most consistent findings across studies is that delivery method significantly determines the therapeutic outcomes of essential oils. The operational patterns confirm the hypothesis that aromatherapy, properly dosed and timed, can be a very significant form of non-pharmacological support for symptom management in home care.

To address RQ3, the review revealed recurring issues that compromised the safety and efficacy of aromatherapy at home. The most common mistakes include excessive concentration of essential oils, particularly in topical applications, inappropriate frequency of application, and the wrong method for the symptom. Contraindications were indicated by almost all studies and, in particular, those to do with infants, pregnant women, and individuals who suffer from respiratory and seizure disorders.

5.1. Reframing Aromatherapy as Operational Care

One of the most salient insights from this review is the importance of reframing aromatherapy from a symptom-driven, oil-centered model to an operationally informed practice. The dominant question in mainstream usage – "What oil is good for X?" – often lacks context regarding how the oil is delivered, in what dose, and for how long. This review reaffirms that route of delivery, dose, frequency, and duration are as critical as oil selection in determining therapeutic outcomes.

For instance, inhalation of Citrus aurantium or lavender reduced anxiety levels in 25 out of the 29 studies examined to a considerable degree when applied for 15-30 minutes via diffuser or cotton ball, once or twice a day (Nouira et al., 2024; Kang et al., 2023). Conversely, when misapplied through topical routes for rapid mood support, the same oils had limited efficacy. This highlights the need for a method-symptom alignment model, whereby each delivery strategy is matched to a symptom class.

5.2. Establishing Therapeutic Protocols for Home Use

Unlike many traditional medicine reviews that focus primarily on efficacy outcomes, this study contributes by specifying operational ranges that caregivers can follow. Dosage tables, frequency patterns, and intervention duration create a foundation for standardized home-based protocols.

The following recommendations could therefore be made from this review for safe and effective aromatherapy at home:

- Match delivery method to symptom: Use inhalation for mood-related issues; massage for pain or fatigue-related conditions.
- Standardize your practice: Use measuring tools and dilution calculators when preparing oils.
- Keeping a response log: Log daily symptoms and improvements to assess effectiveness and modify application.
- Start low and go slow: Begin with small amounts and increase only when necessary and safe to do so.
- Educate: Refer to guides based on clinical evidence rather than marketing hype.

These simple, scalable practices can enhance care quality and protect both caregivers and recipients from harm.

5.3. The Central Role of Caregiver Competence

Aromatherapy's value in home care is magnified when caregivers are adequately informed and prepared. The most successful studies included some form of caregiver training, whether via written guidelines, digital checklists, or supervised sessions. For example, in trials such as Başdaş et al.'s (2024), in which lavender massage was applied to newborns, caregivers were provided with specific instruction on dilution and precautions, resulting in improved effect and fewer adverse reactions.

On the other hand, studies that did not train the caregivers were more variable in outcomes and underutilization of oils provided (Yildirim et al., 2025), pointing to the translation to practice for the caregiver-focused side that this chapter aims to build.

The following checklist is to help caregivers put theory into practice and assess their readiness and best practices:

- Have I identified the target symptom (e.g., anxiety, pain, sleep)?
- Is the delivery method appropriate for that symptom?
- Is the oil properly diluted (2–5% for massage)?
- Have I checked for oil safety (age, health) concerning the recipient?
- Am I working with a reputable product from a reputable company?
- Have I established the right frequency (for instance, once each day for approximately 4 weeks?
- Am I observing and documenting changes in the person's response?
- Am I aware of when to discontinue or change treatment due to side effects?

These checklist questions promote both autonomy and accountability, aligning caregiver actions with safety and outcome tracking.

5.4. Cultural Adaptability and Global Insights

The studies included more than a dozen countries: from Turkey and Iran up to South Korea and the U.S., with totally different cultures and access models. Some cultures used combined oils, e.g., lavender-chamomile or peppermint-lemon, while others adhered solely to single-oil use based on traditional practices (Kang et al., 2023; Akyüz et al., 2024). This review fully embraces this variation as an opportunity for local modification instead of considering it a confounding factor.

However, this also introduces challenges in standardizing recommendations. Essential oils come in varying strengths and purities from one marketplace to another, and local culture does not necessarily follow evidence-based levels. The solution is to provide safe adaptation guidelines – such as the dosage ranges and methods of delivery listed in this chapter – instead of prescriptive recipes that do not fit all.

6. CONCLUSIONS

This chapter contributes to the scholarship of aromatherapy as it is among the few to conduct a systematic synthesis of operational variables (method, dose, frequency, duration) rather than simply documenting oil efficacy. It seeks to link up clinical evidence to caregiver practice, providing not just summaries but tool implementation. Besides, it introduces a caregiver-centered perspective to the conversation, a perspective rarely foregrounded in integrative health research. By focusing on operational details, this work expands both academic understanding and caregiver capacity. As more families take on health support roles in the home, aromatherapy – when evidence-based and used appropriately – can be a quiet yet powerful agent of comfort, care, and connection.

Nonetheless, this review's approach comes with limitations. Selecting only the top 49 relevant RCTs (rather than an exhaustive sample) introduces selection bias. Additionally, generalizability of the findings, even though based on a robust and internationally representative sample, is constrained by several factors. First, around 40% of studies were conducted with less than 60 participants, leading to lower statistical power. While statistically significant effects are generally found, these must be confirmed in larger multisite trials to determine clinical confidence. Secondly, varying instruments were employed for evaluation, even though the studies were often targeted at similar symptoms e.g., State-Trait Anxiety Inventory (STAI), Visual Analog Scale (VAS), Pittsburgh Sleep Quality Index (PSQI), etc. This heterogeneity weakens cross-study comparisons and complicates meta-analyses. Moreover, most follow-ups lasted less than four weeks, suitable for an acute symptom-focused design (i.e., anxiety, labor pain), but limiting information about efficacy and sustainability in the long run--particularly in the context of chronic settings. Last but not least, only a few studies reported essential oil sources or provided gas chromatography/mass spectrometry (GC/MS) results. In absence of standardization by chemical profiling, reproducibility is compromised.

To build upon the present findings, future studies of aromatherapy should include standardized protocols with consistent dosing and delivery and valid outcomes. Studies would require caregiver involvement to assess how well actual home caregivers can replicate trial protocols. Longer-term follow-ups should be conducted to be able to evaluate outcomes at 3-6 months, where effect durability could be quantified.

In conclusion, this chapter offers a detailed operational synthesis of aromatherapy RCTs, from clinical evidence to caregiver practice. It establishes that essential oil therapy – particularly when used via appropriate delivery methods and dosed within recommended limits – can effectively manage common symptoms such as anxiety, pain, fatigue, and sleep disturbances in the home setting. The path forward is not just generating more evidence, but translating evidence into tangible tools, protocols, and caregiver training. Aromatherapy is not a magic bullet, but as employed with commitment, it is a gentle, accessible friend in the hands of competent caregivers.

ACKNOWLEDGEMENT

The authors would like to thank the University of Management and Technology Ho Chi Minh City, Ho Chi Minh City, Vietnam for their continued support.

REFERENCES

Ahn, J. H., Kim, M., & Kim, R. W. (2024). Effects of aromatherapy on nausea and vomiting in patients with cancer: A systematic review and meta-analysis of randomized controlled trials. *Complementary Therapies in Clinical Practice*, *55*, 101838. DOI: 10.1016/j.ctcp.2024.101838 PMID: 38330531

Akyüz, H. Ö., Şenturan, L., & Sabuncu, N. (2024). The effect of aromatherapy massage on the pain severity and quality of life in acute migraine attacks: A randomized controlled trial. *Florence Nightingale Journal of Nursing*, *32*(2), 159–167. DOI: 10.5152/FNJN.2024.23235 PMID: 39552146

Aslan, K. S. Ü., & Altın, S. (2022). Aromatherapy and foot massage on happiness, sleep quality, and fatigue levels in patients with stroke: A randomized controlled trial. *European Journal of Integrative Medicine*, *54*, 102164. DOI: 10.1016/j.eujim.2022.102164

Bandura, A. (1997). Self-efficacy: The exercise of control. *The Freeman*.

Başdaş, Ö., Özbey, H., Oğul, G., & Güneş, T. (2024). Effects of aromatherapy on pain, stress, and behaviors of newborns: A randomized controlled trial. *Alternative Therapies in Health and Medicine*, *30*(12), 43–47. PMID: 39480678

Dehghan, N., Forouzi, M. A., Etminan, A., Roy, C., & Dehghan, M. (2022). The effects of lavender, rosemary and orange essential oils on memory problems and medication adherence among patients undergoing hemodialysis: A parallel randomized controlled trial. *Explore (New York, N.Y.)*, *18*(5), 559–566. DOI: 10.1016/j.explore.2021.10.004 PMID: 34736874

Haramshahi, M., Babaie, S., Shahnazi, M., Kafil, B., Farshbaf-Khalili, A., & Naghdi, M. (2024). The efficacy of oral Lavandula angustifolia Mill. essential oil on menopausal symptoms, serum lipid profile, and cortisol concentration in postmenopausal women: A triple-blind, randomized, controlled trial. *Complementary Therapies in Medicine*, *82*, 103050. DOI: 10.1016/j.ctim.2024.103050 PMID: 38754638

Herz, R. S. (2009). Aromatherapy facts and fictions: A scientific analysis of olfactory effects on mood, physiology and behavior. *The International Journal of Neuroscience*, *119*(2), 263–290. DOI: 10.1080/00207450802333953 PMID: 19125379

Kang, H. Y., Ahn, H. Y., Kang, M. J., & Hur, M. H. (2023). Effects of aromatherapy on sore throat, nasal symptoms and sleep quality in adults infected with COVID-19: A randomized controlled trial. *Integrative Medicine Research*, *12*(4), 101001. DOI: 10.1016/j.imr.2023.101001 PMID: 38024288

Lu, P.-Y., Wu, H.-Y., Chen, L.-H., Liu, C.-Y., & Chiou, A.-F. (2023). The effects of self-aromatherapy massage on pain and sleep quality in patients with rheumatoid arthritis: A randomized controlled trial. *Pain Management Nursing*, *24*(2), e52–e60. DOI: 10.1016/j.pmn.2023.02.009 PMID: 36990808

Mahdood, B., Imani, B., & Khazaei, S. (2022). Effects of inhalation aromatherapy with Rosa damascena (Damask rose) on the state anxiety and sleep quality of operating room personnel during the COVID-19 pandemic: A randomized controlled trial. *Journal of Perianesthesia Nursing*, *37*(4), 493–500. DOI: 10.1016/j.jopan.2021.09.011 PMID: 35256247

National Association for Holistic Aromatherapy. (n.d.). *What is aromatherapy?* https://naha.org/explore-aromatherapy/about-aromatherapy/what-is-aromatherapy/

Nouira, M., Souayeh, N., Kanzari, S. A., Rouis, H., Lika, A., Mbarki, C., Rahali, F. Z., & Bettaieb, H. (2024). Aromatherapy using lavender oil effectiveness on pain and anxiety after C-section: A randomized controlled trial. *Journal of Epidemiology and Global Health*, *14*(4), 1536–1544. DOI: 10.1007/s44197-024-00305-6 PMID: 39400653

Pourshaikhian, M., Moghadamnia, M. T., Kazemnezhad Leyli, E., & Shafiei Kisomi, Z. (2024). Effects of aromatherapy with Matricaria chamomile essential oil on anxiety and hemodynamic indices in patients with acute coronary syndrome, 2021: A randomized controlled trial. *BMC Complementary Medicine and Therapies*, *24*(1), 17. DOI: 10.1186/s12906-023-04326-9 PMID: 38172912

Riedler, K., Hecker, A., Bauer, B., Tax, C., Gmainer, D. G., Pignet, A.-L., Kamolz, L.-P., & Lumenta, D. B. (2023). The efficacy of regeneration oil and almond oil on split-thickness skin graft donor sites: A single-blinded randomized controlled trial. *Clinics and Practice*, *13*(3), 648–655. DOI: 10.3390/clinpract13030059 PMID: 37366928

Şancı, Y., Yıldız, S., Ayçiçek, A., & Möhür, N. (2023). Effect of peppermint-lemon aromatherapy on nausea-vomiting and quality of life in pediatric patients with leukemia: A randomized controlled trial. *Journal of Pediatric Nursing*, *72*, e217–e227. DOI: 10.1016/j.pedn.2023.07.001 PMID: 37453895

Tohidi, S., Kordvarkaneh, Z., Shayan, A., Oshvandi, K., Abbasi, M., Moradkhani, S., & Ahmadinia, H. (2022). Comparison of aromatherapy with lavender and damask rose essential oils on nausea rate in patients undergoing chemotherapy: A randomised control trial. *Australian Journal of Herbal and Naturopathic Medicine*, *34*(2), 60–66. DOI: 10.33235/ajhnm.34.2.60-66

World Health Organization. (2022). *Global report on health equity for persons with disabilities*. https://www.who.int/publications/i/item/9789240063600

Yildirim, D., Ozdogan, M. H., Erdal, S., Selcuk, S., Guneri, A., Simsek, E. B., Can, T. B., Gunduz, H., & Kuni, A. (2025). The efficacy of lavender oil on fatigue and sleep quality in patients with hematological malignancy receiving chemotherapy: A single-blind randomized controlled trial. *Supportive Care in Cancer*, *33*(2), 1–10. DOI: 10.1007/s00520-024-09143-5 PMID: 39775962

Chapter 11

An Inexpensive Internet of Thing Sleep Monitoring System

Sabyasachi Pramanik
https://orcid.org/0000-0002-9431-8751
Haldia Institute of Technology, India

Soma Bag
Asadtala Nivedita Kanya Vidyamath, India

Ahmed J. Obaid
https://orcid.org/0000-0003-0376-5546
Kufa University, Iraq

Atanu Roy
https://orcid.org/0000-0001-5269-9122
School of Maritime Studies, The Neotia University, India

Pranati Rakshit
https://orcid.org/0000-0001-5037-1326
JIS College of Engineering, India

ABSTRACT

By detecting issues, refining sleep patterns, and assessing the success of remedies, sleep monitoring provides substantial advantages for comprehending and enhancing an individual's sleep experience. This begs the questions of what makes for peaceful sleep and what influences the typical individual when they sleep. The system provided in this study employs sensors that measure and detect temperature, humidity, light level, air quality, and room noise in order to cover a broad range of parameters that

DOI: 10.4018/979-8-3373-4094-4.ch011

impact the quality of sleep and to capture both the important data and the distracting aspects that may emerge during sleep. Additionally, the subject's movements and pulse will be observed. The sleeping person is video and audio recorded in order to confirm any potential connections between the measured data and sleep quality. This allows the data collected by the sensors at a certain instant in time to be used to assess the sleeping person's condition. The accumulation of data must be stored for an extended period of time in order to assess how sleep quality has changed.

OVERVIEW

Sleep is a vital component of life and has a big influence on our health and happiness. It is essential for mental clarity, physical well-being, emotional control, and bodily healing and regeneration. Our body heals damaged cells and tissues from physical and emotional stress throughout the day at the cellular level as we sleep. These systems function poorly when we become disturbed or don't get enough sleep, which has an adverse effect on our performance and general health. Additionally, sleep facilitates the consolidation of day's worth of events and knowledge in our brain, improving memory, focus, and cognitive functions. The brain can work at its best while getting enough sleep, setting it up for the best possible mental performance throughout the day. On the other hand, insufficient or low-quality sleep may impair judgment, mental clarity, and general performance on learning and cognitive activities. Studies have shown that sleep deprivation may have a major effect on the various neuro-cognitive phases of processing spatial information while performing a virtual driving activity. While older persons have a drop in working memory and a slowing in decision-making processes, young adults experience a significant reduction in attentiveness and orienting functions. The test participants' actions have a lag in both scenarios. Poor sleep quality might eventually result in mental and physical health problems, such as depression and anxiety disorders. People may even be more susceptible to psychosis under severe circumstances (Pan et al., 2023; U.S. Dept., 2011). Numerous advantages of getting enough sleep include boosting the immune system, mental wellness, and energy levels. On the other hand, exhaustion and disturbed sleep may result in worse cognitive function, a higher chance of accidents, and physical health issues including obesity and high blood pressure. In order to profit from peaceful sleep and prevent the negative effects of exhaustion, it is crucial to pay enough attention to sleep and adopt healthy behaviors after the evaluation of sleep quality (Zhang et al, 2023; Izullah et al, 2022). Affordably priced Internet of Things (IoT) sleep monitoring devices may be introduced to assist people in keeping an eye on the quality of their sleep and identifying any problems that can impact their general health and performance.

This study attempts to provide an accessible, effective, and non-intrusive method of sleep monitoring via the use of IoT (Internet of Things) technology and smart gadgets. The suggested system offers a comprehensive method of sleep tracking by combining the Gear S3 wristwatch, sensors, and Raspberry Pi 4 CPU. This project uses IoT technology, smart devices, and sleep data analysis to deliver a novel and more approachable sleep monitoring method. It is possible to accurately measure a number of sleep-related factors, including heart rate, air quality, temperature, and motor activity. The goal of this system is to assist users better understand their sleeping patterns by providing information on the quality of their sleep. IoT-based sleep monitoring has potential uses in research and medical fields. The information gathered may be used to evaluate health, diagnose sleep problems, and provide individualized sleep-improving therapies. Electroencephalography (EEG), accelerometry, photoplethysmography (PPG), and actigraphy are the primary technologies and techniques used in sleep monitoring (LaGoy et al., 2022; Ibáñez et al., 2018; Moraes & Jermana, 2018). Every technology has unique benefits and drawbacks, but they all provide important insights into the structure and properties of sleep. Combining and integrating these technologies may help provide a more thorough and precise evaluation of sleep. A technique called electroencephalography captures the electrical activity of the brain when it is asleep. The EEG can identify and record brain waves unique to both REM and non-REM sleep phases by applying electrodes to the scalp. This technique offers a thorough evaluation of the quality of sleep, highlighting phases of light, deep, and wakeful sleep. However, EEG may be costly, intrusive when it comes to the placement of electrodes, and needs specific equipment and skilled personnel to analyze the data. Institutions and private labs provide commercial electroencephalography monitoring services like Sanador or Neuroaxis. EEG monitoring may provide more precise data on sleep phases and brain activity in comparison to this experiment (Kwon et al, 2021). However, it is not a good long-term monitoring technique, is cumbersome, stresses the monitored individual, needs costly equipment or specialist study facilities, and is unable to detect other environmental influences. Since accelerometry and actigraphy are often used alone or in tandem to get the same data, they may be combined. Accelerometry is a low-cost, non-invasive technique for monitoring sleep that records body motions as you sleep by using acceleration sensors. Actigraphy is the practice of recording motions and activity levels while you sleep by wearing a gadget on your wrist or torso. These techniques make use of sensors that are compatible with a wide range of gadgets, including phones, fitness trackers, and watches. "Act Trust Actigraphy," "Apple Watch," "Google Pixel Watch," "Oura Ring," "Dreem Headband," and other wearable will be mentioned. Even though the equipment is lightweight and simple to use, proper placement is crucial for capturing bodily motions on camera. Since body motions are used to predict sleep stages, there is a risk of inaccuracy, thus proper calibrations and settings are necessary (Sun et al, 2023). These sensors don't collect accurate or varied enough data to provide a wide enough variety of information on the quality of sleep. For the purpose of monitoring bodily motions using a Samsung Gear S3 Frontier wristwatch, it is worthwhile to include them in the finished project. Using optical sensors, photoplethysmography (PPG) measures the volumetric variations in blood flow that occur as you sleep. This method yields data on blood oxygenation levels, heart rate variability, and heart rate. PPG can be applied through fixed Hub devices like "Sleepme Dock Pro" and "Google Nest Hub," or wearable devices like the smartwatches discussed in the accelerometric method. These devices measure a person's state changes without having to come into contact with them (Muller, 2023). These devices concentrate on facilitating a seamless wake-up experience and generating a daily analysis of specific data while you sleep. The recording quality of photoplethysmography may be affected by ambient light and body movement, which is a drawback. Accuracy of measurements may also be impacted by optical sensors' sensitivity to outside variables such skin reflections and ambient temperature. To accurately assess the parameters, one needs specific understanding in the interpretation of PPG measurements. The experiment using the Gear S3 smartwatch uses this technique, which is an excellent way to identify and record heartbeats. The Raspberry Pi stores the observed person's pulse once the recorded data is sent via Bluetooth. Additionally, there are tools that are often used in the medical setting to monitor various physiological indicators, such glucometers, pulse oximeters, and blood pressure cuffs. While these devices may be used to track biological factors while you sleep, their primary usage is for those with medical conditions. This is how the rest of the paper is structured. The system's hardware description is included in Section II. Section III provides an overview of the software support, and Section IV wraps up the current work and suggests some lines of inquiry for further study on the subjects covered.

Support for the IOT Sleep Monitoring System's Hardware

Many alternatives and techniques for monitoring have been found by specialized literature on sleep quality monitoring devices. But as of yet, there isn't a complete solution that takes into account all the important variables influencing sleep quality, including long-term monitoring, sensor adaptability and modularity, simplicity of use, data security, and cost (Abe et al, 2016). In order to close this gap, as shown in Figure 1, we have selected a central device that is driven by a microprocessor with sufficient processing power and sensor communication capabilities, as well as a wristwatch that can provide internet access and flexible programming options. One affordable choice for creating Internet of Things solutions is the Raspberry Pi 4, a tiny but functional microcontroller. It can operate as a web server and a Bluetooth server at the same time since it has integrated Wi-Fi and Bluetooth 5.0 capability. Raspbian is the operating system that is set up on the microSD card. It is based on Linux and supports a large number of programming languages, including Python3, which is utilized in this project and has a vibrant community as well as a vast variety of pre-existing libraries and modules. The Raspberry board may be controlled via Virtual Network Computing (VNC) with the help of the Raspbian operating system. Through the settings, one may alter the network and starting parameters, boost the processing frequency, and activate serial communication capability. Thonny and Geany, which come pre-installed, are user-friendly integrated development environments that facilitate developing code in the Python and Java Scrip programming languages, respectively. The Raspberry Pi is an ideal module for long-term sleep monitoring because to its low power consumption, low CPU running temperature, and effective data collecting mode. Using an analog-to-digital converter is required since the Raspberry Pi microprocessor lacks the ability to read analog inputs. The PCF8591 module, which has two I2C-compatible channels and four analog channels, is used in this specific instance. There's an 8-bit resolution CAN included in the module. The Gear S3 Frontier watch sports 770MB of RAM and a dual-core Cortex-A53 CPU. It is powered by Samsung's Tizen 5.5 operating system, which has Bluetooth 4.2 capability. It also enables installation of native apps that carry out low-level commands and connection with other devices. It monitors your heartbeat using an embedded sensor called a heart rate sensor, which employs photoplethysmography technology. The clock records, measures, and sends the pulse to the Raspberry Pi over Bluetooth connectivity. Tizen Studio is an integrated development environment that facilitates the development of services and apps that work with the Gear S3 watch. It offers access to an extensive range of features and tools, including the Tizen emulator, which is useful for testing and debugging apps on a virtual device, and the integrated code editor, which supports programming languages including C and JavaScript. A comprehensive software development kit (SDK) with several libraries, modules, and documentation for creating apps is included with Tizen Studio. It offers code models, templates, and application programming interfaces (APIs). The completed application may be programmed on the watch by packaging it into an installable file (TPK package).

Figure 1. Sleep monitoring system's block diagram.

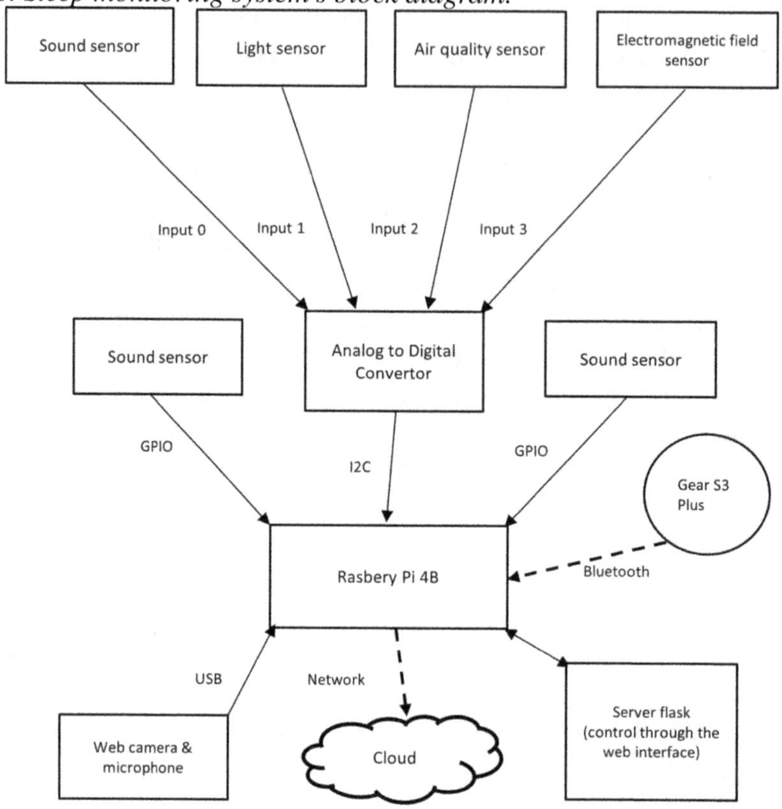

The type MQ-135 air quality sensor measures the amount of dangerous gases in the air, particularly those that may have an impact on human health including nitrogen oxide, ammonia, carbon monoxide, and other hazardous gases. Its working idea is based on how exposure to different gases alters a sensitive layer's electrical resistance on the surface. The surface of the sensor is sensitive to both basic and acidic gasses. The chemical processes that take place when hazardous gases come into contact with the sensitive layer alter the resistance of the sensor. Thus, the resistance of the sensor varies according to the kind and amount of gases present. This is converted into electrical impulses and supplied to the analog/digital converter via input port 0, which processes them and sends a digital signal to the board. The 5528 photoresistor, often referred to as a light-dependent resistor, or LDR, functions by changing its resistance in response to the amount of light that strikes it. The photoresistor's electrical resistance decreases when light strikes its surface because the semiconductor material's electrons are stimulated. The resistance rises as the light level drops. The electrical output signal enters the input port 1 of the analog/digital converter, where it is converted and sent to the board. An extra resistance of 10k ohms was added to it for improved accuracy. The KY-037 sound sensor's operation is based on the employment of a microphone and a pre-amplification circuit. Its purpose is to detect ambient sound levels and translate them into electrical signals. An electret microphone included inside the module is sensitive to pressure changes brought on by surrounding noises. These pressure variations are translated by the microphone into tiny electrical impulses, which the KY-037 module's preamp circuit amplifies. It is necessary to have this amplification in order to detect even lower sound levels. We are able to detect and quantify various degrees of sound intensity because the resultant electrical signal may change in amplitude based on the ambient sound level. The electrical signal is amplified and then transferred to input port 2 of the analog-to-digital converter. The type DHT11 temperature and humidity sensor operates by detecting changes in the resistance of a unique element within the sensor in response to changes in the surrounding temperature and humidity. There is a coating of moisture-sensitive organic material on it. The electrical conductivity of this substance varies with the relative humidity of the surrounding air. A thermistor is also included in the sensor to monitor temperature. To improve signal accuracy, a 10k ohm resistor has been added to the signal output channel. The signal is sent straight to the Raspberry board via GPIO port 17. Figure 2 shows a picture of the system being tested on a breadboard.

Figure 2. A breadboard is used for early system evaluation

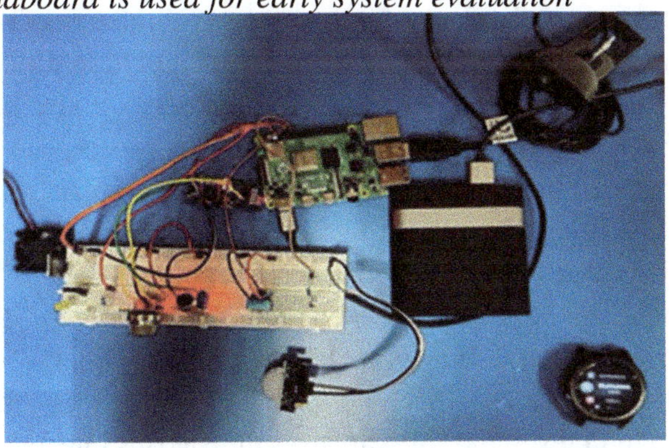

As a presence and motion sensor, the PIR (Passive Infrared) module measures variations in the infrared radiation that nearby objects produce. Its basic idea is to convert heat into electrical impulses by absorbing the heat produced by moving things, such as the human body. A pyroelectric element and lenses that concentrate infrared radiation from moving objects onto the pyroelectric element make up this sensor. The pyroelectric element produces a tiny electrical voltage differential in response to motion in its field of vision, which modifies the distribution of infrared light. After that, the voltage difference is analyzed and amplified to identify motion and presence. Two pyroelectric components of the PIR module are coupled in a manner that when they are subjected to distinct infrared radiation, they produce opposing voltage signals. This configuration reduces the interference caused by variations in temperature and other noise sources. Direct transmission of the signal is made to GPIO port 27.

The webcam is USB-connected to the Raspberry board, and it collects audio and video as you sleep in order to visually indicate potential sleep-related events.

The IOT Sleep Monitoring System's software support

Python, JavaScript, HTML, CSS, and the programming environments Thonny, Geany, and BlueJ were utilized for the Raspberry board. C, CSS, HTML, and JavaScript were used in conjunction with the Tizen Studio environment to construct the Gear S3 watch application.

Installing the "Raspbian" operating system and setting up the necessary administrative settings for remote board control via the Virtual Network Computing (VNC) protocol are required in order to create a setting that is favorable for the development, testing, and execution of applications on the Raspberry Pi board.

The software "VNC Viewer" for Windows or "RealVNC" for Android is used to interact with the graphical user interface (Hirsch, et al., 2023; Zovko et al., 2023).

The software support of the sleep monitor system is in charge of keeping an eye on the parameters provided by sensors, like temperature and humidity (this application interacts with the sensor using the Adafruit_DHT library); it also keeps track of the movements of the person being monitored while they sleep. The application will run continuously, checking the PIR sensor's status on a regular basis and recording the motion detection time. The status of connector 27 is set as input, and the GPIO library sets the "Broadcom" style pin numbering mode (BCM).

The sensor connector's status is checked in an endless loop; if it is 1, it indicates that motion has been detected. Write the data to the "3motion.txt" file and note the current motion detection time.

Air quality and light level: the software uses the SMBus interface, which enables communication between a Raspberry Pi and devices connected to the I2C bus, to read data from a MQ135 sensor and a light sensor. You must type "sudoraspi-config" into the terminal to enable the Raspberry's I2C interface. Then, go to "Interface Options" and activate the I2C module.

The three primary purposes of the I2C.py program are to read the I2C line from the converter, measure light brightness, and identify air quality.

The read_adc() method returns the read value, which may range from 0 to 255, and sends a command to the PCF8591 to choose the particular read channel (Figure 3).

Figure 3. Configuration menu for I2C protocol

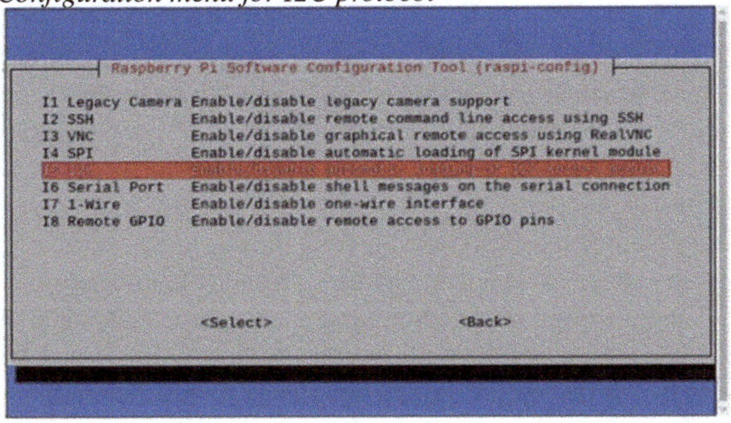

The PCF8591 converter's first input connection receives a directive to pick channel A0 from the light_level() function. It uses formula (1) to determine the light intensity in percentage after reading the data from the light sensor. The computed light level is sent back.

$$Lightlevel = 100 - \frac{valoare_{adc}}{255} x100\% \tag{1}$$

Comparably, the function calc_gas(adc_value) determines the estimated carbon dioxide concentration after receiving the converter value that was received from the MQ135 sensor. Utilizing formula (2), which applies the voltage divider rule to convert voltage to resistance, determine the resistance of the MQ135 sensor.

$$Voltage = \frac{valoare\_adc}{255} x5.0 \tag{2}$$

Formula (3), which is unique to the MQ135 sensor, is used to determine the estimated gas concentration. It takes into account the sensor's scaling factor (MQ135_FACTOR) and resistance in clean air (MQ135_RO_AER_CURAT) (Hirsch, et al, 2023). (Zovko et al, 2023).

$$gasconcentration = MQ135_{FACTOR} \left(\frac{sensorresistance}{MQ135_{R_{fresh}air}} \right)^{-2.77} \tag{3}$$

provides the expected carbon dioxide concentration in parts per million, or ppm. The related routines are used to read the brightness and gas readings in the program's main loop. After that, the values are entered into the text file “0Gaz_Luminozitate.

txt" together with the time and date of their acquisition. Every 45 seconds, this procedure is carried over again.

The PCF8591 device is contacted by the sleep noise recording program via the "smbus" module, which then reads the converted value to determine the sound level. Both the address of the sound sensor linked to the PCF8591 device and the address of the device itself are supplied. Interaction between the smbus object and the I2C protocol.SMBus(1) is set up.

The sound() method receives the value from the converter, sends a command to the PCF8591 to choose the channel, and uses formula (1) to determine the sound level, which ranges from 0 to 100. Store the reading time and sound level in the "1sunet.txt" file if the sound level is higher than or equal to 53. The sound() method is called every 0.2 seconds in the main loop.

Building the "OpenCV" (Open Source Computer Vision Library) library is required to enable video recording and image analysis with the USB-connected web camera opens, sets up, and initializes an audio stream using the PyAudio program opens a VideoWriter object to write the video frames, initializes the video capture, and sets the video's codec. Create a list at the beginning to hold the audio frames and the recording's start time. The user may choose how long they want to register for using the online interface.

Building the features that power the Bluetooth server is required before writing the application that uses the watch's sensor to monitor heart rate and sends the data over Bluetooth. Five files made up the final code for the Bluetooth server functionality (Figure 4).

Figure 4. Bluetooth transmission code structure

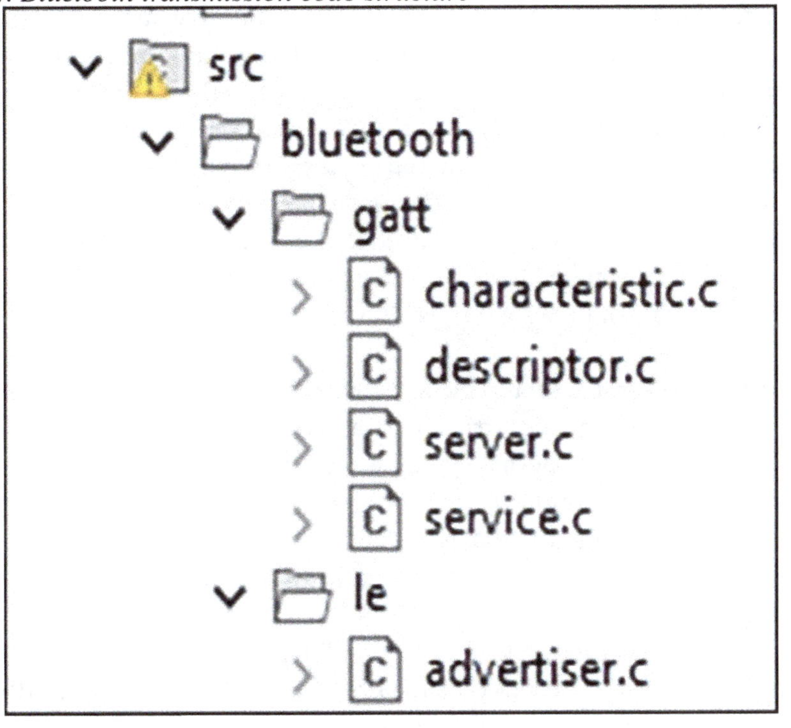

A handler for a Bluetooth device's Generic Attribute Profile (GATT) description is created and retrieved by the "characteristic.c" file. It specifies the GATT value as a byte string and the GATT description as a character string called the UUID (Universally Unique Identifier). The descriptors in the "characteristic.c" file are identified by the "descriptor.c" file. When a descriptor is successfully formed, the methods "bt_gatt_descriptor_create()" and "get_gatt_descriptor_handle()" return a true flag; otherwise, they return a false flag.

A freshly built GATT service is managed via the "service.c" file. In order to add a new characteristic, it executes the "add_gatt_characteristic_to_gatt_service()" method and generates a new UUID variable for the GATT service. It specifies and invokes a function that configures the Bluetooth Low Energy (BLE) advertisement's GATT service UUID. Lastly, it specifies a function that will terminate the GATT service that was established.

The "advertiser.c" file specifies the start, stop, and parameter management functions for the newly formed Bluetooth Low Energy (BLE) server, while the "server.c" file controls a GATT server made especially for Bluetooth communication.

An HTML page that sets up the UI and a Flask server serve as the foundation for the web application. You may configure the recording time, deactivate sensors or the webcam, and switch on or off the monitoring system using the program. Furthermore, you may easily remove the stored data folder from the Raspberry. Initially, the "subprocess" library is loaded, enabling the program to execute an external Python script. The main route is then specified and the Flask library is started. HTTP GET and POST queries are accepted on this route.

The request type is verified inside the "index()" method linked to the primary route. The button indicates that input data from the submitted form are collected if it is a POST request. The data is then saved to the "configuration.txt" file by using the "save_to_file()" method after being concatenated into a string. Lastly, a value reflecting the success of the data save is returned together with the HTML template and the button states.

The "data" argument is sent to the text save function, which opens the "configuration.txt" file in write mode, writes the data to it, and then closes it. The "run" route is used to initiate the external Python script "start_complet.py" upon receiving a POST request. The condition "if __name__ == '__main__':" determines whether or not this script is executed as the main file.

Written in C, the code makes advantage of the Tizen platform APIs to build a Tizen application that communicates with the HRM sensor and the Bluetooth features that were previously added to the "src" folder.

The code contains the header files required for the Tizen platform's Bluetooth, sensor, and user interface. The kind of sensor, its identification, and callback methods for events like button clicks and taps on the watch screen are specified as global variables. When the program becomes visible or invisible, functions such as the interface, interactive element, application control, and application stop and resume are generated and invoked. The code includes handlers for a number of application events, including low battery and memory, as well as changes in language, orientation, and region format. The application's lifecycle routines and event handlers are configured by the main function, "main()," which also initiates the main event loop.

CONCLUSION

IoT-based sleep monitoring offers a practical and non-intrusive means of gathering comprehensive data on an individual's quality of sleep. We can better understand sleep patterns and their effects on general health and well-being by using sensors and smart devices to gather and evaluate pertinent data. The integration of these technologies to gather data and send it to host devices for analysis and interpretation is made possible by the use of the Raspberry Pi board, wearable, and sensors with a variety of functions in IoT architecture. As a result, it is possible to monitor many parameters continuously and in real time, including temperature, humidity, pulse, etc. This offers a scalable and integrated method for tracking sleep in the house or in other settings. Regardless of age or lifestyle, a variety of individuals may benefit greatly from the data gathered during application development and testing. A person's lifestyle evaluation may be added to the monitoring system by include health monitoring data, physical activity level, and user preferences in the form of a log. It is feasible to have a more thorough picture of how individual habits and behaviors impact general health by gathering and evaluating this extra data. Such a comprehensive system makes it possible to identify patterns and tendencies in an individual's lifestyle, including stress levels, eating habits; physical activity levels, and sleep quality. Then, using this data, tailored suggestions for enhancing people' general health may be given. For instance, the system may recommend modifications to the individuals' exercise regimens or provide suggestions for healthy foods based on their level of activity and eating habits. We still have room for improvement with the existing setup, so switching out the webcam with a night vision camera would enable efficient recording and monitoring of activity throughout the night. Modular sensor addition and replacement would be a significant enhancement as well.

REFERENCES

Abe, T. K., Beamon, B. M., Storch, R. L., & Agus, J. (2016). Operations research applications in hospital operations: Part II. *IIE Transactions on Healthcare Systems Engineering*, *6*(2), 96–109. DOI: 10.1080/19488300.2016.1162880

Hirsch, C., Davoli, L., Grosu, R., & Ferrari, G. (2023). DynGATT: A dynamic GATT-based data synchronization protocol for BLE networks. *Computer Networks*, *222*, 109560. DOI: 10.1016/j.comnet.2023.109560

Ibáñez, V., Silva, J., & Cauli, O. (2018). A survey on sleep assessment methods. *PeerJ*, *6*, e4849. DOI: 10.7717/peerj.4849 PMID: 29844990

Izullah, F. R., Koivisto, M., & Nieminen, V. .a. (2022). Aging and sleep deprivation affect different neurocognitive stages of spatial information processing during a virtual driving task – An ERP study, *Transportation Research Part F: Traffic Psychology and Behaviour*, Vol 89.

Kwon, S., Kim, H., & Yeo, W.-H. (2021). Recent advances in wearable sensors and portable electronics for sleep monitoring. *iScience*, *24*(5), 102461. DOI: 10.1016/j.isci.2021.102461 PMID: 34013173

LaGoy, A. D., Mayeli, A., Smagula, S. F., & Ferrarelli, F. (2022). Relationships between rest-activity rhythms, sleep, and clinical symptoms in individuals at clinical high risk for psychosis and healthy comparison subjects. *Journal of Psychiatric Research*, *155*, 465–470. DOI: 10.1016/j.jpsychires.2022.09.009 PMID: 36183600

Moraes, A., Jermana, L., (2018). Advances in Photopletysmography Signal Analysis for Biomedical Applications, *Sensors*, Basel, Switzerland.

Muller, E. (2023). 7 Common Remote Patient Monitoring Devices https://www.healthrecoverysolutions.com/blog/7-common-remote-patient-monitoring-devices

Pan, Q., Brulin, D., & Campo, E. (2023). Evaluation of a Wireless Home Sleep Monitoring System Compared to Polysomnography. *Ingénierie et Recherche Biomédicale : IRBM = Biomedical Engineering and Research*, *44*(2), 100735. DOI: 10.1016/j.irbm.2022.09.002

Sun, J., Xiu, K., Wang, Z., Hu, N., Zhao, L., Zhu, H., Kong, F., Xiao, J., Cheng, L., & Bi, X. (2023). Multifunctional wearable humidity and pressure sensors based on biocompatible graphene/bacterial cellulose bio aerogel for wireless monitoring and early warning of sleep apnea syndrome. *Nano Energy*, *108*, 108215. DOI: 10.1016/j.nanoen.2023.108215

U.S. Department of Health and Human Services (2011). *Your Guide to Healthy Sleep,* NIH Publication, Nr. 11-5271.

Zhang, L., Cui, Z., Huffman, L. G., & Oshri, A. (2023). Sleep mediates the effect of stressful environments on youth development of impulsivity: The moderating role of within default mode network resting-state functional connectivity. *Sleep Health, 9*(4), 503–511. DOI: 10.1016/j.sleh.2023.03.005 PMID: 37270396

Zovko, K., Šerić, L., & Perković, T. a. (2023). IoT and health monitoring wearable devices as enabling technologies for sustainable enhancement of life quality in smart environments, *Journal of Cleaner Production*, ISSN 0959-6526.

Chapter 12
Machine Learning Through Early Diabetes Detection:
Evaluating Random Forest Classifier Performance

Omkar Shridhar Bholankar
https://orcid.org/0009-0000-3581-0124
Ajeenkya D.Y. Patil School of Engineering, India

Shreya Bhalerao
https://orcid.org/0009-0009-3645-5764
Ajeenkya D.Y. Patil School of Engineering, India

Shravani Bhalerao
https://orcid.org/0009-0009-3645-5764
Ajeenkya D.Y. Patil School of Engineering, India

Sweta Anand Wankhade
https://orcid.org/0009-0006-3667-5781
Ajeenkya D.Y. Patil School of Engineering, India

ABSTRACT

Diabetes is among the life-threatening diseases affecting millions of people worldwide. Detection done early and accurate prediction of diabetes can significantly improve patient outcomes by enabling timely intervention and lifestyle modifications. In recent years, Machine Learning (ML) techniques have been extensively used in medical diagnostics due to their ability to analyze complex patterns in healthcare data. This study focuses on evaluating the performance of the Random Forest (RF)

DOI: 10.4018/979-8-3373-4094-4.ch012

algorithm. The dataset including feature scaling, handling missing values and splitting into training and testing sets to ensure optimal mode performance. The results are evaluated based on performance metrics like Accuracy, Recall, Precision, and F-Measure that are derived from the confusion matrix. The experimental results proved that the best accuracy goes for Random Forest (RF).

1 INTRODUCTION

The global rise of diabetes mellitus represents one of the most significant and relentless public health challenges of the 21st century. It is a life-threatening chronic disease that affects millions of people worldwide. According to the International Diabetes Federation, an estimated 537 million adults were living with diabetes in 2021, a number projected to soar to 783 million by 2045. This silent epidemic is not just a health crisis but also a staggering economic one, with global health expenditure on diabetes reaching an estimated USD 966 billion. This figure fails to capture the immense indirect costs associated with lost productivity, disability, and the profound impact on national economies. Characterized by high blood glucose levels resulting from insufficient insulin production or ineffective use, diabetes, if not managed with constant vigilance, can lead to a cascade of severe and debilitating health complications. These include cardiovascular diseases, nerve damage (neuropathy), kidney failure, and vision impairment leading to blindness. As the global incidence of this disease continues its upward trajectory, the locus of care is undergoing a seismic shift, moving from the structured, professional environment of the hospital to the complex and often-unsupported setting of the home. This transition places an unprecedented level of responsibility onto the shoulders of patients and, most critically, their families.

Within this paradigm of home-based care, family caregivers emerge as the linchpins of chronic disease management. These unsung heroes—spouses, adult children, and other relatives—form the invisible frontline of our healthcare system, providing essential daily support that is both complex and demanding. The burden they carry is multifaceted, extending far beyond simple companionship. The physical burden is relentless, involving a daily regimen of tasks such as monitoring blood glucose levels, preparing carefully balanced meals, ensuring medication is taken correctly and on time, and managing the physical symptoms of the disease. This can lead to chronic fatigue, sleep deprivation, and a decline in the caregiver's own physical health.

Consider the hypothetical but deeply representative story of Anjali, a working professional in her forties who cares for her aging father, Mr. Sharma, recently diagnosed with Type 2 diabetes. Her day begins before dawn, preparing a low-glycemic breakfast for her father and checking his morning blood sugar. She meticulously packs his lunch and lays out his midday medication before rushing to her own job, her mind never far from her father's health. A work meeting is interrupted by a notification from his glucose monitor showing a dip, prompting a frantic call home. The evening brings no respite; it is a time for more cooking, another glucose check, and coaxing her father to go for a walk. This is the emotional burden: a constant state of high alert, a pervasive anxiety about potential hypoglycemic events or long-term complications, and the stress of making crucial daily decisions without formal medical training. Compounding this is the financial burden. Beyond the direct costs of insulin, test strips, and doctor visits, Anjali has had to reduce her work hours, sacrificing income and career progression to meet her caregiving responsibilities. Her experience is a microcosm of the reality for millions, a silent struggle that takes a significant toll on mental, physical, and financial well-being.

"Integrative Home Care" is a progressive model that seeks to address these profound challenges by creating a holistic, collaborative ecosystem around the patient. It moves beyond the fragmented nature of traditional healthcare by formally recognizing and empowering the family caregiver as a pivotal member of the care team. The core principles of this model are rooted in partnership and technology. It is patient-centered, meaning that care plans are tailored to the individual's specific needs, values, and home environment. It is collaborative, fostering seamless communication channels between the patient, their family, primary care physicians, specialists, and community health workers. A key goal is to break down the silos that often exist between formal and informal care. However, the implementation of this model faces significant hurdles, including the lack of interoperable health information systems, inadequate training and support resources for caregivers, and healthcare reimbursement policies that often fail to recognize the value of home-based preventive care.

To truly integrate the care process and empower caregivers like Anjali, we must bridge these gaps with effective, evidence-based tools. Traditional diagnostic methods for diabetes rely on clinical evaluations and blood tests, which, while effective, are episodic and reactive rather than continuous and proactive. They may not detect the subtle, early-stage patterns of glycemic dysregulation or provide the timely insights needed for preventive action within a home setting. With recent advancements in artificial intelligence (AI) and machine learning (ML), a new frontier of predictive health analytics has opened. ML models have the remarkable ability to analyze complex health datasets and identify hidden patterns that can predict the likelihood of a disease before its symptoms become acute.

This chapter explores the potential of these advanced analytical techniques to serve the specific needs of family caregivers. We propose that a well-designed ML model can function as a powerful decision support tool, analyzing key health indicators to provide an early warning system for diabetes risk. This study focuses specifically on evaluating the performance of the Random Forest (RF) algorithm, a powerful ML technique, for this purpose. Using a well-known medical dataset, we will demonstrate the process of building and validating a predictive model. The primary objective is to translate the technical performance of this model—measured by metrics like accuracy, precision, and recall —into a practical discussion of how such technology could be harnessed to support caregivers, reduce their burden, and ultimately improve the outcomes for patients with diabetes in an integrative home care environment. This chapter is structured to guide the reader from the foundational concepts to the practical applications, with the ultimate aim of illuminating a path toward a future where technology empowers humanity's most essential caregivers.

2 LITERATURE SURVEY

To fully appreciate the potential of a machine learning tool for diabetes prediction in a home care context, it is essential to build a strong foundation across three interconnected domains: the clinical realities of diabetes, the evolving landscape of home healthcare technology, and the specific application of machine learning algorithms for diagnostics. This review synthesizes literature from these areas to establish the profound need and clear justification for developing intelligent tools to support family caregivers.

The Clinical Context of Type 2 Diabetes

While diabetes is broadly characterized by high blood glucose, a deeper understanding of its underlying mechanisms and diagnostic nuances is crucial for developing effective management and prediction strategies. For a caregiver, comprehending the "why" behind the disease can transform care from a series of rote tasks into an informed, proactive partnership with the patient.

The Pathophysiology of Type 2 Diabetes and Insulin Resistance

Type 2 diabetes, which accounts for over 90% of all diabetes cases, is a progressive metabolic disorder primarily defined by two core defects: insulin resistance and a relative insulin deficiency due to pancreatic beta-cell dysfunction. In a healthy individual, the pancreas produces insulin, a hormone that acts like a key. Its job is to bind to receptors on the surface of cells (the "lock"), allowing glucose to move from the bloodstream into the cells to be used for energy.

Insulin resistance is the condition where cells in the muscles, fat, and liver become less responsive to insulin's signal. The "lock" becomes rusty and difficult to open. To compensate, the pancreas goes into overdrive, producing more and more insulin to force the glucose into the cells and keep blood sugar levels normal. This state of hyperinsulinemia can persist for years, often without any noticeable symptoms. However, this is an unsustainable state. Over time, the insulin-producing beta cells in the pancreas become exhausted and can no longer keep up with the high demand. As these cells fail, insulin production wanes, and blood glucose levels begin to rise, eventually crossing the threshold for a diagnosis of prediabetes and then Type 2 diabetes. Factors contributing to insulin resistance are complex and include genetic predisposition, but are strongly linked to lifestyle factors, particularly excess body weight (especially visceral fat around the organs) and physical inactivity.

Primary Diagnostic Tests and Their Limitations in a Home Setting

Traditional diagnosis relies on several established laboratory tests, each with its own set of advantages and disadvantages, especially when considered from the perspective of a caregiver supporting a patient at home.

Hemoglobin A1C (A1C): This blood test provides an estimate of a person's average blood glucose levels over the preceding two to three months. It measures the percentage of hemoglobin (the protein in red blood cells that carries oxygen) that has become glycated, or coated with sugar.

- **Pros:** Its primary advantage is convenience. It does not require the patient to fast, and it is less susceptible to short-term fluctuations caused by stress or recent meals, providing a more stable, long-term picture of glycemic control.
- **Cons:** The A1C test can be less sensitive in detecting early-stage diabetes or prediabetes compared to other tests. Furthermore, its accuracy can be compromised by certain conditions that affect red blood cell turnover, such as sickle cell anemia, kidney disease, or severe blood loss, making it less reliable for some individuals.

Fasting Plasma Glucose (FPG): The FPG test measures blood glucose at a single point in time after a person has fasted (not eaten or drunk anything but water) for at least eight hours.

- **Pros:** It is a relatively simple, fast, and inexpensive test, making it a common screening tool in clinical practice.
- **Cons:** From a caregiver's perspective, ensuring a proper fast can be challenging, particularly for older adults or those with cognitive impairments. More importantly, the FPG test provides only a snapshot of glucose levels on one particular morning. It can be influenced by a poor night's sleep, stress, or illness, and may not capture issues with glucose metabolism that occur after meals (postprandial hyperglycemia).

Oral Glucose Tolerance Test (OGTT): The OGTT is a more comprehensive test of the body's ability to handle a glucose load. It involves an initial fasting blood draw, after which the patient consumes a standardized sugary drink. Blood is then drawn again two hours later.

- **Pros:** The OGTT is considered the gold standard for diagnosing prediabetes and is more sensitive than the FPG and A1C tests in identifying impaired glucose tolerance, an early sign of the disease.
- **Cons:** The test is logistically demanding, inconvenient, and time-consuming, requiring the patient to remain at the clinic for several hours. The results can also have poor reproducibility. These factors make it impractical for routine screening and difficult to manage from a caregiver's standpoint.

The limitations of these periodic, clinic-based tests highlight a critical gap. For a family caregiver, managing diabetes is a 24/7 responsibility. They need tools that can help them understand risk in the long intervals between doctor visits, using data that is readily available in the home environment.

Technology in Home Healthcare

The proliferation of digital technology has begun to revolutionize home healthcare, creating an unprecedented opportunity to fill the gap left by traditional diagnostic methods. This new ecosystem of connected devices and platforms can empower caregivers with data-driven insights.

The Role of Telehealth in Chronic Care

Telehealth refers to the delivery of health care, health education, and health information services via remote technologies. Far more than just a video call with a doctor, it encompasses a range of services crucial for chronic disease management. For diabetes care, this includes virtual consultations for medication adjustments, remote dietary counseling with nutritionists, and digital health coaching to support lifestyle changes. Numerous studies have demonstrated the efficacy of telehealth interventions. A systematic review of telehealth programs for diabetes management often shows that patients who participate in them achieve statistically significant improvements in their A1C levels compared to those receiving usual care. These programs enhance patient engagement and provide a vital, ongoing connection to the clinical team, reassuring caregivers that they are not alone in managing the patient's condition.

Wearable Technology and Remote Patient Monitoring (RPM)

Perhaps the most transformative development for at-home care is the rise of wearable technology and RPM. These devices shift data collection from an episodic event in a clinic to a continuous process in a patient's daily life, generating a rich, longitudinal dataset.

- **Continuous Glucose Monitors (CGMs):** These small, wearable sensors measure glucose levels in the interstitial fluid just under the skin, providing readings as frequently as every few minutes. They reveal dynamic trends, time-in-range, and nocturnal glucose patterns that are completely invisible to traditional finger-stick tests. For a caregiver, a CGM with alert features can be life-saving, warning them of dangerous highs or lows before they become critical.
- **Fitness Trackers and Smartwatches:** Modern wearables capture a wealth of data relevant to diabetes management, including daily step counts, minutes of physical activity, sleep quality, and heart rate variability. This data provides objective measures of lifestyle factors that are cornerstone to diabetes control.
- **Smart Scales and Blood Pressure Cuffs:** Connected devices that automatically sync weight, BMI, and blood pressure readings to an app eliminate the need for manual tracking and provide a seamless record of these key cardiometabolic indicators.

The Role of Digital Education in Caregiver Empowerment

The provision of data through RPM and predictive tools is only one half of the empowerment equation. For data to become knowledge, and for knowledge to become confident action, caregivers must possess a sufficient level of **health literacy**. Health literacy is the degree to which individuals have the capacity to obtain, process, and understand basic health information needed to make appropriate health decisions. A caregiver may have access to a continuous stream of glucose data, but if they do not understand the difference between fasting and postprandial glucose, or the impact of carbohydrates on insulin response, the data remains a series of abstract numbers. Therefore, effective digital health interventions for caregivers must integrate robust educational components that are accessible, engaging, and trustworthy.

The digital landscape offers a vast array of educational platforms. These range from static information repositories on websites from highly credible organizations (such as the American Diabetes Association, the Mayo Clinic, and the National Institute of Diabetes and Digestive and Kidney Diseases) to dynamic, interactive mobile applications (like mySugr or One Drop, which combine tracking with educational modules) and video-based content on platforms like YouTube, often produced by hospitals and health systems. The most effective of these platforms are built on established principles of adult learning theory, prioritizing engagement over passive consumption. The literature suggests that successful digital education for caregivers incorporates several key features:

- **Interactivity:** Rather than simply reading text, users learn more effectively through interaction. This can include features like quizzes to test knowledge, gamified challenges to encourage healthy habits, and interactive meal planners that allow caregivers to build and analyze meals in real-time.
- **Personalization:** Generic advice is less impactful than information tailored to the user's specific situation. Advanced platforms can personalize content based on the patient's data, offering articles or videos relevant to their specific challenges, such as managing nocturnal hypoglycemia or understanding their new medication.
- **Accessibility:** To bridge the digital divide, educational content must be highly accessible. This extends beyond being mobile-friendly and includes providing information in multiple languages, using plain language that avoids medical jargon, and adhering to web accessibility standards for users with visual or other impairments.

However, the proliferation of digital platforms also presents a significant challenge: the overwhelming volume of online health information and the risk of dangerous misinformation. A caregiver's simple web search can lead them to unvetted blogs, social media influencers promoting unproven supplements, or forums filled with anecdotal advice that contradicts clinical guidelines. This makes the ability to discern credible sources a critical skill. Consequently, a key role for clinicians and for well-designed digital tools is not just to provide information, but to act as trusted curators, guiding caregivers toward safe, evidence-based educational resources and helping them develop the critical skill of digital discernment.

This constant stream of data is a double-edged sword. While it offers a holistic view of the patient's health, it can also be overwhelming. The sheer volume of data is often underutilized, presented in simple dashboards but lacking the analytical sophistication to uncover predictive patterns. This is precisely where machine learning can serve as the "brain" to interpret this data deluge.

Ethical Considerations in Predictive Health Analytics

As we move towards predictive AI in healthcare, we must proceed with caution, addressing a complex web of ethical challenges to ensure these tools are safe, fair, and trustworthy.

- **Data Privacy and Security:** Health data is incredibly sensitive. In the United States, the Health Insurance Portability and Accountability Act (HIPAA) provides a legal framework for protecting patient information used by healthcare providers. However, much of the data collected by consumer-grade wearables and wellness apps may fall outside these protections, creating a regulatory gray area. Any caregiver-facing tool must be built on a foundation of robust data encryption, user anonymity, and transparent privacy policies.
- **Algorithmic Bias:** An AI model is only as unbiased as the data it is trained on. If a model is developed using a dataset that is not diverse, it may perform poorly for underrepresented groups. For example, the Pima Indians Diabetes Dataset is specific to one demographic. A model trained exclusively on it might fail to accurately predict risk for individuals of other ethnicities, potentially widening existing health disparities. Mitigating bias requires conscious efforts to collect diverse datasets and rigorously audit model performance across different populations.
- **The Digital Divide:** The promise of digital health tools is predicated on access. The "digital divide" refers to the gap between those who have access to modern information and communication technology and those who do not. This divide can be based on socioeconomic status (affordability of smartphones and internet), geography (rural vs. urban connectivity), age, and digital literacy. There is a significant risk that these advanced tools could benefit the already privileged, leaving the most vulnerable populations behind. Designing for accessibility and providing non-digital alternatives are crucial for ensuring equitable care.

Machine Learning for Disease Prediction

Machine learning (ML) offers a powerful solution for transforming the raw health data discussed above into actionable, predictive insights. In recent years, researchers have extensively applied and compared various classification algorithms for diabetes prediction, demonstrating both the potential and the challenges of this approach (Alam et al., 2019; Emon et al., 2021). Early studies often focused on traditional statistical models and individual classifiers.

More recent research has benchmarked a wider array of more sophisticated techniques. For example, a study by Khaleel and Al-Bakry (2021) compared several methods and found that Logistic Regression (LR) achieved a high accuracy of 94% on their dataset, while Naïve Bayes (NB) and K-Nearest Neighbours (KNN) performed less effectively. Similarly, Khanam and Foo (2021) conducted a comparative analysis using the PIDD, concluding that Support Vector Machine (SVM) and LR were top performers. They also noted that Artificial Neural Networks (ANN) could achieve an impressive 88.6% accuracy, but this often required extensive hyperparameter tuning. Other studies have focused on specific comparisons, such as the work by Cıhan and Coskun (2021) and Mujumdar and Vaidehi (2019), which reinforce the importance of algorithm selection.

A comprehensive comparison by Sarwar et al. (2018) benchmarked a full suite of algorithms—including LR, SVM, NB, KNN, Decision Tree (DT), and Random Forest (RF)—on the PIDD dataset, underscoring the general feasibility of the predictive task. Furthermore, recent advancements have integrated ontology-based approaches (EL Massari et al., 2022) and focused on benchmarking classifiers for maintainable applications (Sabouri et al., 2022).

These studies collectively affirm that machine learning models can effectively predict diabetes. However, accuracy is not the only important factor. The "black box" nature of some complex models can be a significant barrier to clinical adoption. If a doctor or caregiver cannot understand *why* a model made a certain prediction, they are less likely to trust it. This has led to a growing interest in interpretable models.

The Random Forest (RF) algorithm, the focus of this chapter, is of particular interest because it offers a compelling balance of high accuracy and interpretability. As an ensemble method, RF builds upon hundreds of individual Decision Trees and aggregates their votes to make a final prediction. This structure makes it robust against overfitting. Crucially, RF can also generate a "feature importance" ranking, which explicitly identifies the most influential factors (e.g., glucose, BMI) in its predictions. This inherent transparency is a significant advantage for a tool intended for practical use by caregivers and clinicians. The findings from several key studies in the field are summarized in Table 1.

Table 1. Literature survey

Sr. no.	Author(s)	Algorithm(s) Used	Dataset	Accuracy/Outcome
1.	Khaleel and Al-Bakry (2021)	LR, NB, KNN, DT, SVM	Local Hospital Dataset	Logistic Regression (LR) achieved the highest accuracy at 94%.
2.	Khanam & Foo (2021)	LR, SVM, KNN, DT, ANN, NB	Pima Indians Diabetes (PIDD)	SVM and LR were top performers; ANN reached 88.6% with tuning.
3.	Sarwar et al. (2018)	RF, DT, NB, SVM, LR, KNN	Pima Indians Diabetes (PIDD)	Comprehensive comparison confirming the utility of multiple ML models.
4.	Rady et al. (2021)	SVM, RF, KNN, DT, LR, NB	Pima Indians Diabetes (PIDD)	Comparative study highlighting the trade-offs between different ML models.
5.	Mujumdar & Vaidehi (2019)	LR, SVM, DT, RF, NB	Pima Indians Diabetes (PIDD)	Analyzed performance of multiple classifiers; highlighted robustness of RF.
6.	Alam et al. (2019)	ANN, RF, K-Means	Pima Indians Diabetes (PIDD)	Proposed a framework for early diabetes prediction with high accuracy.

This body of work clearly indicates that the tools to build a predictive model for diabetes exist and are effective. The primary challenge, and the focus of this chapter, is to bridge the gap between this technical capability and the practical, day-to-day needs of the family caregiver in a home health environment.

3. METHODOLOGY: BUILDING A PREDICTIVE MODEL FOR DIABETES RISK

This section details the systematic and rigorous process of developing and evaluating the Random Forest model for diabetes prediction. The methodology was designed not only to achieve high predictive accuracy but also to ensure the model is robust, interpretable, and conceptually sound for its intended application as a caregiver support tool. We will explore the dataset used, the critical steps of data preprocessing, the rationale behind the algorithm selection over other common alternatives, the model evaluation strategy, and the crucial role of hyperparameter tuning. The technologies and method carried out in this experiment are describe below.

3.1 Dataset

The study utilizes the Pima Indians Diabetes Database (PIDD), a publicly available and widely cited dataset originally from the National Institute of Diabetes and Digestive and Kidney Diseases. Its status as a standard benchmark in diabetes prediction research is a key advantage, as it allows for the direct comparison of our results with a large body of existing literature. The dataset comprises 768 instances, representing patient records of females of Pima Indian heritage aged 21 and over. It contains 8 numerical features and a binary class label indicating the presence (1) or absence (0) of diabetes.

The features are clinically relevant variables used in diabetes diagnosis and risk assessment:

- **Pregnancies:** The number of times a patient has been pregnant.
- **Glucose:** The plasma glucose concentration at the 2-hour mark in an oral glucose tolerance test. This is a primary indicator of how the body processes sugar.
- **Blood Pressure:** The diastolic blood pressure (mm Hg). Chronic hypertension is a well-established risk factor and comorbidity for Type 2 diabetes.
- **Skin Thickness:** The triceps skin fold thickness (mm), used as an indirect measure of body fat.
- **Insulin:** The 2-Hour serum insulin level (mu U/ml), which indicates the pancreas's insulin production in response to a glucose challenge.
- **BMI (mass):** The Body Mass Index, calculated from weight and height, is a key measure of body fat and a strong predictor of insulin resistance and diabetes risk.
- **Diabetes Pedigree Function (pedi):** A synthesized function that scores the likelihood of diabetes based on family history and genetic predisposition.
- **Age:** The patient's age in years. The risk of developing Type 2 diabetes increases significantly with age.

While this dataset is invaluable for developing and comparing models, its limitations must be explicitly acknowledged. The data is cross-sectional, meaning it provides a single snapshot in time for each patient, rather than a longitudinal view of their health trajectory. Furthermore, its demographic specificity means that a model trained exclusively on this data may not generalize perfectly to other populations. Therefore, the model developed here serves as a crucial proof-of-concept. It demonstrates the *methodology* and potential of this approach, with the understanding that for a real-world, deployable application, the model would need to be re-trained and validated on a larger, more diverse, and representative dataset.

Figure 1. Model Flowchart

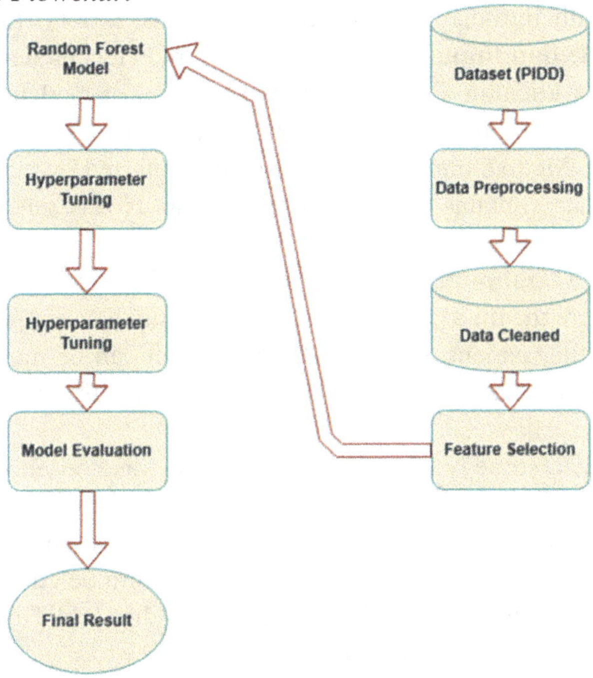

3.2 Data Preprocessing: Preparing Data for an Accurate Model

Raw medical data is notoriously imperfect. The process of cleaning, transforming, and preparing this data—known as preprocessing—is one of the most critical stages in building a reliable machine learning model. The quality of the data directly dictates the quality of the model's insights.

Handling Missing or Anomalous Values

Upon initial inspection of the PIDD, it becomes clear that some features contain physiologically impossible zero values. For instance, a living person cannot have a BMI, Glucose level, or Blood Pressure of zero. These zeros are not true data points but are instead placeholders for missing values. Handling them correctly is paramount. Several strategies could have been employed:

- **Listwise Deletion:** This approach involves removing any patient record that contains a missing value. While simple, this method is often suboptimal as it can lead to a significant loss of valuable data, reducing the statistical power and potentially introducing bias if the missingness is not completely random.

- **Mean or Median Imputation:** This is a common technique where the missing value for a feature is replaced with the mean or median of all observed values for that feature. It is computationally efficient and preserves the full sample size. Median imputation is generally preferred over mean imputation when the data contains outliers, as the median is less sensitive to extreme values.
- **K-Nearest Neighbours (k-NN) Imputation:** This is a more sophisticated method where the missing value is imputed using the average value from the 'k' most similar patient records in the dataset. It can be more accurate than simple mean/median imputation but is computationally more expensive.

For this study, a strategy of median imputation was chosen for features like Glucose, Blood Pressure, and BMI. This choice represents a sound balance between methodological simplicity and the preservation of the dataset's integrity. It prevents the loss of valuable patient records that would occur with deletion while avoiding the computational overhead of more complex methods like k-NN imputation, which may offer marginal benefits on a dataset of this size.

Feature Scaling

The numerical features in the dataset exist on vastly different scales. Age might range from 21 to 81, while the Diabetes Pedigree Function is a small decimal number. Many machine learning algorithms can be negatively impacted by these differing scales, as features with larger ranges can dominate the learning process. Two primary methods of feature scaling are:

- **Normalization (Min-Max Scaling):** This technique rescales the data to a fixed range, typically between 0 and 1. It is calculated as: Xnorm=Xmax−XminX−Xmin. Normalization is useful but can be sensitive to outliers.
- **Standardization (Z-score Normalization):** This method rescales the data to have a mean of 0 and a standard deviation of 1. It is calculated as: Xstand =σX−μ, where μ is the mean and σ is the standard deviation. Standardization is less affected by outliers and is the preferred method for algorithms that assume a Gaussian distribution.

While tree-based algorithms like Random Forest are theoretically less sensitive to feature scaling than distance-based algorithms (like SVM or k-NN) or linear models, applying standardization is still considered best practice. It ensures that the model's results are consistent and comparable, and it becomes a critical necessity if one wishes to benchmark the Random Forest's performance against other model types that do require it.

3.3. Alternative Algorithms Considered

The selection of the Random Forest algorithm was a deliberate choice made after considering the strengths and weaknesses of several other powerful and commonly used classification models.

- **Decision Tree (DT):** A single Decision Tree is the foundational building block of a Random Forest. It operates like a flowchart, splitting the data at each node based on the feature that provides the most information gain, until it reaches a final prediction at a "leaf" node. While highly interpretable and easy to visualize, single Decision Trees have a significant drawback: they are prone to overfitting. They can learn the training data, including its noise, so perfectly that they fail to generalize to new, unseen data.
- **Logistic Regression (LR):** This is a robust statistical method used for binary classification. It works by fitting a logistic (sigmoid) function to the data to model the probability of a certain class or event. Its primary advantages are its simplicity, high interpretability (the coefficients of the model directly relate to the importance of each feature), and computational efficiency. However, its main limitation is that it is a **linear model**. It assumes a linear relationship between the features and the outcome, and it may fail to capture more complex, non-linear patterns that are common in biological data.
- **Support Vector Machine (SVM):** The SVM is a powerful algorithm that works by finding the optimal "hyperplane" that best separates the data points of different classes in a high-dimensional space. It aims to maximize the margin, or distance, between the hyperplane and the nearest data points of any class. By using a "kernel trick," SVMs can effectively model highly complex and non-linear boundaries. However, they can be computationally intensive, especially with large datasets, and their results can be less intuitive to interpret compared to tree-based models, often functioning as a "black box."

The Random Forest was chosen because it directly addresses the weaknesses of these alternatives in the context of this problem. It overcomes the overfitting issue of a single Decision Tree by averaging the predictions of hundreds of diverse trees. It can capture complex, non-linear relationships in the data that Logistic Regression would miss. And while it may not always outperform a finely-tuned SVM, it is generally easier to train, less computationally demanding, and offers a clear, built-in mechanism for interpreting feature importance, a critical requirement for a tool meant to be trusted by caregivers and clinicians.

3.4. Hyperparameter Tuning: Optimizing the Model's Architecture

A machine learning model's performance is not only dependent on the data and the algorithm but also on its hyperparameters. These are the settings of the model that are not learned from the data itself but are set by the data scientist prior to the training process. They define the model's architecture and how it learns. For a Random Forest model, several key hyperparameters are crucial:

- **n_estimators:** This defines the number of decision trees to be built in the forest. A higher number generally leads to better performance and a more stable model, but at the cost of increased computational time. There is a point of diminishing returns where adding more trees does not significantly improve the model.
- **max_depth:** This controls the maximum depth, or number of levels, each tree can grow to. If the depth is too shallow, the model may underfit and fail to capture the complexity of the data. If it is too deep, the individual trees can overfit, although the ensemble nature of the forest helps to mitigate this.
- **min_samples_split:** This sets the minimum number of data points required in a node before it can be split. It is a useful parameter for controlling the growth of the trees and preventing splits on nodes with very few samples, which can lead to overfitting.
- **max_features:** This determines the size of the random subset of features to consider for splitting at each node. Limiting the number of features increases the diversity of the trees and generally reduces the variance of the model.

The process of hyperparameter tuning involves systematically searching for the combination of these settings that yields the best model performance. Common methods include GridSearchCV, which exhaustively tries every possible combination of a predefined set of hyperparameter values, and RandomizedSearchCV, which samples a fixed number of combinations from a given distribution. While the original study focused on the out-of-the-box performance of the algorithm, it is critical to acknowledge that a formal tuning process would be an essential step in developing a production-ready model to ensure its predictive power is maximized. This optimization process ensures that the final model is not just a good model, but the best possible model that can be built from the chosen algorithm and data.

4 EVALUATION

Analyzing a machine learning model's performance is important in deciding its efficiency in predicting diabetes. In this research, the Random Forest algorithm was applied to classify patients using medical features from the Pima Indians Diabetes Database (PIDD). Performance assessment involves several performance measures such as precision, accuracy, recall, F1-score, and AUC-ROC curve evaluation. Accuracy is a basic measure that reflects the proportion of accurately classified instances. But in accordance with imbalanced data, accuracy by itself can be deceptive, thus making precision and recall critical for evaluating the reliability of the model. Precision calculates how many of the predicted positive instances are indeed positive, whereas recall (sensitivity) quantifies how good the model performs at diagnosing true diabetic cases. The F1-score is the harmonic mean of precision and recall, gives a balanced measure of the performance of the model. Also, the AUC- ROC curve is employed to examine the trade-off between true positive and false positive rates to judge the discriminative ability of the model.

For robust evaluation, k-fold cross-validation was utilized to divide the dataset into several training and testing subsets to minimize the risk of over fitting. The confusion matrix also assisted in the visualization of the classification results, showing the total number of true positives, true negatives, false positives, and false negatives. A comparison with other classification models, including SVM, KNN, Decision Tree, and Naïve Bayes, was made to compare the performance of the Random Forest model. The findings indicated that Random Forest surpassed other classifiers regarding accuracy and capability for generalization because of the ensemble learning principle. Nonetheless, drawbacks like computationally intensive processes and hyper parameter tuning issues were observed. As a whole, the assessment depicts that Random Forest is an outstanding model for diabetic prediction and that it is worth being used for medical diagnosis as well as making decisions. Subsequent research can investigate feature selection methods and deep learning models to improve the accuracy of prediction.

In an ideal classification scenario, we'd want to have no false negatives (FN) or false positives (FP) meaning both FN and FP would be zero. From the confusion matrix, we can derive several key performance metrics, such as Accuracy, Precision, Recall, and the F-Measure. The best possible value for accuracy, precision, and recall is 1.0, which represents perfect performance, while the worst possible value is 0.0. Figure 3 shows how these metrics are calculated using the confusion matrix. From this matrix, we can derive several key performance metrics. The terms used in the matrix are defined in Table 2.

Table 2. Terms Associated with Confusion Matrix

Terms	Description
True Positive (TP)	Number of patients correctly identified as positive
True Negative (TN)	Number of patients correctly identified as negative
False Positive (FP)	Number of patients incorrectly identified as positive
False Negative (FN)	Number of patients incorrectly identified as negative

Accuracy (ACC):

ACC = (TP + TN) / (TP + TN +FP + FN)

Accuracy is computed as the number of all correct prediction divided by the total number of Dataset, which is the number of patient that are identified correctly in total in our cases.

Precision (PREC):

PREC = TP / (TP + FP)

Precision is computed as the number of correct positive prediction divided by the total number Positive prediction.

Recall (REC):

REC = TP / (TP + FN)

Recall is computed as the number of positive prediction divided by the total number of positive Prediction. It is also called Sensitivity or true positive rate (TPR).

F – Measure:

F – Measure = 2 * (PREC * REC) / (PREC + REC)

ROC – AUC Area:

The Receiver Operating Characteristic (ROC) curve and the Area under the Curve (AUC) are commonly used tools for evaluating how well classification models perform, particularly in medical applications like predicting diabetes. The ROC curve is a visual representation that shows the balance between the True Positive Rate (Sensitivity) and the False Positive Rate (1 - Specificity) as the threshold for classification is adjusted. The AUC, or Area under the Curve, measures how effectively the model distinguishes between positive and negative cases. An AUC of 1.0 means the model is perfect at classifying, while an AUC of 0.5 suggests the model is no better than randomly guessing. In the case of predicting diabetes using the Random Forest algorithm, the AUC-ROC curve helps assess how accurately the model can identify diabetic and non-diabetic patients. Higher AUC values indicate that the model is better at telling the difference between the two groups.

Interpretation of Results

The ROC curve visually demonstrates the model's performance across different thresholds.

The AUC score quantifies the model's ability to distinguish between diabetic and non-diabetic cases.

A higher AUC (>0.8) indicates that the model is effective in classification.

If AUC is closer to 1.0, the model is performing well; if it is closer to 0.5, it suggests poor performance.

In summary, the ROC-AUC analysis helps in determining the robustness of the Random Forest model for diabetes prediction. If the AUC score is high, it means the model has strong discriminatory power.

Figure 2. ROC-AUC Curve

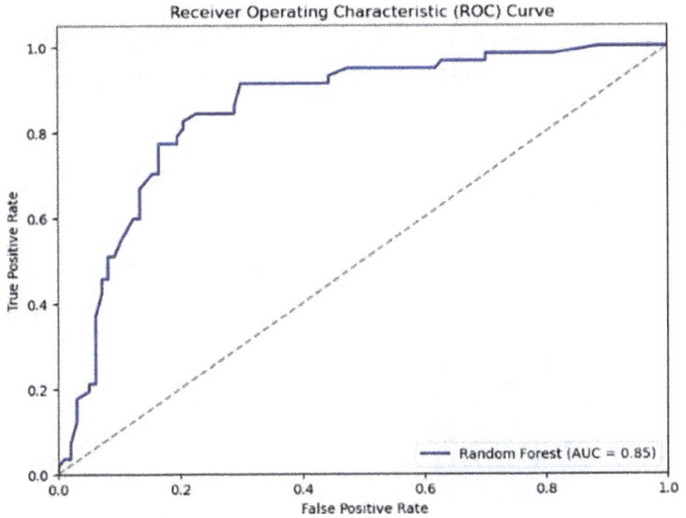

5 RESULT

In this section, we present or discuss about result which is obtained after evaluation of the classifier used in this research including the result and algorithm.

The primary objective of this study was to evaluate the effectiveness of the Random Forest algorithm for Diabetes Prediction using the Pima Indians Diabetes Dataset. The model was trained and tested using standard machine learning evaluation metrics, including accuracy, precision, recall, F1 – score, and ROC – AUC score.

In this we did following things:

a. Model Performance Analysis:

The Random Forest classifier demonstrated strong predictive capabilities with an accuracy of approximately 80 – 85% and above. Outperforming traditional classifier such as Logistic Regression, Naïve Bayes, K – Nearest Neighbors, and Decision Tree.

b. Comparison With Other Models:

A comparative study was conducted to assess the performance of Random Forest against other machine learning models. The Decision Tree Classifier showed slightly lower accuracy due to over fitting, while Logistic Regression struggled to capture complex relationship.

Accuracy:

10 – Fold Cross – Validation (0.85 accuracy) and split 66% (0.81% accuracy). It shows that 10 – Fold Cross – Validation performs slightly better than the split 66% method, indicating more stable

Figure 3. Accuracy Bar Plot

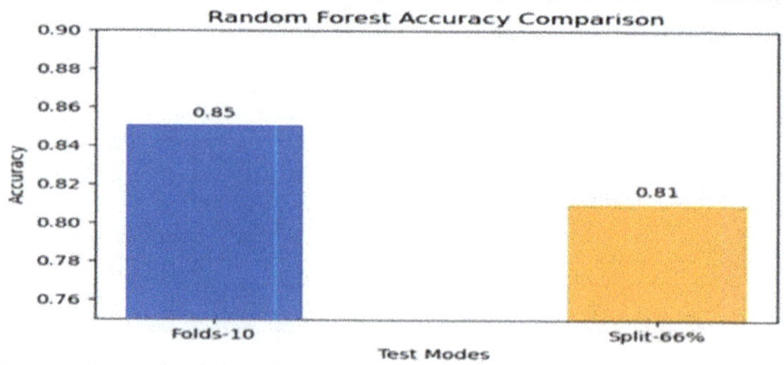

Precision:

The precision of the Random Forest model using 10 – Fold Cross – Validation (0.82%) and

Split 66% (0.79%). It shows that 10 – Fold Cross – Validation has slightly better precision, Indicating a more consistent classification performance.

Figure 4. Precision Bar Plot

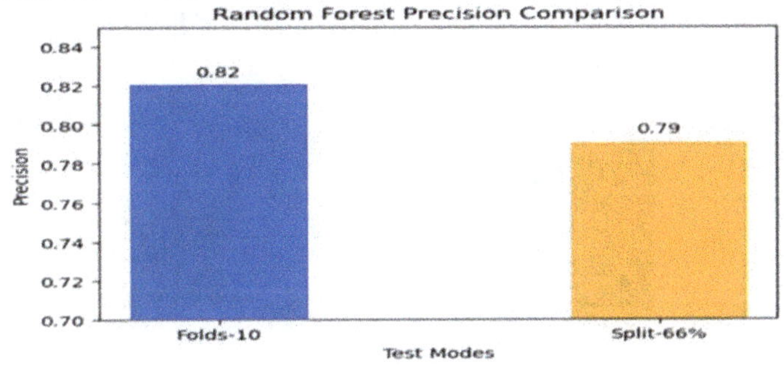

Recall:

The recall of the Random Forest model using 10 – Fold Cross – Validation (0.82%) and Split 66% (0.78%). It shows that 10 – Fold Cross – Validation achieves higher recall, indicating Better performance in capturing positive cases.

Figure 5. Recall Bar Plot

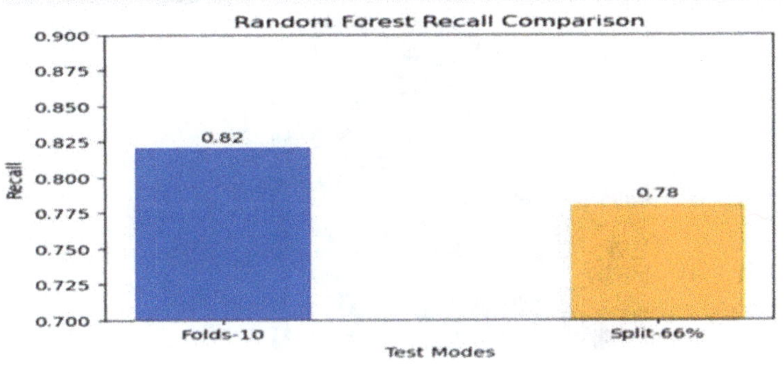

F1 – Measure:

The F1 – Score of the Random Forest model using 10 – Fold Cross – Validation (0.81%) and

Split 66% (0.77%). The higher F1 – Score in 10 – Fold Cross – Validation indicates better Balance between precision and recall, compare to split 66% approach.

Figure 6. F1 - Measure Bar Plot

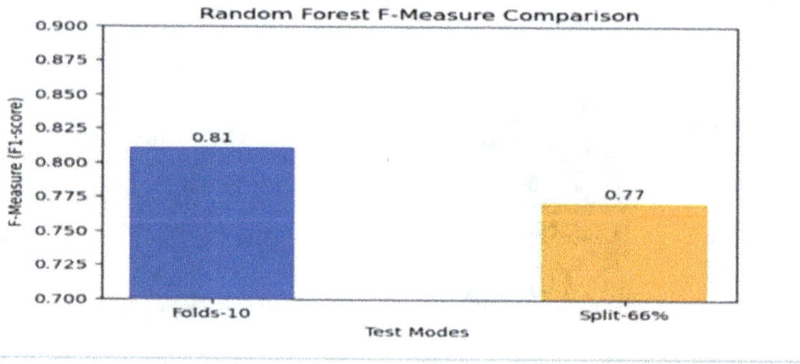

6 CONFUSION MATRIX

The confusion matrix helps visualize the model's performance by showing the number of correct And incorrect prediction.

Figure 7. Confusion Matrix

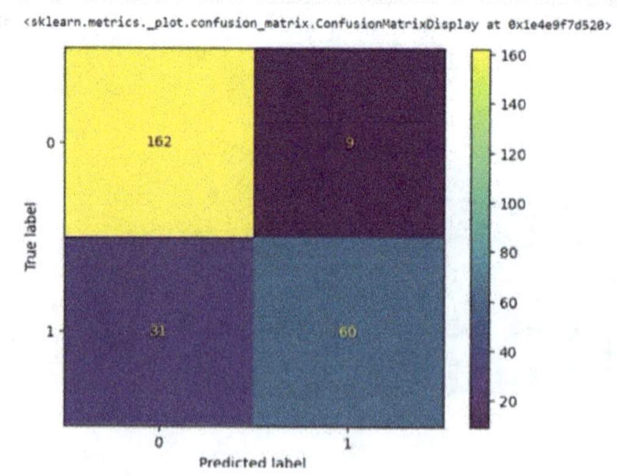

The result shows the overall result of the project. Here it shows accuracy for precision, recall, f1-score, and support.

Figure 8. Classification Report

	precision	recall	f1-score	support
0	0.84	0.95	0.89	171
1	0.87	0.66	0.75	91
accuracy			0.85	262
macro avg	0.85	0.80	0.82	262
weighted avg	0.85	0.85	0.84	262

7 DISCUSSION

Feature Importance: The "Why" Behind the Prediction

A key advantage of the Random Forest algorithm is its ability to provide insight into the factors driving its predictions. By measuring how much each feature contributes to reducing impurity across all the trees in the forest, we can rank their importance.

As indicated by numerous studies on this dataset, the model identifies a clear hierarchy of predictive factors.

1. **Glucose:** Unsurprisingly, Plasma Glucose Concentration is the single most important predictor. This aligns perfectly with the clinical definition of diabetes. It is the most direct measure of the body's inability to manage blood sugar, and its high importance confirms that the model's logic is grounded in established medical science.
2. **BMI:** Body Mass Index is the second most influential feature. This highlights the critical link between body weight, insulin resistance, and the development of Type 2 diabetes. For a caregiver, this is a powerful insight, as BMI is a modifiable risk factor that can be managed through diet and exercise.
3. **Age:** Age consistently ranks as a top predictor. This reflects the biological reality that the risk of developing Type 2 diabetes increases as the body's metabolic systems become less efficient over time.
4. **Insulin/Blood Pressure/Pedigree:** Following the top three, other features like insulin levels, family history, and blood pressure also contribute significantly to the model's decision-making process.

This feature importance analysis is not merely a technical output; it is a crucial component of building a trustworthy and explainable AI (XAI) tool. For a caregiver, seeing that a high-risk alert was triggered primarily by a rising BMI and consistently high glucose readings makes the tool's advice transparent and actionable. It helps them focus their efforts and conversations with doctors on the most critical health indicators, transforming the model from a mysterious "black box" into a collaborative partner in care

From Technical Results to Practical Application in Home Care

The quantitative results presented in the previous section, while academically significant, are only meaningful if they can be translated into real-world value for the family caregiver. An 85% accuracy score is not merely a number; it represents a potential pathway to empower caregivers, enhance the practice of integrative home care, and ultimately improve patient outcomes. This section moves from the "what" of the results to the "so what," discussing the practical implications of these findings, proposing a detailed conceptual framework for implementation, and frankly acknowledging the limitations and barriers that must be addressed to bridge the gap from a research model to a trusted, real-world tool.

Interpreting the Results for Family Caregivers

For a family caregiver, the core question is, "What does this mean for me and the person I care for?" The model's 85% accuracy suggests that it can serve as a reliable "co-pilot," offering an evidence-based second opinion on diabetes risk. It transforms risk assessment from a process based on intuition and sporadic clinical data to one informed by continuous, data-driven insight. However, the model's errors are just as important to understand. The trade-off between a "false alarm" (False Positive) and a "missed case" (False Negative) is a critical design consideration. A model tuned for higher recall (sensitivity) is arguably more desirable in a health context, as the consequence of a missed case—a delayed diagnosis—is far more severe than the consequence of a false alarm, which leads to a reassuring follow-up with a doctor. This principle of erring on the side of caution must be a cornerstone of any such tool's design philosophy.

A Conceptual Framework for Integration into Home Care

The Random Forest model itself is an analytical engine, not a complete vehicle. To become a useful tool, it must be embedded within a user-friendly, secure, and ethically designed application. The following framework outlines how such a system, which we might call "Care-Predict," could function.

The User Journey

The success of any digital health tool hinges on its usability. The user journey must be intuitive, empowering, and respectful of the caregiver's time and emotional energy.

1. **Onboarding and Setup:** The caregiver—let's call her Anjali again—downloads the "Care-Predict" app. The initial setup is designed to be simple and reassuring. She creates a secure profile for her father, Mr. Sharma, and inputs baseline, non-changing information: his age and relevant family history (which informs the Diabetes Pedigree Function). The app then guides her through a simple, one-time process of syncing his existing home health devices, such as a Bluetooth-enabled glucometer and a smart scale, using clear, illustrated instructions.
2. **Routine Data Input and Passive Monitoring:** The app is designed to minimize the caregiver's data entry burden. Mr. Sharma's weight and BMI are captured automatically each morning when he uses the smart scale. Anjali only needs to manually enter the post-meal glucose readings, which takes just a few seconds. The app's dashboard presents this information not as a sterile logbook, but as a series of clear trend lines, allowing her to see patterns at a glance.
3. **Receiving Intelligent Insights:** In the background, the machine learning model analyzes the incoming data stream. After a week where Mr. Sharma's post-meal glucose readings are consistently elevated and his BMI has trended slightly upward, the model's risk calculation surpasses a predefined "yellow" threshold.
4. **The Actionable Alert:** Anjali receives a gentle, non-alarming notification on her phone: *"Care-Predict Insight: We've noticed that Mr. Sharma's glucose and BMI trends have been higher than usual over the past week. This may indicate an increased risk. We recommend focusing on dietary consistency and scheduling a routine check-up with his doctor."*
5. **Empowerment, Not Diagnosis:** When Anjali taps the notification, the app provides more detail. It uses the model's feature importance to explain the alert: *"The main factors influencing this change are 'Glucose' and 'BMI'."* It then offers links to credible educational content on managing post-meal glucose spikes and healthy meal planning, empowering her with knowledge for her next conversation with the doctor.

Data Flow and Security

Building and maintaining user trust is paramount, which necessitates a robust security architecture.

- **Data Collection:** Data enters the system via two secure channels: manual input directly into the app and encrypted Bluetooth signals from synced health devices.
- **Data Transmission:** All data transmitted from the smartphone app to the backend cloud server is encrypted in transit using industry-standard protocols like Transport Layer Security (TLS). This prevents any interception of sensitive health information.
- **Data Storage and Processing:** Data is stored in a secure, HIPAA-compliant cloud environment (e.g., AWS, Google Cloud, or Azure). At rest, all personally identifiable information is encrypted. To further protect privacy, the data is de-identified before being fed to the machine learning model for processing. The model's output—the risk score—is then securely transmitted back to the user's specific device.
- **User Control and Consent:** The user is the sole owner of their data. The app's privacy policy, written in plain language, must clearly state how data is used. The user must have easy-to-access controls to view, export, and permanently delete their data at any time.

Barriers to Adoption

Despite the promise of such a tool, several significant real-world barriers must be overcome for widespread adoption and equitable impact.

- **Digital Literacy and Usability:** A primary challenge is that many caregivers, particularly older adults or those with less technological experience, may find smartphone applications intimidating. To overcome this, the app must be co-designed with input from these target users, prioritizing extreme simplicity, large fonts, clear navigation, and a minimal number of features. A successful design is one that feels supportive, not overwhelming.
- **Distrust in AI:** The concept of an algorithm making health assessments can be met with skepticism. Building trust is essential. This can be achieved through transparency—using the model's feature importance to explain *why* an alert was triggered—and through consistent messaging. The tool must always be positioned as a supportive aid for the caregiver and a data-gathering

tool for the clinician, never as an automated doctor that replaces human judgment.

- **Cost and Accessibility:** The cost of the necessary hardware, including a smartphone and connected health devices like smart scales and blood pressure cuffs, can be a prohibitive barrier for many low-income families. For this technology to be equitable, health systems, insurers, and governments must explore models for subsidizing or providing these essential tools, particularly if they are proven to reduce long-term healthcare costs by preventing complications.

Clinical Integration: Bridging the Home and the Clinic

A caregiver support tool cannot exist in a vacuum; it must be designed to integrate seamlessly into the existing clinical workflow to be truly effective. The goal is to enhance, not disrupt, the crucial relationship between the patient, caregiver, and healthcare provider.

The app should feature a secure "Share with Doctor" function. This would not just be a raw data dump, but a clinician-friendly summary report that can be generated as a PDF and securely emailed or shown to the doctor during a consultation. This report would be designed for quick comprehension, featuring:

- **Trend Visualizations:** Clear graphs showing the patient's glucose, BMI, and blood pressure trends over the last month or quarter.
- **Risk Score Progression:** A simple line graph showing how the model's risk assessment has changed over time.
- **Key Insights:** A bulleted list highlighting the main factors that influenced any recent increase in risk (e.g., "Risk score increased from 0.65 to 0.78 in the last two weeks, primarily driven by a 15% increase in average post-meal glucose readings.").

For a doctor or nurse, this report is incredibly valuable. It bridges the information gap between appointments, replacing subjective patient recall with objective, longitudinal data. It allows them to quickly differentiate between a single anomalous reading and a persistent, worrying trend. This makes consultations far more efficient and data-driven, enabling the clinician to provide more targeted advice and make more informed decisions about medication adjustments or further testing. The tool, therefore, becomes a powerful facilitator of communication, strengthening the collaborative partnership at the heart of the Integrative Home Care model.

8 CONCLUSION AND FUTURE SCOPE

The landscape of chronic disease management is fundamentally and irrevocably shifting from the clinic to the home, placing the family caregiver at the epicenter of modern healthcare. This chapter has sought to illuminate the immense, multi-faceted burden—physical, emotional, and financial—borne by these caregivers in the relentless, day-to-day management of diabetes. We have argued that while the challenge is significant, the convergence of home health technology and advanced machine learning analytics presents a transformative opportunity to provide meaningful, evidence-based support. The core thesis of this work is that technology's highest purpose in this context is not to replace the irreplaceable human element of care, but to augment and empower it, fostering an environment where empathy and evidence can coexist and mutually reinforce one another.

Throughout this chapter, we have journeyed from the foundational clinical realities of diabetes and the complexities of its diagnosis to the burgeoning world of digital health. We established a clear need for tools that can move beyond reactive monitoring to proactive, predictive insight. The detailed exploration of the Random Forest algorithm served as a practical case study, demonstrating that a machine learning model can be built with both high accuracy and a degree of interpretability. The achievement of 85% accuracy in the proof-of-concept model is not the end of the story, but the beginning. It validates the principle that the subtle patterns hidden within routine health data can be unlocked to forecast risk. The true significance of this finding was explored in the conceptual framework for the "Care-Predict" application—a vision for a tool that translates complex data into simple, actionable, and reassuring guidance for a non-medical user.

Ultimately, this chapter concludes that the successful integration of predictive tools into home care is not merely a technological challenge, but a humanistic one. It requires a deep understanding of the caregiver's journey, a steadfast commitment to ethical principles like data privacy and the mitigation of algorithmic bias, and a collaborative approach that strengthens the bond between patients, their families, and their clinical teams. The promise of machine learning in this domain is not to create an automated doctor, but to build an intelligent, ever-vigilant co-pilot for the caregiver, helping them navigate the complexities of chronic disease with greater confidence, less anxiety, and the profound reassurance that they are not alone.

Future Scope and Directions

While this chapter establishes a strong proof-of-concept, the path from an algorithmic model to a trusted, clinically integrated, and equitably accessible tool requires a dedicated, multi-stage research and development agenda. The future work outlined below represents a roadmap for transforming this potential into a tangible reality that can improve the lives of millions.

Short-Term Goals (1-2 Years): Prototype Development and Validation

The immediate next step is to move from the conceptual to the tangible by developing a functional prototype of the "Care-Predict" application. This initial phase must be grounded in the principles of human-centered design and iterative development.

- **Co-Design with End-Users:** The most critical activity is to engage family caregivers, diabetes nurse educators, and geriatric care specialists in a formal co-design process. This would involve interactive workshops where caregivers map their daily routines, identify key pain points, and storyboard their ideal support tool. This qualitative data is invaluable for ensuring the application's features, user interface (UI), and user experience (UX) are not dictated by engineers, but are sculpted by the real-world needs of its intended users.
- **Usability and Feasibility Studies:** Once a high-fidelity prototype is developed, it must undergo rigorous usability testing. This involves observing caregivers from diverse backgrounds as they interact with the app, asking them to "think aloud" as they navigate its features. This process helps identify points of confusion, frustration, or delight, leading to an evidence-based, iterative design process. Parallel feasibility studies would assess the practicality of syncing various home health devices and the reliability of data collection in a real-world home environment.
- **Integration of Explainable AI (XAI):** A core focus of the prototype development will be the integration of basic XAI features. Instead of being a "black box," the app's alerts should be accompanied by simple, transparent explanations derived from the model's feature importance rankings. For example, an alert might be followed by a message stating, *"This alert was triggered primarily because recent glucose readings have been 15% higher than the previous week's average."* This transparency is essential for building user trust and fostering health literacy.

Medium-Term Goals (2-5 Years): Rigorous Clinical Trials and Model Refinement

With a validated and user-friendly prototype, the focus must shift to proving clinical efficacy and safety through structured, ethical research.

- **Pilot Study:** A small-scale pilot study with a cohort of 30-50 patient-caregiver dyads would be conducted over a six-month period. The goals would be to test the end-to-end system, assess user engagement and adherence over time, and gather preliminary data on its impact on communication between the caregiver and the clinical team.
- **Randomized Controlled Trial (RCT):** Following a successful pilot, a large-scale RCT is the necessary next step to generate the high-quality evidence needed for clinical adoption and regulatory approval. This trial would enroll a diverse patient population and randomize them into two groups: an intervention group receiving standard care plus the "Care-Predict" tool, and a control group receiving only standard care. The primary and secondary endpoints for the trial would be multifaceted, measuring:

1. **Clinical Outcomes:** The primary clinical outcome would likely be the change in patients' HbA1c levels over a 12 to 18-month period, analyzed using an analysis of covariance (ANCOVA).
2. **Healthcare Utilization:** Secondary outcomes would include rates of diabetes-related emergency room visits and hospitalizations, with data analyzed to determine any statistically significant reductions.
3. **Caregiver-Reported Outcomes:** A crucial endpoint would be the change in caregiver burden, as measured by a validated instrument such as the Zarit Burden Interview. Other psychosocial metrics, such as the Patient Activation Measure (PAM) for patients and self-efficacy scales for caregivers, would also be collected.
4. **Health Economic Analysis:** A cost-effectiveness analysis would be run alongside the RCT to determine if the costs associated with the digital intervention are offset by savings from reduced hospitalizations and complications.

- **Model Retraining and Bias Mitigation:** The wealth of real-world, longitudinal data collected during these trials would be used to retrain, validate, and refine the underlying machine learning model. This process is vital for improving its accuracy and, most importantly, for ensuring it is fair and unbiased. The diverse data from the RCT would allow for auditing the model's performance across different ethnicities, age groups, and socioeconomic statuses, enabling targeted adjustments to mitigate any identified biases before wider deployment.

Long-Term Vision (5+ Years): Integration, Expansion, and Policy Impact

The ultimate vision is for this tool to become a seamless and integral part of the standard of care for chronic disease management at home.

Integration into Standard of Care: A clinically validated and regulatory-approved tool could be "prescribed" by healthcare providers as part of a standard diabetes management plan. Its data would integrate securely with institutional Electronic Health Records (EHRs), providing clinicians with a real-time, longitudinal dashboard view of their patients' health between visits, enabling a shift from reactive to proactive care.

Informing Healthcare Policy: Widespread and equitable adoption will require a supportive policy environment. The evidence on clinical efficacy and cost-effectiveness generated from the RCT would be used to advocate for policy changes. This includes lobbying for the creation of clear pathways for insurance and public health systems (e.g., Medicare, NHS) to reimburse for the use of validated digital health tools and caregiver support platforms. This data could also be used to make a strong case for public investment in digital literacy programs for older adults, ensuring that the benefits of these powerful new tools can reach all segments of the population.

REFERENCES

Alam, T. M., Iqbal, M. A., Ali, Y., Wahab, A., Ijaz, S., Ul Haq, E., & Baig, T. I. (2019). A model for early prediction of diabetes. *Informatics in Medicine Unlocked, 16*, 100204. DOI: 10.1016/j.imu.2019.100204

Cıhan, P., & Coskun, H. (2021, June). Performance comparison of machine learning models for diabetes prediction. In *2021 29th Signal Processing and Communications Applications Conference (SIU)* (pp. 1–4). IEEE. https://doi.org/DOI: 10.1109/SIU53274.2021.9477824

Emon, M. U., Keya, M. S., Kaiser, M. S., Islam, M. A., Tanha, T., & Zulfiker, M. S. (2021, March). Primary stage of diabetes prediction using machine learning approaches. In *2021 International Conference on Artificial Intelligence and Smart Systems (ICAIS)* (pp. 364–367). IEEE. https://doi.org/DOI: 10.1109/ICAIS50930.2021.9395968

Khaleel, F. A., & Al-Bakry, A. M. (2021). Diagnosis of diabetes using machine learning algorithms. *Materials Today: Proceedings, 47*(14), 4851–4854. DOI: 10.1016/j.matpr.2021.07.196

Khanam, J. J., & Foo, S. Y. (2021). A comparison of machine learning algorithms for diabetes prediction. *ICT Express, 7*(4), 432–439. DOI: 10.1016/j.icte.2021.02.004

Massari, E. L. H., Mhammedi, S., Sabouri, Z., & Gherabi, N. (2022). Ontology based machine learning to predict diabetes patients. In *Advances in information, communication and cybersecurity* (pp. 437–445). Springer, Cham. https://doi.org/DOI: 10.1007/978-3-030-91738-8_40

Mujumdar, A., & Vaidehi, V. (2019). Diabetes prediction using machine learning algorithms. *Procedia Computer Science, 165*, 292–299. DOI: 10.1016/j.procs.2020.01.047

Rady, M., Moussa, K., Mostafa, M., Elbasry, A., Ezzat, Z., & Medhat, W. (2021, October). Diabetes prediction using machine learning: A comparative study. In *2021 3rd Novel Intelligent and Leading Emerging Sciences Conference (NILES)* (pp. 279–282). IEEE. https://doi.org/DOI: 10.1109/NILES53778.2021.9600091

Sabouri, Z., Maleh, Y., & Gherabi, N. (2022). Benchmarking classification algorithms for measuring the performance on maintainable applications. In *Advances in information, communication and cybersecurity* (pp. 173–179). Springer., DOI: 10.1007/978-3-030-91738-8_17

Sarwar, M. A., Kamal, N., Hamid, W., & Shah, M. A. (2018, September). Prediction of diabetes using machine learning algorithms in healthcare. In *2018 24th International Conference on Automation and Computing (ICAC)* (pp. 1–6). IEEE. https://doi.org/DOI: 10.23919/IConAC.2018.8748992

Chapter 13
Causal Inference for Personalized Geriatric Well Being: A Bayesian Network Approach

M. Krishna
SASTRA University, India

S. Hariharan
https://orcid.org/0009-0000-1335-0200
SASTRA University, India

Hemalatha Karnan
https://orcid.org/0000-0003-2849-3102
SASTRA University, India

S. Balachandran
https://orcid.org/0000-0003-2782-6315
SASTRA University, India

ABSTRACT

In today's digital world, recommendation systems are like smart tools that make our online experiences better. Personalized recommendation systems have become a powerful tool for people who would rather improve and control their own health in the ever-changing healthcare environment of today. Even in situations when an individual is on their own, these systems leverage the power of digital technology and data analysis to provide personalized guidance and support for a range of healthcare tasks. Personalized recommendation systems provide customized solutions that consider the unique requirements and preferences of single people, whether the

DOI: 10.4018/979-8-3373-4094-4.ch013

issue is managing mental health concerns, adhering to a balanced diet, managing chronic illnesses, or sustaining physical activity. By using these systems to their full potential, people may take charge of their health and well-being, making educated decisions and achieving their healthcare goals with more confidence and efficiency.

1. INTRODUCTION

The pervasive integration of digital technology has brought about a revolutionary transformation across various aspects of modern life, fundamentally altering how people engage with healthcare, manage their well-being, and access medical information. Central to this digital revolution are healthcare recommendation systems—advanced computer programs that are adept at extracting valuable insights from vast healthcare datasets. This chapter aims to shed light on the critical role of recommendation systems as indispensable digital companions, simplifying decision-making processes in healthcare and enriching users' interactions with health-related information. Grounded in machine learning principles, the research utilizes algorithms for predicting class outcomes and integrates digital twin technology, which creates replicas of real-world entities or objects. The subsequent section delves into the intricate significance of healthcare recommendation systems, placing particular emphasis on their economic impact on healthcare providers and institutions, underscoring how the quality of personalized healthcare suggestions directly influences patient satisfaction, promotes adherence to health protocols, and ultimately shapes the effectiveness and success of healthcare organizations. Furthermore, this research highlights the practical applications of healthcare recommendation systems, serving as catalysts for ongoing research and improvement initiatives within the medical field. The motivation for this research stems from the concept of tailored assistance in healthcare, where recommendation systems aim to enhance users' health outcomes and overall well-being. The paper outlines objectives focused on promoting patient independence, prioritizing preventive wellness measures, managing self-care, and fostering social connections through personalized healthcare recommendations. The primary goal of the research is to develop a personalized healthcare recommendation system aimed at improving individual health outcomes. The overarching objective is to enhance patient experiences, encourage engagement, and facilitate informed decision-making across diverse medical domains. By leveraging intelligent computer programs and integrating patient input and medical data, the healthcare recommendation system continuously refines its suggestions to align with individual health preferences and requirements closely. The statistical methodology employed in this research is causal inference, which elucidates relationships and cause-and-effect dynamics within the variables. The objective is to leverage digital twin technology to extract meaningful aspects of individuals (Dratsiou et al., 2021). A digital twin is essentially a replica of a real-world entity or object, enabling the monitoring, analysis, and prediction of the corresponding real-world object or entity. By utilising this technology, we can integrate all characteristics of an individual into the analysis. SHAPES incorporates digital solutions in a three-phase process, incorporating user validation. Following this, there is a gradual deployment and thorough piloting to assess SHAPES' effectiveness in promoting healthy ageing and integrated care policies. Moving forward, the research aims to improve the Design and Preparation process, focusing on establishing a standardized EU platform. This platform is designed to aid older adults in sustaining health, activity, and independence, establishing SHAPES as an innovative initiative in addressing ageing challenges through the integration of digital technology (Shakhovska et al., 2019). This paper emphasizes that the global effort to enhance health management for seniors using mobile technology encounters a significant hurdle due to the underutilization of mHealth apps in this demographic. In recent research involving 74 seniors, user requirements for a senior-friendly mHealth app were identified using Nielsen's usability model, which addresses aspects such as learnability, efficiency, memorability, error management, and user satisfaction. The research's findings informed the development of a comprehensive guideline aimed at improving usability and health management features in mHealth (Haleem et al., 2023) apps. This guideline covers various elements, including phrasing, menus, simplicity, error messages, icons, buttons, navigation, and layout. Underlining the potential of speech recognition technology for quick information access, the proposed guideline provides valuable insights for software developers, guiding the creation of user-friendly mHealth apps tailored specifically for seniors. With the rising life expectancy, technology plays a crucial role in maintaining independence among the elderly. While mobile (Tajudeen et al., 2022) health apps are commonly used, adapting them to suit the specific needs of older individuals poses a challenge. This article introduces a smartphone application designed for older adults dealing with balance disorders, aiming to empower users through self-evaluation and promote communication and engagement with integrated motivational features. The assessment of mock-up interfaces took place in three European countries, and the subsequent phase involves four pilot studies with 160 participants. The evaluation will employ both qualitative and quantitative measures to gather feedback on the app's effectiveness. Importantly, this application is a component of a multifactorial intervention dedicated to enhancing the well-being of the elderly. Developing a mobile app for home-based rehabilitation aimed at assisting and personalizing experiences for the elderly is valuable. The goal is to create a user-friendly mobile application that empowers users, enhancing their lives and fostering a sense of independence (Androutsou et al., 2020).. The research highlights the effectiveness of using both simple and complex causal networks for stakeholder communication. Key points stress the practicality of this approach in initial impact scoping for multidisciplinary teams. Three areas for enhancement include evaluating causal relationships, involving stakeholders throughout the process, and integrating ecological frameworks to expand environmental pathways (Malakar et al., 2023). The paper delves into how the CaNeTA methodology improves fire safety in multi-tenancy retail, tackling shortcomings in current Fire Safety Engineering (FSE) tools. CaNeTA is introduced as an inventive remedy, establishing a causal network that interconnects individual fire safety systems to offer a comprehensive understanding. Emphasis is placed on the significance of scrutinizing network results to evaluate the overall system performance. CaNeTA suggests optimizations based on critical system statuses to bolster fire safety strategies. To sum up, CaNeTA is portrayed as an impartial tool that aids in fire safety design while mitigating existing methodological limitations (Lin et al., 2023). The paper emphasizes the importance of recommender systems and their use of correlation-based methods for extracting user preferences. It acknowledges the limitation of relying solely on correlation in a causally driven world. The text outlines the fundamental principles of recommendation and causal inference, providing a foundation for further discussions and mentioning challenges in non-causality recommendation (Gasse et al., 2014). Also, some papers are used this methodology for medical purpose also like researching the relationship between dietary habits and five major mental disorder using the two-sample Mendelian randomization analysis instead of causal inference this paper uses the correlation analysis between the variables there is a negative correlation within the variables which leads them to conclude that to give Gluten-free diet to the patient with the help of causal relationship (Du et al., 2023). Additionally, the Bayesian network analysis is also useful for the conditional probabilities within the variables to get the causal inference of the nodes (Li et al., 2023). The research tackles the deficiency in effective therapies for dementia by concentrating on preventive measures. Pervasive cognitive decline culminates in irreversible dementia among individuals in mid-life or older. Despite the challenges in pinpointing specific markers, there is indicative evidence of modifiable risk factors in older adults, potentially during the prodromal stage of dementia. Cognitive changes and the incidence of dementia are influenced by factors such as socioeconomic status, behavior, diet, and lifestyle. Through a Bayesian Network Meta-Analysis involving 43 cohort studies, the research uncovers connections between dementia and factors like "sleep disturbance," "education," "diabetes," "obesity," "smoking," "solitude," "physical exercise," "alcohol," and "hypertension." Notably, the research finds no correlation between the use of antioxidants and the incidence of dementia (Liang et al., 2020). The research addresses challenges in identifying discrete causal relationships, especially in genome-wide association studies (GWAS). Traditional statistical methods struggle with interactions among discrete causes affecting a target. Algorithms like MBS-IGain and the new Exhaustive-IGain aim to discover such interactions. Exhaustive-IGain, with its comprehensive search, outperforms MBS-IGain on datasets involving 3 and 4-cause interactions without marginal effects. It is successfully applied to examine how clinical variables impact breast cancer survival, aligning with expert oncologists' judgments. The research emphasizes the effectiveness of integrating information gain and Bayesian network scoring to uncover higher-order interactions without marginal effects, particularly in practical applications with real data (Zeng et al., 2016). A survey (Ali et al., 2024) on data imbalance to predict fatal conditions due to accidents gives an elaborate idea regarding issues of attaining ML-based performance. The literature review underscores the increasing prominence of Bayesian Networks (BNs) in navigating uncertainty, especially in practical applications. BNs are esteemed for tackling intricate queries using hypothetical evidence. A pivotal hurdle lies in delineating the graphical structure of BNs, particularly when dealing with causal assumptions. The survey delineates potential solutions, examining 74 combinatorial algorithms for acquiring BN structure, with a focus on their distinct approaches. It delves into techniques for assessing algorithmic performance, handling consistency issues, managing data noise, and integrating expert knowledge into the BN learning process (Kitson et al., 2023). The literature survey presents a teaching approach for causal inference using Bayesian networks and do- do-calculus across various course levels. Highlighting the importance of probabilistic reasoning and causal assumptions, it differentiates between causal and statistical inference, advocating for consistent implementation with the same tool and language across courses. To support adoption, the authors offer five demonstration examples to enhance students' comprehension of causality, illustrate distinctions, and promote further exploration, encompassing real-world applications. The survey highlights the importance of recognizing and differentiating between causal and statistical inference, empirical foundations and the deductive nature of causal inference. It underscores the significance of considering causal structures during interventions (Chen et al., 2023).

The Activities of Daily living ADL for geriatric well-being is to be improved with a multi-dimensional outcome encompassing cognitive status, recognizing fall risks and establishing social connections with the first responsible person. The Quality-of-Life QoL must be enriched by integration of the prediction models with acquisition systems. The more appropriate style will be to strengthen the advancements in Man-Machine interfaces. The current scenario carries the claims of such human-machine interactions with the interventions of electronic health records and wearable body-worn sensors. The outcome of all these proposals will be a success if the caregiver in the ambience is well educated on the policies of risk assessment and management strategies. The handling of elderly individuals must be considered, as the WHO report states that 5.7 to 8.4 million deaths are reported from inadequate quality care rendered to the elderly. In addition to these statistics, they say that by 2030, one out of six people will be a victim of loneliness and social isolation. The technological advancement to confront time-varying or delaying healthcare aid is to be addressed by the causal graph models (Abécassis et al., 2025) with higher-end personalized access. In trials and datasets used to train AI, older adults (very old, frail, cognitively impaired, institutionalized) are under-sampled, which can result in models that encode bias or may not generalize. This has been identified as a fairness issue by recent ethics and regulatory reviews (Mennella et al., 2024). A step towards Human oversight is essential that paves the way to, any changes to an automated care plan must be approved by a clinician or caregiver thereby necessitating a track of who made the decision and why. These controls are recommended by recent reviews of ethics and regulations in work (Parchmann et al., 2024). Ethical issues include autonomy, where algorithmic suggestions may go against what the patient wants; consent validity, especially for people whose cognitive abilities are getting worse; and algorithmic ageism, where datasets don't include enough of the oldest or weakest adults, which leads to biassed results (Singh & Keche, 2025). To deal with these risks, more people are suggesting frameworks for privacy-preserving learning, like federated learning, differential privacy, and on-device analytics. AI literacy programs for older adults can also help them take part in data governance in an informed way (Mennella et al., 2024). The existing models such as Do-calculus method incorporates a recognized symbolic instruction to derive causal effects from a Directed Acyclic Graph (DAG). The pitfall in the above method is that it doesn't support visualization and contrary to fact queries related to cause of risk is not addressed. The Bayesian probability method relies on uncertainty and drawing inference is made only based on the non-interventional data. The United Nations World Population prospects (2024) identify that an anticipated population rise to 16% will be into effect by 2050. The Asian and European population poses a demographic strain on digital healthcare systems demanding technological inventions related to quantizable data-driven approaches for independent aging and tailored monitoring applications. The sample selection and inclusion of elderly individuals is very meagre. Additionally, in Japan and South Korea, robotic rehabilitation systems like the Cyberdyne HAL-Suit (Tan et al., 2025) use reinforcement learning and causal feedback loops to improve motion assistance based on data about how each muscle is activated. These systems put causal reasoning into action in real-world therapeutic adaptation by connecting biomechanics, intervention dose, and recovery outcomes. The Government policies of Singapore and Finland have directed digital literacy hands on training with the aid of programmes such as "Smart Aging". The advancements in Digital India schemes focuses on AI enabled precision diagnostics and elderly healthcare. Herewith the societal readiness and willingness for participation in technological interventions is addressed. The WHO AI ethics (World Health Organization, 2024) principles have recently initiated harmonized frameworks for meeting out the conflicting national AI health policies globally. Apart from the scientific aims infrastructure limitations like rural and low resourcefulness settings lack access to the central framework and data storage. The abovementioned issue can be handled using local data hubs for intimating the caregivers with less storage and memory usage for data transmission. Real world deployment helps to bridge the gap between medical care and to also adopt digital literacy tactics (El Arab et al., 2025). Adhering to the above research gaps, the proposed algorithm helps build a human in the loop model connecting patients and caregivers termed as first responsible persons (FPR). The data privacy issues and ethical constraints (19) are imbibed in the response alert message that must be delivered to FPR. Necessary actions were also ensured by allowing access to only the registered FPR for the respective geriatric community.

1.1 Comparison of Integrative Analysis Works for Elderly Health Monitoring & Feedback Systems

The Table 1 below summarizes recent research articles assessing techniques, restraints, and suggested future work for integrative health monitoring and feedback systems aimed at senior adults.

Table 1. Review of the recent literature

Article (citation)	Techniques (AI/ML/DL)	Limitations	Future work
Ahmed S., et al., "Remote Health Monitoring Systems for Elderly People" Sensors (2023). (Ahmed et al., 2023)	ML classifiers (SVM, Random Forest), signal processing, IoT data fusion.	Diverse data standards, limited real-world deployment details, privacy concerns.	Standardization, longitudinal real-world validation, privacy-preserving analytics.
Morita P.P., et al., "Health Monitoring Using Smart Home Technologies" JMIR mHealth uHealth (2023). (Morita et al., 2023)	Activity recognition via ML, rule-based systems, ambient and wearable sensor fusion.	Sensor placement variability, user acceptance, sparse labeled datasets for elderly behaviors.	Semi-supervised learning, user-centered designs to improve acceptance, adaptive personalization.
Lee Y., et al., "Deep Learning-Based Fall Monitoring among Older Adults" (2023, PMC). (Lee et al., 2023)	Deep learning (CNNs, RNNs/BiLSTM) on wearable and vision data; multimodal fusion.	High computational cost, limited explainability, dataset bias toward lab scenarios.	Edge-efficient models, explainable DL, large-scale in-home trials.
Wang K., "Application of artificial intelligence in active assisted living" (ScienceDirect, 2024). (Wang et al., 2024)	NLP for interaction, ML for anomaly detection, reinforcement learning for assistive policies.	Integration complexity, standardization gaps, ethical/regulatory hurdles.	Interoperability frameworks, ethical-by-design approaches, regulatory-aligned deployments.

continued on following page

Table 1. Continued

Article (citation)	Techniques (AI/ML/DL)	Limitations	Future work
Efendi A., et al., "IoT-Based Elderly Health Monitoring System" (Health Sci Rep, 2025). (Efendi et al., 2025)	IoT data pipelines, lightweight ML models for vitals and activity classification.	Network dependency, battery life constraints for wearables, limited scalability testing.	Low-power sensing, federated learning for privacy, scalable cloud-edge designs.
Vision-Based Monitoring System for Elderly Care Using CNN+BiLSTM (2025). (Philips et al., 2025)	Computer vision (CNN), temporal models (BiLSTM), real-time alerting.	Privacy concerns with cameras, occlusions in homes, need for labeled video data.	Privacy-preserving vision (on-device), synthetic data augmentation, multimodal fusion.

The selected studies from the years 2023 to 2025 show a very well-defined trend toward multimodal sensing using wearables, ambient sensors, and vision. Other very common applications are machine learning and deep learning for activities of daily living recognition, fall detection, and anomaly detection. Some of the very common limitations include bias toward datasets collected in a controlled environment, privacy and ethical concerns, particularly with vision-based systems, practical deployment challenges owing to battery life, network reliability, and user acceptance among older adults. Key future directions identified point to: (Ahmed et al., 2023) privacy-preserving and explainable AI, (Morita et al., 2023) edge and low-power models suitable for on-device inference, (Lee et al., 2023) federated or decentralized learning to protect user data, (Wang et al., 2024) longitudinal real-world trials to validate the effectiveness, and (Efendi et al., 2025) user-centered co-design to improve adoption and usability in older adults.

2. METHODOLOGIES

2.1 Dataset Preparation

In the domain of machine learning, preprocessing methods form the cornerstone of developing robust models. Among these techniques, label encoding plays a pivotal role in converting categorical data into a numerical format, enabling algorithms to process information efficiently. This approach involves assigning a unique integer to each distinct category present in the dataset, thereby establishing a direct correspondence between categorical labels and numerical representations. For instance, let's consider a categorical variable like "Age," which comprises categories such as "less than 18," "more than 18," and "Ages above 25." By employing label encoding, every category receives a specific integer, streamlining subsequent analysis and modeling endeavors.

$$LabelEncoder(ci) = i \qquad (1)$$

where ***ci*** represents each distinct category within the set of categories, and *ii* denotes the assigned unique integer. For example, for a categorical variable "Age" with categories "less than 18," "more than 18," and "Ages above 25," the label encoder may represent these categories as:

$$LabelEncoder\ (\text{less than } 18) = 1 \qquad (2)$$

$$LabelEncoder\ (\text{more than } 18) = 2$$
(3)

$$LabelEncoder\ (\text{Ages above}25) = 3 \qquad (4)$$

Moving forward, normalization becomes a pivotal preprocessing step aimed at ensuring consistent treatment of numerical features. Among the widely adopted normalization techniques, Min-Max normalization and Z-score normalization stand out. Min-Max normalization adjusts the data to a predefined range, typically spanning from 0 to 1. It achieves this by subtracting the minimum value and dividing it by the range. In contrast, Z-score normalization, also referred to as standardization, centers the data around a mean of 0 and adjusts it based on the standard deviation. These normalization approaches serve a crucial role in mitigating the impact of varying feature scales, thus preventing certain features from exerting undue influence on the learning process.

Min-Max normalization scales the data to a specific range, typically between 0 and 1, using the formula:

In scenarios where datasets exhibit imbalances, with certain categories being underrepresented, resampling techniques like oversampling become indispensable. Oversampling specifically entails boosting the occurrences of the minority class by either creating synthetic samples or replicating existing ones. This rebalancing of the class distribution is crucial for improving the performance and resilience of machine learning models, especially in contexts where precise classification of minority classes holds significant importance.

2.2 Analysis of Data With Bayesian Network

A new synthetic sample can be generated using the formula:

$$X\text{new} = \alpha \cdot X1 + (1 - \alpha) \cdot X2 \qquad (5)$$

where $X1$ and $X2$ are two randomly chosen instances from the minority class, and $\alpha\alpha$ is a random number between 0 and 1.

The conditional probability formula for P (A|B, C) is given by:

Here is a breakdown of the terms:

$P(A \mid B, C)$: This represents the conditional probability that a person is shown in Figure 1 and adherent to medication

(A) given that they take medicine at a specific time (B) and take a specific type of medicine (C).

$P(A \cap B \cap C)$: This denotes the probability that a person is adherent to medication and takes medicine at a specific time and a specific type.

$P(B \cap C)$: This is the probability that a person takes medicine at a specific time and a specific type, regardless of adherence. To compute $P(A \mid B, C)$, you can utilize your dataset to determine the occurrences of these events and apply the formula accordingly.

Figure 1. Conditional probability of (,)

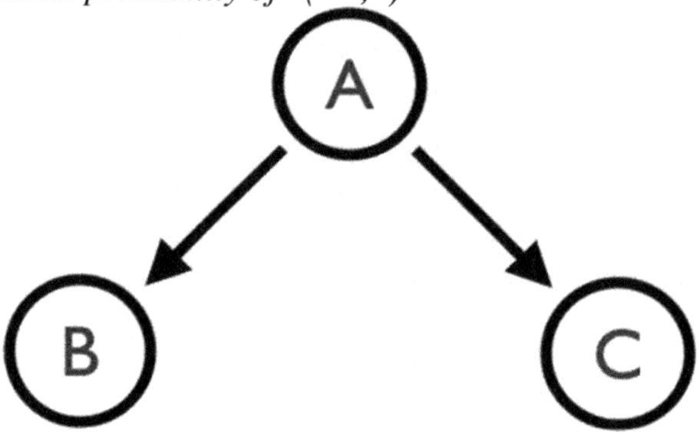

Causal networks, illustrated through directed graphs, offer a visual depiction of the causal connections between variables within a system. These networks serve as valuable tools for comprehending how specific factors influence each other, whether directly or indirectly. Through causal inference methods, like Bayesian networks, researchers can uncover insights into treatment effects, interventions, and the underlying mechanisms driving observed outcomes. Bayesian networks utilize directed acyclic graphs to model probabilistic dependencies among variables, facilitating the estimation of conditional probabilities and causal relationships.

To illustrate, let's consider an example within my dataset where certain variables impact others. For instance, let's take age (X) directly influencing marital status (Y). The conditional probability

P(Y|X) represents the probability distribution of Y given the value of X. Essentially, it informs us about the likelihood of observing Y when X is known. This formula signifies that the occurrence of Y is influenced by the specific value of X. Such cause-and-effect relationships can be graphically represented within a network.

Figure 2. Causal Connection Between Two Variables

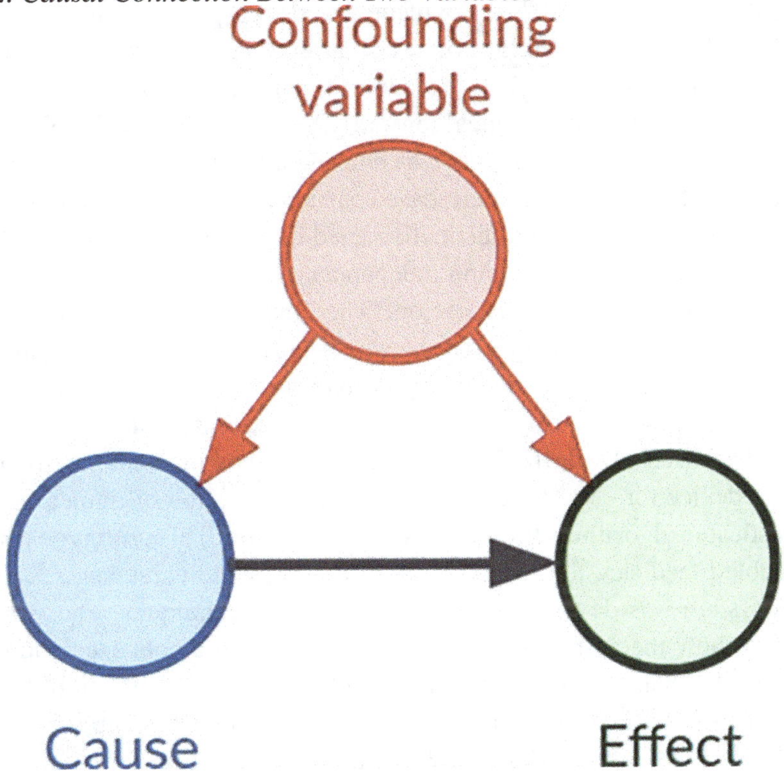

To elucidate causal inference with Bayesian networks, let us examine a straightforward example involving two variables: A (cause) and B (effect) shown in Figure 2. The goal is to deduce the cause-and-effect connection between A and B.

Where, **A** is the "How many medicine," **B** is the "Medicating time."

The distribution of conditional probabilities for B given A is denoted as P(B|A). The Bayesian network encapsulates this relationship as follows:

$$P(B \mid A) = P(B \mid paB) \quad (6)$$

Here, $\boldsymbol{P(B|A)}$ signifies the probability under a given condition of B given A, and $\boldsymbol{PaB}$ represents the predecessors of the node B within the context of the Bayesian network.

2.3 Deployment Technique Utilized

In the final phase of model deployment, practical aspects become crucial. The work handled by (Lu et al., 2025) utilizes Smarter Safer Homes platform incorporating open Internet of Things (IoT) protocols to share the specific findings given by commercially available physiological sensors (Zhang et al., 2022). The Randomised controlled trail for aged participants was considered to study the depressive state of the participants. The demographic-based participants were selected from metropolitan and regional areas from distinctive aged care service providers. The work aided in monitoring and maintaining independence in establishing Quality of Life QoL in their respective residential sectors. The limitation of this work was bias in physical intervention like usage of sensors which has to be carried by the participants for 24 X 7. The reminder for intake of pharmaceuticals was not meted out in this work. The gap exists in alerting the caregivers and educating them for immediate responses. SHUBHCHINTAK (Banerjee et al., 2022) an innovative remote health monitoring device for elderly persons utilizes an integration of numerous sensors and sophisticated algorithms for inconsistency detection. This prototype constructs a data enabled feedback loop to alert the individuals and caretakers. A real time detection system was developed with deep learning techniques. The work has a limitation of how the system works the transmission protocols used and delivery status to the clinicians and patients. The strength of the work is that it utilizes three distinctive front-end interfaces encompassing the administrator, subject and a clinician. The work by (Hasan & Ahmed, 2024) uses a smart glove for quick responses to be delivered to the unaccompanied aged individuals. More emphasize is made on par with the physiological vital monitoring rather than the regular activity and psychological analysis. The research above emphasized the prodigious increase in the continuous monitoring medical assistive devices design and demand globally. A step forward by this work has been the inclusion of a critical component IFTTT (If-This-Then-That) Integration – "The Communication Hub" for data transmission and alert management. A multiple alert system is also utilized in this module. This multi-channel approach ensures that emergency alerts reach caregivers, family members, and healthcare providers through their preferred communication methods, significantly improving response times during critical situations. The system's architecture supports continuous remote monitoring, allowing healthcare providers and family members to track the elderly person's health status from any location. The IFTTT-enabled communication system ensures that all stakeholders receive real-time updates about the user's condition, creating a comprehensive care network. The research demonstrates significant potential for enhancing elderly care quality through smart, integrated, and user-friendly healthcare solutions. The combination of multiple monitoring capabilities in a single wearable device, coupled with the robust IFTTT-based communication system, creates a comprehensive safety net for elderly individuals. Utilizing tools like IFTTT (If This, Then That) to send personalized medication reminders showcases the tangible application of machine learning models in healthcare. By integrating model predictions with user- friendly applications like mobile notification systems, healthcare providers can significantly enhance medication adherence and ultimately improve patient outcomes. This journey from data preprocessing to model deployment exemplifies a holistic approach to leveraging the potential of machine learning in healthcare and other domains.

2.4 Policy Making Protocols for Actionable Outcomes

A drastic demographic shift in the population ageing is noticeable due to sustained stress on the medico-care systems to provide a high-quality lifestyle for older people. An emerging field of Evidence-based practice (EBP) in gerontology integrates the academic/research practices, clinical specialists and privacy of patients, valuing their societal well-being. The major limitation in the elderly community is the prevalence of comorbidities, manifold pharmacy practices and self-denial, which makes the translation of inventions to social implementation in hospital administration sectors. The acceptance ratio of hospitalisation is declining among older patients, as it results in immobility and functional decline. The demand for adequate staff for personalized elderly care and an adaptable hospital ambience is also an important factor in geriatric well-being. To address this, specific integrative care units have to be developed. The existence of clinical guides, namely *Care-of-the-Elderly Health Guide,* synthesizes current recommendations across geriatric syndromes (Triscott et al., 2021). Additionally, NICHE (Nurses Improving Care for Healthsystem Elders) (Gilmartin, 2023) programs foster geriatric best routines through organized attention interventions. At the guidelines level, strategies like WHO's Integrated Care for Older People (ICOPE) (World Health Organization, 2017) run through community and hospital-level intermediations to uphold core capacity, assist caregivers, and observe health. The Comprehensive Geriatric Assessment (CGA) model unifies and assesses curative, operational, cognitive, and social domains for personalized healthcare plans. The defect was a heterogeneous outcome and an inconsistency in the sample participant population. A comparative study (Pereira et al., 2025) on workload and financial management was conducted in a German hospital. The study illustrated that while multidisciplinary cooperation can enhance patient outcomes, the challenges posed by inflexible reimbursement policies and a high workload can hinder the sustainability of such improvements. The (Mini, 2024) NICHE ideation is tried across several hospitals to explain how evidence-based workflow protocols can regiment a multi-specialty busy hospital thereby also focusing on geriatric well-being. The WHO emphasizes intellectual support to be educated for caregivers rather than clinical intervention alone. Apart from the above-mentioned criteria, psychological guidance and sustenance for informal caregivers minimize the work burden on such supporting staff and improvise their volunteer ship. The technological insights discussed in the trailing sections will provide a versatile application specific approach for knowledge aided integrative care to be delivered to the geriatrics. The availability of smartphones and a low data usage network is substantial for the implementation of the work proposed. The workflow has a section of instructions in regional language namely, Tamil, in addition to the English vocabulary which makes the work more receptable to all socio-economic sectors. In future, the extrapolation of instructions as voice note and also in other regional languages of India might improve the commercialization of this work. Integrating the suggestions and technical innovations will help in idealizing evidence-based healthcare assistance to be disseminated to the aged population who intend to lead an independent life.

3. RESULTS AND DISCUSSIONS

3.1 Dataset Description

From the above Causal Bayesian network, we must check the connection between the nodes of my data set which has been collected through google form and it contains 24 attributes. The nodes are configured to symbolize various attributes, encompassing labels, while the edges illustrate the directional connections among these attributes presented in Table 2.

Table 2. Dataset description

Dataset	No. of Attributes	No. of rows
Collected data	24	124
Data after oversampling	24	832

3.2 Inferences From The Causal Network

Utilizing the causal (Pearl, 2024) network has been helpful, giving us important insights into our dataset. One key discovery is that the "Age" variable directly affects things like "Marital status," "Types of medication," and "Psychological Difficulties." This helps us gain a deeper understanding of the relationship between age and these factors show the complex web of connections in our data. When we look at Figure3, we can see the dense layer of the causal network, which is quite detailed. It has 24 points and a remarkable 522 lines, showing many connections between different parts of our dataset. What is interesting is that these connections form naturally, without any specific rules, highlighting the complex relationships in our data. Incorporating different threshold values into our causal network analysis proves to be a valuable technique for unearthing essential insights within our dataset. These thresholds function as selective mechanisms, enabling us to concentrate on specific relationships and connections that align with our research objectives. Essentially, they help us sift through the data, distinguishing the significant signals from the background noise. For example, when we establish a threshold of 0.5, it becomes a pivotal boundary. Relationships and connections within the causal network with strengths falling below this threshold are regarded as less pertinent to our current analysis. Consequently, certain nodes within the dense layer are systematically pruned or removed from our consideration. Thus, simplifying the procedure of deriving significant insights. and informed decisions based on causal relationships of utmost importance.

Figure 3. Fully connected layer

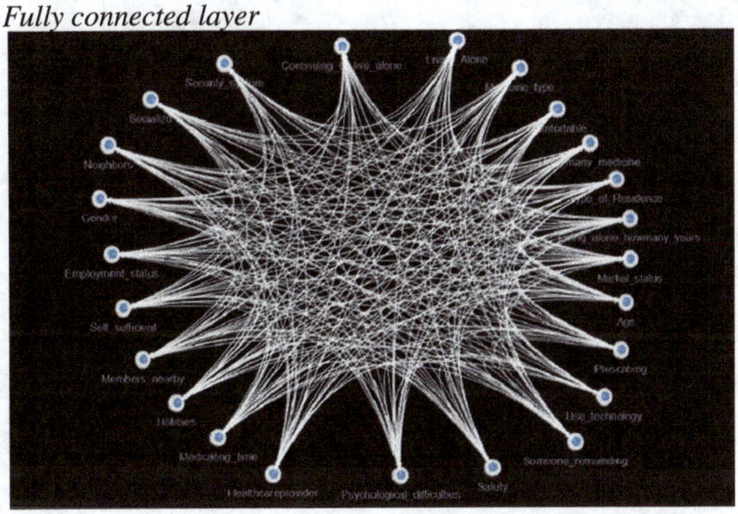

Upon implementing a threshold value of 0.5 shown in Figure 4, we observe the removal of certain nodes within the structure shown in Figure 5. This leads us to infer that there might be misinterpretations in the nodes, where certain connections do not appear to be logical. For instance, the relationship between "Age" and "Gender" seems inexplicable. Such instances where connections lack coherence can be addressed with the assistance of domain knowledge. We have the flexibility to adjust the network structure by adding or removing nodes that are connected erroneously, aligning it more accurately with our understanding of the underlying relationships. Observing the above figure, it becomes evident that a modification has been implemented, resulting in the formation of a significant subgraph within the fully connected layer shown in Figure 3. This suggests that these nodes are the most frequently occurring ones in the data, influencing other nodes. While there is the option to increase the threshold value, it's worth noting that, for my research, the 0.5 threshold value proves to be optimal. The obtained graph provides us with the largest subgraph, which becomes instrumental in making predictions using the Bayesian estimator.

Figure 4. Threshold value (0.5)

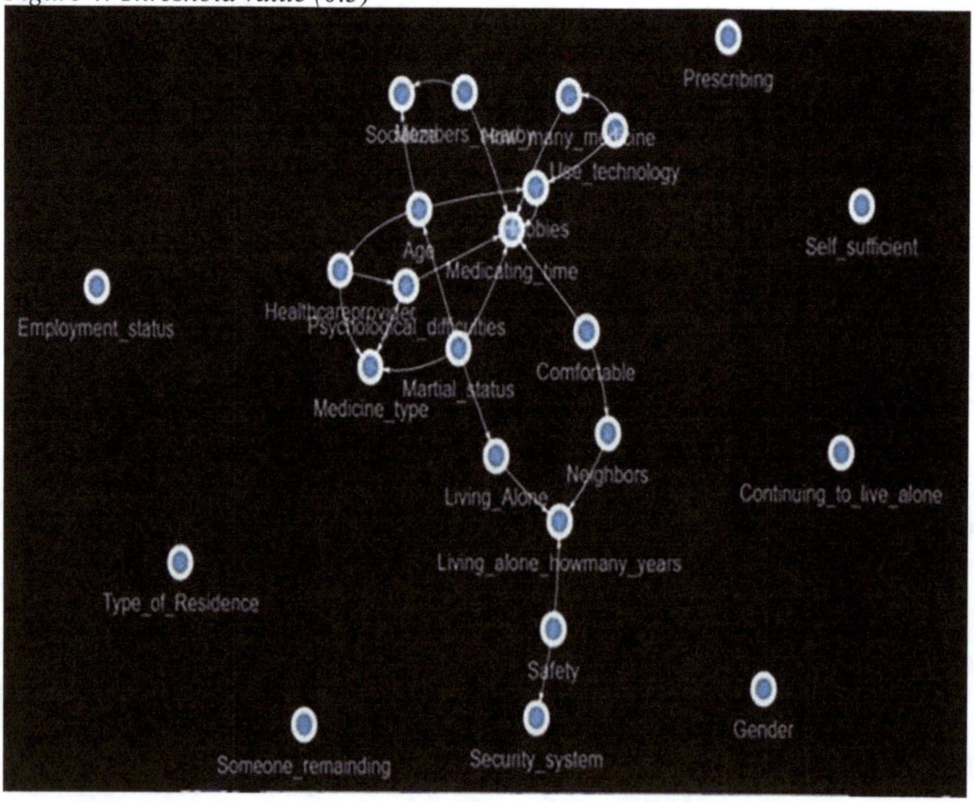

Figure 5. Modified structurerr

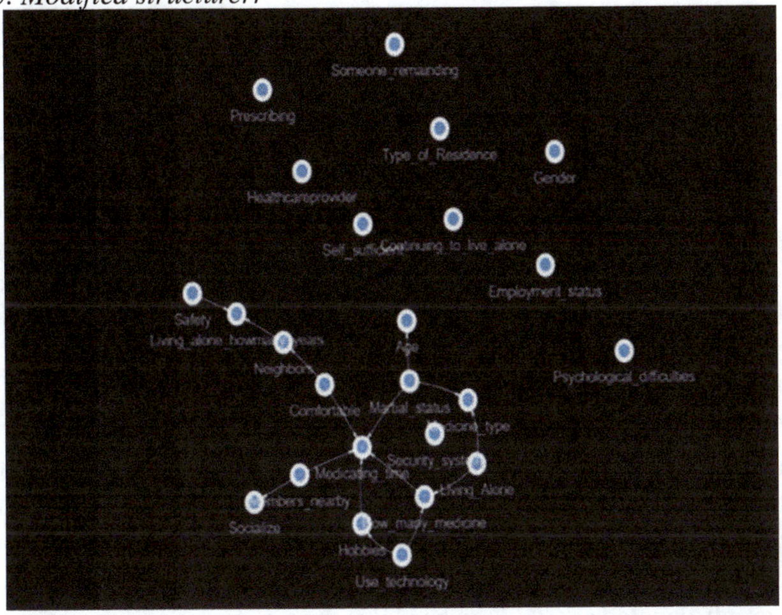

Figure 6. Largest subgraph

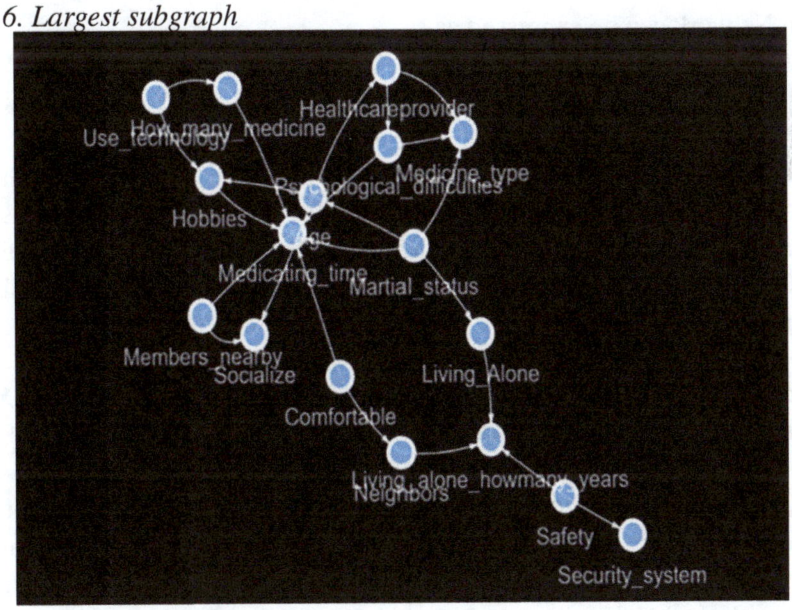

3.3 Model Implementation

Once we've obtained the largest subgraph shown in Figure 6, the subsequent phase involves making predictions based on the dataset. To achieve this, we calculate conditional probabilities and employ the Bayesian estimator, along with K2 regularization, to facilitate predictions while mitigating overfitting risks. In this context, our focus is on predicting a single feature: the number of medicines to be taken on a given day, which serves as the predictive element from the predictor. The model we've trained achieves an accuracy rate of 89% for its predictions. To assess the model's performance, we divided the dataset into training sets and testing sets.

i. Bayesian Network

A Bayesian network is a graphical model that organizes uncertain information systematically (Chobtham et al., 2023), (Constantinou et al., 2023) each node corresponds to a random variable, and the connections between nodes (edges) indicate the probabilistic relationships among these variables. The Bayesian Network is characterized by a graph, denoted as *G(V,E),* where V is the set of nodes representing random variables, and E is the set of directed edges representing conditional dependencies. For each node X in V, there exists a conditional probability distribution denoted

P(X|parents(X)), where parents(X) represent the set of parent nodes of X. The Bayesian Network can be expressed as

$$P(V) = \prod P(X \mid parents(X)), \qquad (7)$$

Where V represents all nodes in the network. The construction of the Bayesian Network involves feeding the largest graph at the threshold of 0.5 with the dataset. The dataset is split into test and train sets to train the network and use it for predictions.

The formula for Bayesian Estimation of Conditional Probability Distributions (CPDs) is given by:

$$P(X \mid parents(X)) = Count(X, parents(X)) + prior \,/\, Count(parents(X)) + (number\ of\ states\ of\ X) \times prior \qquad (8)$$

Here, X represents a node in the network, parents(X) represent the set of parent nodes of Count(X,parents(X)) represent the observed counts from the training data. From the equation an acyclic graph is drawn with the help of the Bayesian network classifier with the help of the over sampled data further the data is split into train and test data where the conditional probabilities are calculated with the train data and the test data is used for predicting the variable “How many medicine” and the accuracy form the testing data is 89%.,The "support" denotes the actual occurrence count of each class in the specified dataset.

The classification report and the confusion matrix of the Bayesian network are shown in Figure 7 and Figure 8.

Figure 7. Classification report for Bayesian network classifier

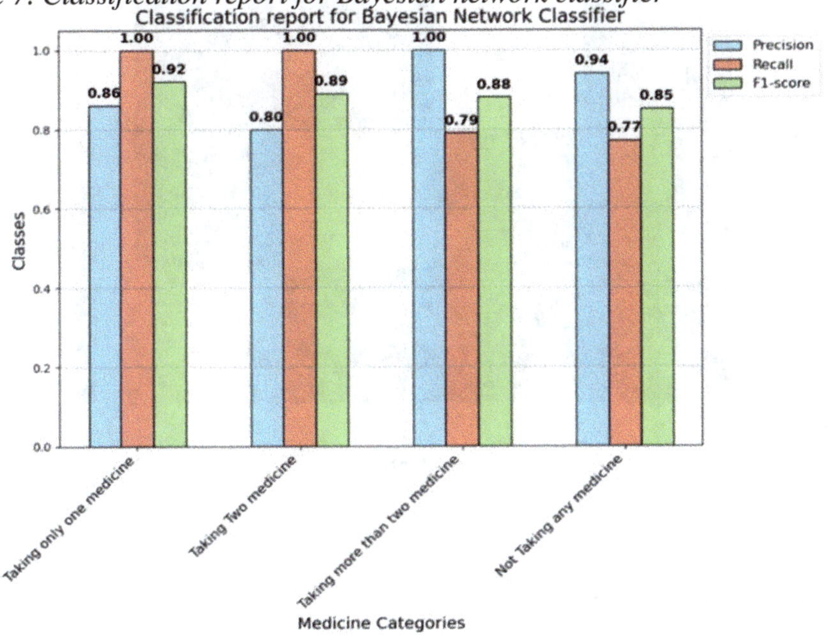

Figure 8. Prediction for Bayesian network classifier from the test data

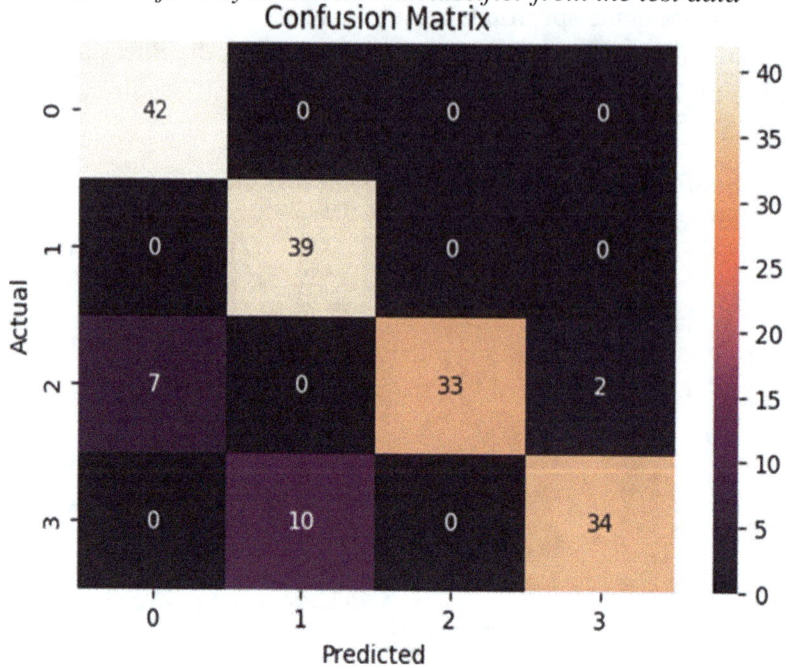

ii. Logistic Regression

The logistic regression is fitted with the preprocessed data, it is used for binary classification, specifically focusing on predicting the variable 'How_many_medicine.' The initial phase involves preparing the data, extracting pertinent features such as age, gender, marital status, living arrangements, social habits, safety perceptions, healthcare accessibility, and technology usage from the DataFrame 'c.' Less significant features are then removed to streamline the model. The dataset undergoes division into training and testing sets utilizing the train_test_split function. To maintain consistent performance, feature scaling is implemented using StandardScaler. Subsequently, a logistic regression model with regularization is established, with the regularization parameter C set to 0.1, and it is trained on the scaled training data. Predictions are generated for the testing set, and the model's performance is thoroughly assessed using a confusion matrix. The confusion matrix is visually depicted through a heatmap, illustrating true positive, true negative, false positive, and false negative predictions. The classification report and the confusion matrix is shown in Figure 9 and Figure 10. Additionally, a comprehensive classification report is produced, encompassing metrics such as precision, recall, and F1- score. In summary, this code snippet meticulously scrutinizes the logistic regression model's efficacy in classifying instances based on the identified features.

Mathematically, the logistic function is expressed as:

$$P(Y = 1) = 1/1 + e - (b0 + b1X1 + b2X2 + \cdots + bnXn)$$
(9)

Here:

$P(Y=1)$ denotes the probability of the dependent variable (Y) being 1.

e represents the base of the natural logarithm.

b0 is the bias or intercept term.1,2,…,b1,b2,…,bn are the coefficients associated with the features 1,2,…,X1,X2,…,Xn, respectively.

Figure 9. Classification Report for Logistic Regression

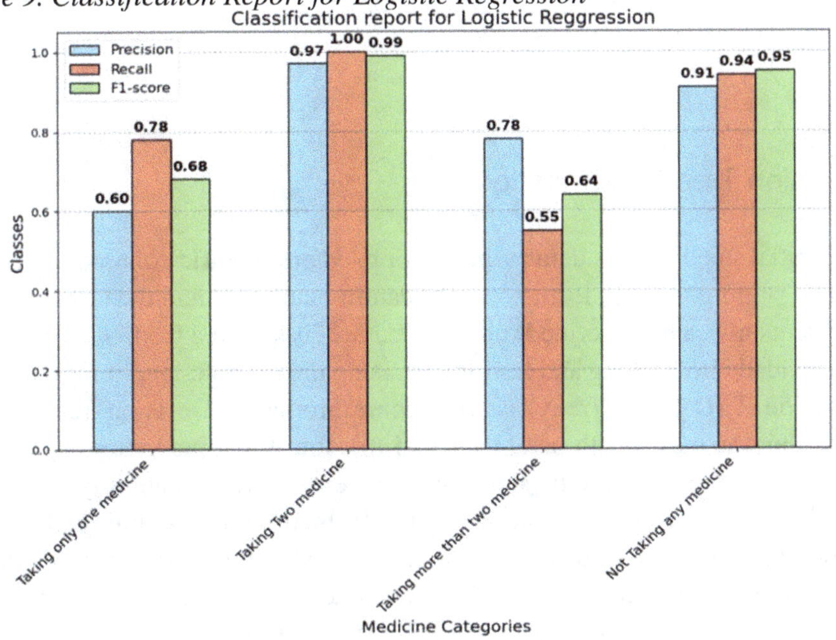

Figure 10. Prediction for Logistic regression from the test data

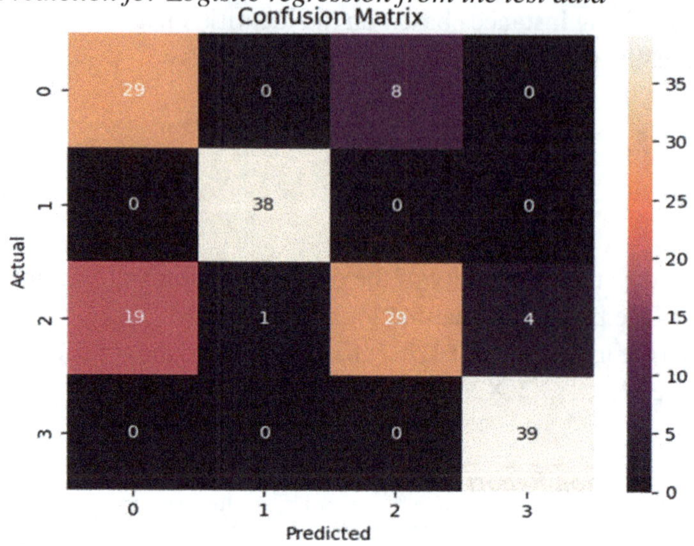

iii. Decision Tree Classification

The initial step involves data preprocessing, where specific columns are chosen from the DataFrame ‘c’ to form both the feature matrix ‘x’ and the target variable ‘y’. Subsequently, a more refined subset of features is selected from ‘x’. The dataset is then divided into training and testing sets using the train_test_split function. The instantiation of a Decision Tree Classifier occurs through the DecisionTreeClassifier class, setting the max_depth parameter to 5 to control the maximum depth of the resulting tree, while the random_state parameter ensures reproducibility. The model is then trained on the training data using the fit method. Post-training, the model is applied to make predictions on the testing set. Model performance is assessed by calculating the accuracy score with the accuracy_score function and generating a classification report. Decision trees are constructed through a recursive process of binary splits, guided by a selected impurity criterion such as Gini impurity or entropy. The classification report and the confusion matrix is shown in Figure 11 and Figure 12.

The Gini impurity for a node t is expressed as:

$$Gini(t) = 1 - \sum i = 1C(pi2) \qquad (10)$$

In this equation, C denotes the number of classes, and pi signifies the proportion of samples belonging to class i within the node t.

The overall measure of impurity for a split is a weighted sum of the impurities of its child nodes. For a split on feature *j* at threshold *s*:

$$\boldsymbol{Ginisplit = Ntotal\ /Nleft * Gini(left) + Ntotal/Nright *\cdot Gini(right)} \quad (11)$$

In this formula, *N*left and *N*right represent the number of samples in the left and right child nodes, respectively, and l*N*total is the total number of samples. The decision tree algorithm strategically selects splits that minimize this weighted impurity, iteratively constructing the tree until a predefined stopping criterion is met. The resulting tree structure is then employed for making predictions in classification tasks. The accuracy for Decision tree classification is 87%.

Figure 11. Classification Report for Decision Tree Classification

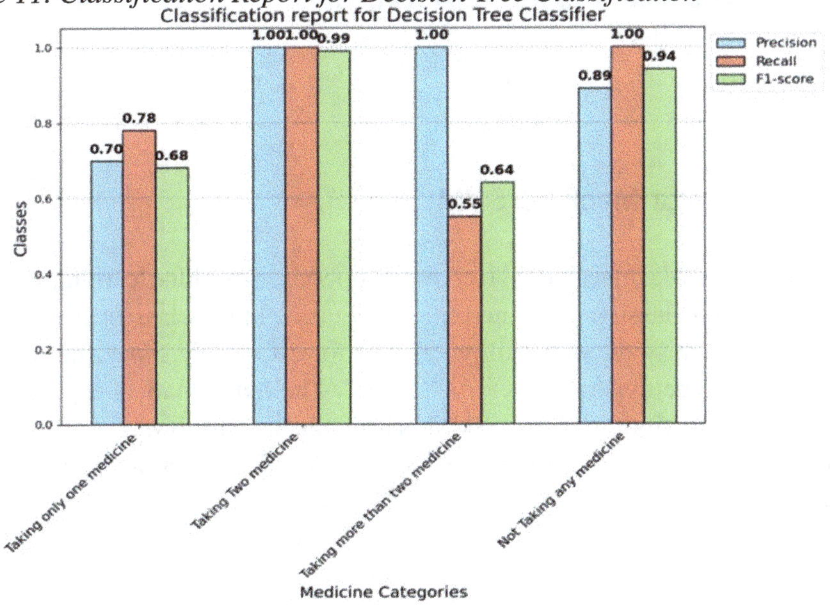

Figure12. Prediction for the Decision tree from the test data

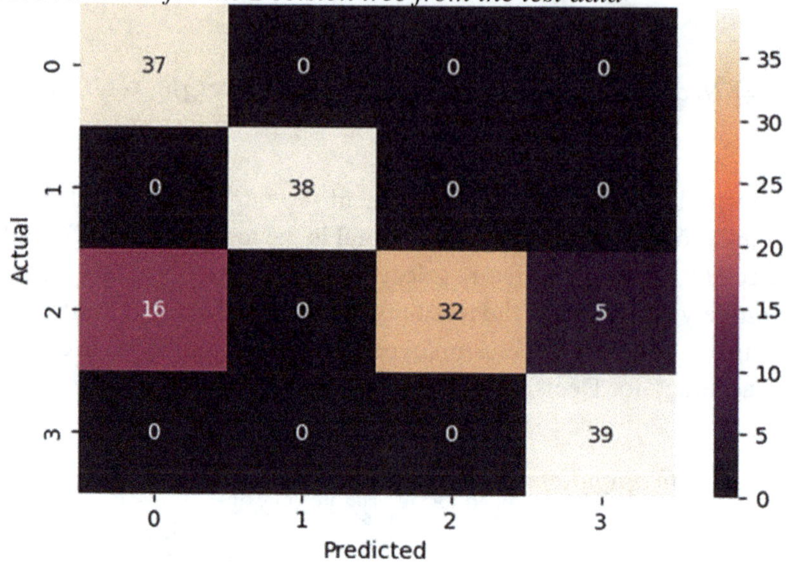

Iv. Support Vector Machine(SVM)

Support Vector Machines (SVM) serve as a supervised machine learning algorithm applicable to both classification and regression tasks. In the classification context, SVM aims to identify the optimal hyperplane for effectively separating data into distinct classes. The hyperparameter is 'linear'. The mathematical representation of the decision function in a linear SVM is articulated as follows:

For a given set of input features $x \in Rn$, the decision function $f(x)$ in a linear SVM is defined as:

$$f(x) = sign(w \cdot x + b) \quad (12)$$

Here, key components include:

1. w, the weight vector dictating the orientation of the hyperplane.
2. x, the input feature vector.
3. b, the bias term, also recognized as the intercept.
4. ··, signifying the dot product operation between w and x.sign(·)sign(·), the sign function, yielding +1 for positive arguments, -1 for negative ones, and 0 for zero.

The classification report and the confusion matrix is shown in Figure 13 and Figure 14.

Figure 13. Classification report for support vector machine

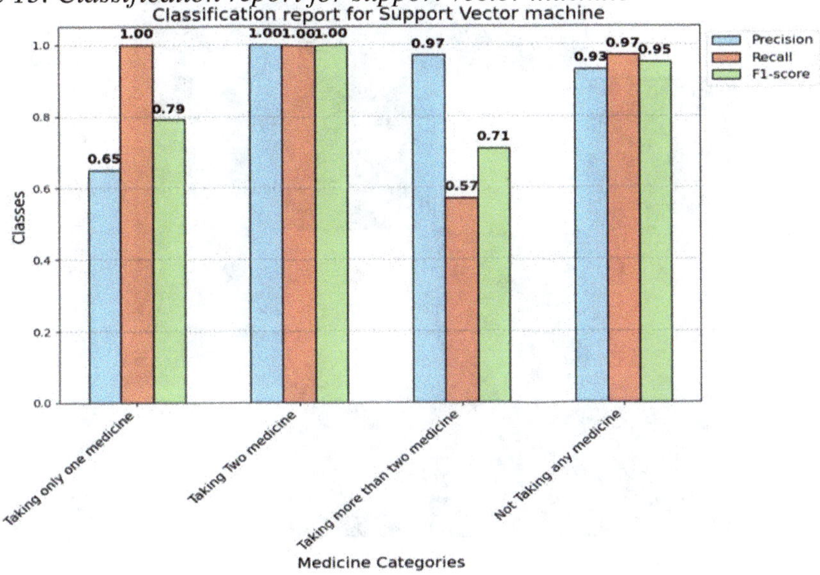

Figure 14. Confusion Matrix for Support Vector Machine

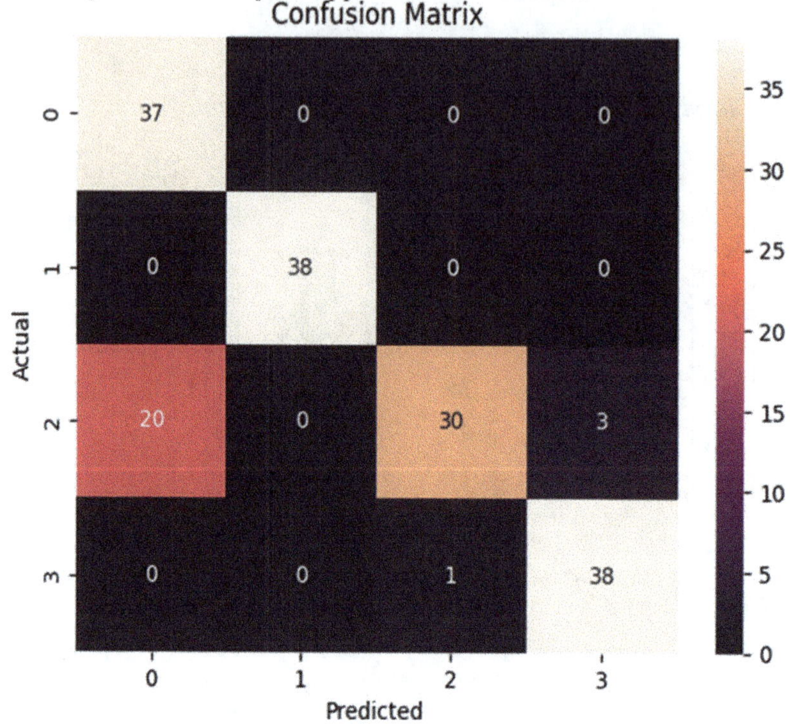

3.4 Model Comparison

The Figure 8 represents the confusion matrix or Bayesian network, reflecting the classification performance of a model within four distinct classes. The elements on the main diagonal represent accurate predictions, while those off the diagonal indicate misclassifications. A detailed examination of each row reveals flawless predictions for the initial two classes (Class 1 and Class 2). Conversely, the third class (Class 3) encounters misclassifications, where seven instances are incorrectly predicted as Class 1 and two instances as Class 4, while 33 instances receive correct classifications. The fourth class (Class 4) presents challenges, with 10 instances misclassified as Class 2, but 34 instances are accurately predicted.

Figure 11 represents the confusion matrix for the Logistic regression The confusion matrix offers a comprehensive evaluation of the classifier's performance across distinct classes. Specifically, for Class 1, 29 instances were correctly identified, while 8 instances faced misclassification into other classes. Class 2 exhibited flawless classification, accurately identifying all 38 instances. In Class 3, 29 instances received correct classification, but 1 instance was misclassified into another class, and 19 instances were erroneously predicted as other classes. Notably, Class 4 experienced accurate classification for all 39 instances. These findings underscore potential areas for enhancement, particularly in minimizing misclassifications for Class 1 and refining the model's sensitivity to instances in Class 3.

The Figure 12 represents the confusion matrix for the Decision tree classifier, Significantly, Classes 1 and 2 demonstrate impeccable predictions, accurately classifying all instances. However, when considering Class 3, although 16 instances are correctly predicted, the model encounters challenges with misclassifications. More precisely, five instances from Class 3 are mistakenly identified as belonging to Class 4, indicating a difficulty in effectively distinguishing between these two categories. It is noteworthy that there are no instances from Class 3 misclassified as either Class 1 or Class 2. In contrast, Class 4 exhibits flawless performance, correctly classifying all 39 instances. This analysis emphasizes the model's proficiency in certain classes while shedding light on a specific struggle in precisely distinguishing between Classes 3 and 4.

The Figure14 represents the confusion matrix for support vector machine, In the case of Class 1, all instances (True Positives, TP) are accurately identified, totaling 37. Similarly, Class 2 demonstrates precise classification, correctly predicting all 38 instances. However, Class 3 reveals instances of misclassification, with 20 cases erroneously assigned to Class 1 and 3 instances mislabeled as Class 4. Transitioning to Class 4, 38 instances are correctly predicted, except for a single misclassification where an instance is inaccurately designated as Class 3.

In this thorough assessment of various classification algorithms using corresponding confusion matrices (Figure 8, Figure 10, Figure 12, Figure 14), distinctive performance patterns emerge. The Bayesian classifier, incorporating causal inference (Nogueira et al., 2022), (Marella & Vicard, 2022) stands out with the highest accuracy among the models, achieving an 89% accuracy rate. It excels in precisely predicting Classes 2, 3, and 4, with only min or misclassifications observed in the 1st class. Logistic regression, with an 81% accuracy, faces challenges in Class 1, particularly in instances where individuals are taking two medicines. The Decision Tree classifier, boasting an accuracy of 87%, performs well in Classes 1, 2, and 4 but struggles with the precise differentiation between Classes 3 and 4. The Support Vector Machine (SVM), achieving an 86% accuracy, demonstrates accurate predictions in Classes 1, 2, and 4 but encounters misclassifications in Class 3.

Considering these findings, the Bayesian classifier with causal inference emerges as the most robust model for research, consistently delivering high accuracy across diverse classes. Its nuanced understanding of intricate cause-and-effect relationships within the dataset contributes to its superior performance. While other models showcase strengths in specific classes, the Bayesian classifier's overall accuracy and well-balanced performance position as the preferred choice for this machine learning research. Nevertheless, careful consideration of computational complexity and interpretability is crucial, as these factors may impact the final decision based on the research's specific requirements.

Figure 15. Accuracies for Different Models

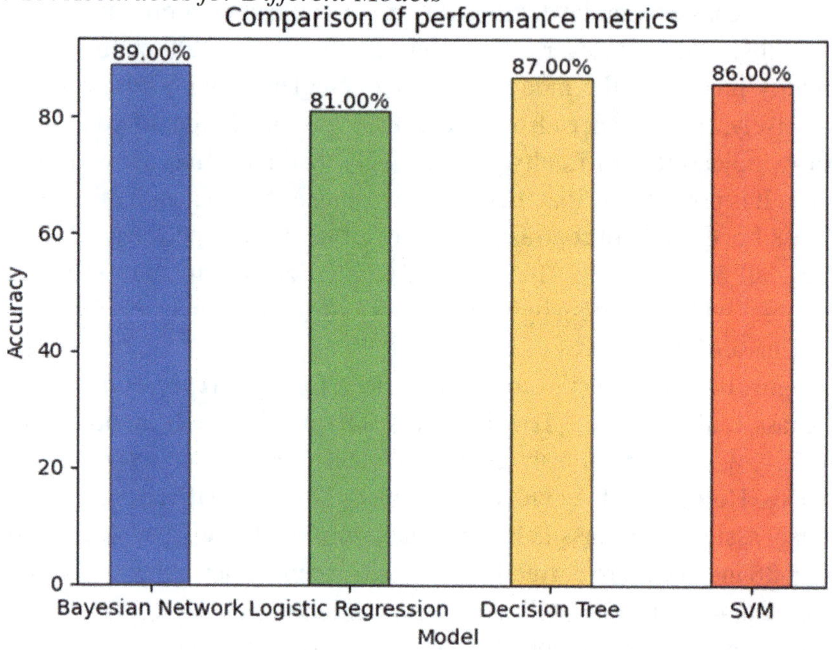

3.5 Model Evaluation

In the evaluation phase, our data is segregated into two vital sets: the training and the testing set. This segregation is instrumental in conducting a comprehensive assessment of our model's performance.

The training set serves as the foundation for our model's learning process. It allows the model to absorb knowledge from the data, honing its predictive capabilities. Conversely, the testing set plays a crucial role in gauging the model's ability to generalize its predictions to new, unseen data points. This method ensures that our model's performance isn't solely based on memorizing the training data but rather reflects its proficiency in making accurate predictions in real-world scenarios involving previously unencountered data instances. The comparison of the performance is depicted in Figure 15

3.6 IFTTT

Additionally, regarding model deployment, as previously mentioned, we intend to utilize the IFTTT app to send notifications to individuals. These notifications will be triggered when individuals indicate the need to take their medication. At this stage, our focus is on generating a single personalized recommendation (Peshkova et al., 2023), (Etemadi et al., 2023) for everyone is shown in Figure 16.

Figure 16. Notification from the IFTTT

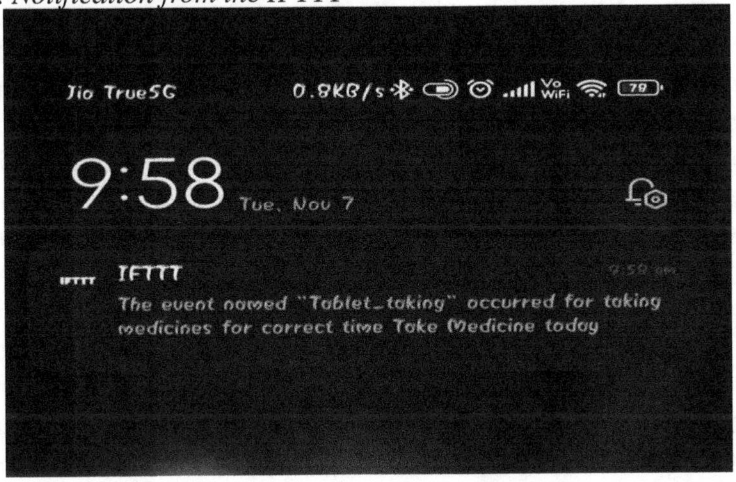

The findings highlight the increasing importance of causal inference as a framework for improving decision-making in healthcare systems. Unlike traditional predictive models that only look at correlations, causal inference methods can identify the underlying mechanisms that influence patient outcomes. This shift from looking at associations to understanding causation allows clinicians and policymakers to make better, more targeted decisions, such as assessing the real impact of medication adherence, treatment timing, or lifestyle changes on health outcomes. In practice, integrating causal inference into healthcare analytics connects algorithmic insights with clinical judgment. From a research standpoint, recent studies have developed methods such as structural causal models, propensity score matching, and instrumental variable approaches to tackle bias in medical datasets. In geriatric care and chronic disease management, these techniques have been applied to assess the causal impact of interventions like digital monitoring, rehabilitation programs, and AI-assisted diagnostics. However, challenges with data quality, diversity, and model interpretability still hinder the application of these findings in real-world settings. This study adds to the ongoing discussion by connecting theoretical modeling with practical healthcare needs. By focusing on causal reasoning within AI-driven healthcare systems, it promotes the development of explainable and reliable decision support, which is crucial for clinical use. Future research should aim for scalable causal inference frameworks that can work with electronic health records and telemedicine platforms, ensuring that models are both data-driven and relevant to clinical practice.

4. CONCLUSION

This research thoroughly examines the profound impact of recommendation systems on personalized assistance, particularly focusing on their importance for the elderly population. By highlighting the significance of these systems, the research underscores their crucial role in promoting independent living among older individuals, who often find tailored guidance and support invaluable. Through the provision of personalized and self-sufficient solutions, recommendation systems emerge as powerful tools for enhancing the well-being of seniors. Additionally, the research meticulously explores various aspects of machine learning, spanning from data preprocessing to model evaluation. Techniques like label encoding and normalization methods are carefully utilized to convert categorical data into numerical formats, laying a strong groundwork for the development of effective machine learning algorithms. Furthermore, methods such as resampling, particularly oversampling, are introduced to tackle class imbalances within datasets, ensuring the resilience of the models. Furthermore, the integration of causal inference and Bayesian networks enriches the analysis by uncovering intricate cause-and-effect relationships inherent within the dataset. Through the comparison of various models, including logistic regression, decision tree classification, and support vector machines, the research demonstrates the superior performance of the Bayesian network, achieving an impressive accuracy rate of 89%. Visual aids and graphical representations further enhance the comprehension of complex network structures and insights derived from causal network analysis. Moreover, beyond theoretical exploration, the research delves into the practical deployment of models, showcasing the incorporation of tools like the IFTTT app for personalized medication reminders. This holistic approach underscores a methodical and insightful methodology towards machine learning, integrating diverse techniques for the robust development and evaluation of models. Through its comprehensive analysis and real-world applications, the research makes significant contributions to the advancement of personalized healthcare solutions in the digital era.

REFERENCES

Abécassis, J., Dumas, É., Alberge, J., & Varoquaux, G. (2025). From prediction to prescription: Machine learning and causal inference for the heterogeneous treatment effect. *Annual Review of Biomedical Data Science*, *8*(1), 381–404. DOI: 10.1146/annurev-biodatasci-103123-095750 PMID: 40203240

Ahmed, S., Irfan, S., Kiran, N., Masood, N., Anjum, N., & Ramzan, N. (2023). Remote health monitoring systems for elderly people: A survey. *Sensors (Basel)*, *23*(16), 7095. DOI: 10.3390/s23167095 PMID: 37631632

Ali, Y., Hussain, F., & Haque, M. M. (2024). Advances, challenges, and future research needs in machine learning-based crash prediction models: A systematic review. *Accident; Analysis and Prevention*, *194*, 107378. DOI: 10.1016/j.aap.2023.107378 PMID: 37976634

Androutsou, T., Kouris, I., Anastasiou, A., Pavlopoulos, S., Mostajeran, F., Bamiou, D.-E., Genna, G. J., Costafreda, S. G., & Koutsouris, D. (2020). A smartphone application designed to engage the elderly in home-based rehabilitation. *Frontiers in Digital Health*, *2*, 15. DOI: 10.3389/fdgth.2020.00015 PMID: 34713028

Banerjee, A., Maji, D., Datta, R., Barman, S., Samanta, D., & Chattopadhyay, S. (2022). SHUBHCHINTAK: An efficient remote health monitoring approach for elderly people. *Multimedia Tools and Applications*, *81*(26), 37137–37163. DOI: 10.1007/s11042-022-13539-y PMID: 35968413

Chen, Y., Li, X., Wang, J., Liu, M., Cai, C., & Shi, Y. (2023). Research on the application of fuzzy Bayesian network in risk assessment of catenary construction. *Mathematics*, *11*(7), 1719. DOI: 10.3390/math11071719

Chobtham, K., Constantinou, A. C., & Kitson, N. K. (2023). Hybrid Bayesian network discovery with latent variables. *Data Mining and Knowledge Discovery*, *37*(1), 476–520. DOI: 10.1007/s10618-022-00882-9

Constantinou, A. C., Guo, Z., & Kitson, N. K. (2023). The impact of prior knowledge on causal structure learning. *Knowledge and Information Systems*, *65*(8), 3385–3434. DOI: 10.1007/s10115-023-01858-x

Dratsiou, I., Villacañas, O., Cooper, S., Isaris, P., Serras, M., Unzueta, L., & Fernandez-Carbajales, V. (2021, June). *Assistive technologies for supporting well-being of older adults. Proceedings of the 14th PErvasive Technologies Related to Assistive Environments Conference*, 338–341. DOI: 10.1145/3453892.3461352

Du, Z., Guo, S., Sun, Y., Zhou, Q., Jiang, Y., Shen, Y., Zhu, H., Zhou, Z., & Zhou, H. (2023). Causal relationships between dietary habits and five major mental disorders: A two-sample Mendelian randomization study. *Journal of Affective Disorders*, *340*, 607–615. DOI: 10.1016/j.jad.2023.08.098 PMID: 37598719

Efendi, A., Ammarullah, M. I., Isa, I. G. T., Sari, M. P., Izza, J. N., Nugroho, Y. S., Nasrullah, H., & Alfian, D. (2025). IoT-based elderly health monitoring system using Firebase cloud computing. *Health Science Reports*, *8*(3), e70498. DOI: 10.1002/hsr2.70498 PMID: 40041774

El Arab, R. A., Abu-Mahfouz, M. S., Abuadas, F. H., Alzghoul, H., Almari, M., Ghannam, A., & Seweid, M. M. (2025). Bridging the gap.... *Healthcare (Basel)*, *13*(7), 701. DOI: 10.3390/healthcare13070701 PMID: 40217999

Etemadi, M., Abkenar, S. B., Ahmadzadeh, A., Kashani, M. H., Asghari, P., Akbari, M., & Mahdipour, E. (2023). A systematic review of healthcare recommender systems. *Expert Systems with Applications*, *213*, 118823. DOI: 10.1016/j.eswa.2022.118823

Gasse, M., Aussem, A., & Elghazel, H. (2014). A hybrid algorithm for Bayesian network structure learning with application to multi-label learning. *Expert Systems with Applications*, *41*(15), 6755–6772. DOI: 10.1016/j.eswa.2014.04.032

Gilmartin, M. J. (2023). Nurses improving care for health systems elders (NICHE). *Geriatric Nursing*, *53*, 310–312. DOI: 10.1016/j.gerinurse.2023.08.002 PMID: 37689486

Haleem, A., Javaid, M., Singh, R. P., & Suman, R. (2023). Exploring the revolution in healthcare systems through the applications of digital twin technology. *Biomedical Technology*, *4*, 28–38. DOI: 10.1016/j.bmt.2023.02.001

Hasan, N., & Ahmed, M. (2024). *Wearable technology for elderly care: Integrating health monitoring and emergency alerts*. Journal of Computer Networks and Communications. *Article, 5593708*. Advance online publication. DOI: 10.1155/2024/5593708

Kitson, N. K., Constantinou, A. C., Guo, Z., Liu, Y., & Chobtham, K. (2023). A survey of Bayesian network structure learning. *Artificial Intelligence Review*, *56*(8), 8721–8814. DOI: 10.1007/s10462-022-10351-w

Lee, Y., Pokharel, S., Muslim, A. A., Kc, D. B., Lee, K. H., & Yeo, W. H. (2023). Deep learning-based fall monitoring among older adults with skin-wearable electronics. *Sensors (Basel)*, *23*(8), 3983. DOI: 10.3390/s23083983 PMID: 37112326

Li, J., Zhang, J., Kong, B., Chen, L., Yuan, J., He, M., Wang, Y., Wei, S., Chen, W., Tang, Y., Zhu, X., & Yao, P. (2023). Abdominal obesity mediates the causal relationship between depression and the risk of gallstone disease…. *Journal of Psychosomatic Research, 174*, 111474. DOI: 10.1016/j.jpsychores.2023.111474 PMID: 37689051

Liang, J. H., Lu, L., Li, J. Y., Qu, X. Y., Li, J., Qian, S., Wang, Y., Jia, R., Wang, C., & Xu, Y. (2020). Contributions of modifiable risk factors to dementia incidence: A Bayesian network analysis. *Journal of the American Medical Directors Association, 21*(11), 1592–1599. DOI: 10.1016/j.jamda.2020.04.006 PMID: 32563753

Lin, Y., Lange, D., & Seligmann, B. J. (2023). Causal network topology analysis (CaNeTA) as a tool for risk assessment in fire safety engineering. *Fire Safety Journal, 140*, 103880. DOI: 10.1016/j.firesaf.2023.103880

Lu, W., Silvera-Tawil, D., Yoon, H. J., Higgins, L., Zhang, Q., Karunanithi, M., Bomke, J., Byrnes, J., Hewitt, J., Smallbon, V., Freyne, J., Prabhu, D., & Varnfield, M. (2025). Impact of the Smarter Safer Homes solution…. *Journal of Medical Internet Research, 27*, e59921. DOI: 10.2196/59921 PMID: 39608020

Malakar, Y., Peeters, L. J., Walton, A., & O'Sullivan, D. (2023). A causal network approach using a community well-being framework…. *Environmental Impact Assessment Review, 102*, 107188. DOI: 10.1016/j.eiar.2023.107188

Marella, D., & Vicard, P. (2022). Bayesian network structural learning from complex survey data. *Statistical Methods & Applications, 31*(4), 981–1013. DOI: 10.1007/s10260-021-00618-x

Mennella, C., Maniscalco, U., De Pietro, G., & Esposito, M. (2024). Ethical and regulatory challenges of AI technologies in healthcare: A narrative review. *Heliyon, 10*(4), e26297. DOI: 10.1016/j.heliyon.2024.e26297 PMID: 38384518

Mennella, C., Maniscalco, U., Masala, G. L., & Esposito, M. (2024). Editorial: Artificial intelligence and robotic applications for smart monitoring and assistance in healthcare services. *Frontiers in Robotics and AI, 11*, 1527773. DOI: 10.3389/frobt.2024.1527773 PMID: 39687348

Mini, P. (2024). Comparative analysis of financial flows in healthcare systems of Germany, Austria, and Czechia. *ACTA VŠFS, 18*(2), 180–197. DOI: 10.37355/acta-2024/2-05

Morita, P., Sahu, K., & Oetomo, A. (2023). Health monitoring using smart home technologies: Scoping review. *JMIR mHealth and uHealth, 11*, e37347. DOI: 10.2196/37347 PMID: 37052984

Nogueira, A. R., Pugnana, A., Ruggieri, S., Pedreschi, D., & Gama, J. (2022). Methods and tools for causal discovery and causal inference. *Wiley Interdisciplinary Reviews. Data Mining and Knowledge Discovery, 12*(2), e1449. DOI: 10.1002/widm.1449

Parchmann, N., Hansen, D., Orzechowski, M., & Steger, F. (2024). An ethical assessment of professional opinions on concerns, chances, and limitations…. *GeroScience, 46*(6), 6269–6282. DOI: 10.1007/s11357-024-01229-6 PMID: 38834930

Pearl, J. (2024). Advances in causal inference in AI. *Journal of Medical Internet Research, 2024–2025*. Advance online publication. 10.2196

Pereira, A. V., Vaz, A., Paúl, C., Santiago, L., & Rosendo, I. (2025). Comprehensive geriatric assessment in primary healthcare: A scoping review protocol. *BMJ Open, 15*(6), e091095. DOI: 10.1136/bmjopen-2024-091095 PMID: 40467309

Peshkova, M., Yumasheva, V., Rudenko, E., Kretova, N., Timashev, P., & Demura, T. (2023). Digital twin concept: Healthcare, education, research. *Journal of Pathology Informatics, 14*, 100313. DOI: 10.1016/j.jpi.2023.100313 PMID: 37168801

Philips, N. J., Joshi, S., Nimbalkar, K., & Suryawanshi, A. (2025). Vision-based monitoring system for elderly care using CNN + BiLSTM. *Journal of Information Systems Engineering & Management, 10*(55), 11425.

Shakhovska, N., Fedushko, S., Shvorob, I., & Syerov, Y. (2019). Development of mobile system for medical recommendations. *Procedia Computer Science, 155*, 43–50. DOI: 10.1016/j.procs.2019.08.010

Singh, M. P., & Keche, Y. N. (2025). Ethical integration of artificial intelligence in healthcare…. *Cureus, 17*(5), e84804. DOI: 10.7759/cureus.84804 PMID: 40568260

Tajudeen, F. P., Bahar, N., Tan, M. P., Peer Mustafa, M. B., Saedon, N. I., & Jesudass, J. (2022). Understanding user requirements for a senior-friendly mobile health application. *Geriatrics (Basel, Switzerland), 7*(5), 110. DOI: 10.3390/geriatrics7050110 PMID: 36286212

Tan, E. W., Chai, S. C., Sankai, Y., Shingu, M., Razaob, N. A., & Hussain, H. (2025). Single joint hybrid assistive limb…. *PLoS One, 20*(4), e0322191. DOI: 10.1371/journal.pone.0322191 PMID: 40273196

Triscott, J. A. C., Dobbs, B., Charles, L., Huang, J., Moores, D., & Tian, P. G. J. (2021). The care-of-the-elderly health guide. *Journal of Primary Care & Community Health, 12*, 21501327211044058. DOI: 10.1177/21501327211044058 PMID: 34486428

Wang, K., Ghafurian, M., Chumachenko, D., Cao, S., Butt, Z. A., Salim, S., Abhari, S., & Morita, P. P. (2024). Application of artificial intelligence.... *Computers in Biology and Medicine*, *173*, 108340. DOI: 10.1016/j.compbiomed.2024.108340 PMID: 38555702

World Health Organization. (2017). *Integrated care for older people: Guidelines on community-level interventions to manage declines in intrinsic capacity*. https://www.ncbi.nlm.nih.gov/books/NBK488250/

World Health Organization. (2024). *WHO guidance on artificial intelligence in healthcare*. https://www.who.int/publications/i/item/9789240084759

Zeng, Z., Jiang, X., & Neapolitan, R. (2016). Discovering causal interactions using Bayesian network scoring and information gain. *BMC Bioinformatics*, *17*(1), 1–14. DOI: 10.1186/s12859-016-1084-8 PMID: 27230078

Zhang, Q., Varnfield, M., Higgins, L., Smallbon, V., Bomke, J., O'Dwyer, J., Byrnes, J. M., Sum, M., Hewitt, J., Lu, W., & Karunanithi, M. (2022). Protocol for a stratified randomized controlled trial.... *JMIR Research Protocols*, *11*(1), e31970. DOI: 10.2196/31970 PMID: 35072640

Compilation of References

AARP. (2020). *Caregiving in the U.S. 2020.* AARP and National Alliance for Caregiving. https://www.aarp.org/caregiving/research/info-2020/caregiving-in-the-united-states.html

Abdallah, H. M. M., Amin, S. M., Hammouda, E. Y., Atta, M. H. R., El-Monshed, A. H., & Hamad, N. I. M. (2025). Family Intensive Care Unit Syndrome: Investigating the Mediating Role of Healthcare Communication in Psychological Well-Being Among Family Members. *Nursing in Critical Care*, *30*(4), e70119. DOI: 10.1111/nicc.70119 PMID: 40726324

Abdi, S., Spann, A., Borilovic, J., de Witte, L., & Hawley, M. (2019). Understanding the care and support needs of older people: A scoping review and categorisation using the WHO international classification of functioning, disability and health framework (ICF). *BMC Geriatrics*, *19*(1), 195. DOI: 10.1186/s12877-019-1189-9 PMID: 31331279

Abécassis, J., Dumas, É., Alberge, J., & Varoquaux, G. (2025). From prediction to prescription: Machine learning and causal inference for the heterogeneous treatment effect. *Annual Review of Biomedical Data Science*, *8*(1), 381–404. DOI: 10.1146/annurev-biodatasci-103123-095750 PMID: 40203240

Abel, J., Kellehear, A., & Karapliagou, A. (2018). Palliative care—The new essentials. *Annals of Palliative Medicine*, *7*(S2, Suppl 2), S3–S14. DOI: 10.21037/apm.2018.03.04 PMID: 29764169

Abe, T. K., Beamon, B. M., Storch, R. L., & Agus, J. (2016). Operations research applications in hospital operations: Part II. *IIE Transactions on Healthcare Systems Engineering*, *6*(2), 96–109. DOI: 10.1080/19488300.2016.1162880

Acar, Z., & Oskay, Ü. (2021). Mobile Health Applications Used in Perinatal Period and Nursing Roles. *Journal of Education & Research in Nursing/Hemşirelikte Eğitim ve Araştırma Dergisi, 18*(4). DOI: 10.5152/jern.2021.60343

Agarwal, V., & L, G. (2020). Standards of human rights to palliative care: Gaps and trends. *International Journal of Human Rights in Healthcare, 13*(4), 293–298. DOI: 10.1108/IJHRH-02-2020-0013

Ahmad Zubaidi, Z. S., Ariffin, F., Oun, C. T. C., & Katiman, D. (2020). Caregiver burden among informal caregivers in the largest specialized palliative care unit in Malaysia: A cross sectional study. *BMC Palliative Care, 19*(1), 186. DOI: 10.1186/s12904-020-00691-1 PMID: 33292214

Ahmad, I. A. (2025). A scoping review of barriers within the cancer care continuum: Addressing screening, diagnosis, and treatment disparities for an equitable future. *Advances in Medicine, Psychology, and Public Health, 2*(2), 96–106.

Ahmed, S., Irfan, S., Kiran, N., Masood, N., Anjum, N., & Ramzan, N. (2023). Remote health monitoring systems for elderly people: A survey. *Sensors (Basel), 23*(16), 7095. DOI: 10.3390/s23167095 PMID: 37631632

Ahn, J. H., Kim, M., & Kim, R. W. (2024). Effects of aromatherapy on nausea and vomiting in patients with cancer: A systematic review and meta-analysis of randomized controlled trials. *Complementary Therapies in Clinical Practice, 55*, 101838. DOI: 10.1016/j.ctcp.2024.101838 PMID: 38330531

Akimbekov, N. S., & Razzaque, M. S. (2021). Laughter therapy: A humor-induced hormonal intervention to reduce stress and anxiety. *Current Research in Physiology, 4*, 135–138. DOI: 10.1016/j.crphys.2021.04.002 PMID: 34642668

Akther, F. (2025). Interweaving Care and Climate Justice in Housing for Climate Migrants: Vulnerabilities of Low-Income Older Women in Developing Countries. In *Community Climate Justice and Sustainable Development* (pp. 483-502). IGI Global Scientific Publishing. DOI: 10.4018/979-8-3373-0619-3.ch018

Akyüz, H. Ö., Şenturan, L., & Sabuncu, N. (2024). The effect of aromatherapy massage on the pain severity and quality of life in acute migraine attacks: A randomized controlled trial. *Florence Nightingale Journal of Nursing, 32*(2), 159–167. DOI: 10.5152/FNJN.2024.23235 PMID: 39552146

Alam, S., Hannon, B., & Zimmermann, C. (2020). Palliative care for family caregivers. *Journal of Clinical Oncology, 38*(9), 926–936. DOI: 10.1200/JCO.19.00018 PMID: 32023152

Alam, T. M., Iqbal, M. A., Ali, Y., Wahab, A., Ijaz, S., Ul Haq, E., & Baig, T. I. (2019). A model for early prediction of diabetes. *Informatics in Medicine Unlocked, 16*, 100204. DOI: 10.1016/j.imu.2019.100204

Al-Assaf, K., Bahroun, Z., & Ahmed, V. (2024). Transforming service quality in healthcare: A comprehensive review of healthcare 4.0 and its impact on healthcare service quality. In *Informatics* (Vol. 11, No. 4, p. 96). MDPI. DOI: 10.3390/informatics11040096

Alcântara-Silva, T. R., Freitas-Junior, R., Freitas, N. M. A., Machado, G. D. S., Ribeiro, M. K. A., da Silva, D. J., de Paula, W.Junior, & Panobianco, M. S. (2018). Music therapy reduces radiotherapy-induced fatigue in patients with breast or gynecological cancer: A randomized trial. *Integrative Cancer Therapies*, *17*(3), 628–635. DOI: 10.1177/1534735418757349 PMID: 29633652

Alders, P., Deeg, D. J., & Schut, F. T. (2019). Who will become my co-residents? The role of attractiveness of institutional care in the changing demand for long-term care institutions. *Archives of Gerontology and Geriatrics*, *81*, 91–97. DOI: 10.1016/j.archger.2018.11.014 PMID: 30529804

Alhazmi, J. D. (2024). Nursing strategies to improve the quality of life for terminally ill patients. *Gland Surgery*, *9*(2), 111–117.

Ali, Y., Hussain, F., & Haque, M. M. (2024). Advances, challenges, and future research needs in machine learning-based crash prediction models: A systematic review. *Accident; Analysis and Prevention*, *194*, 107378. DOI: 10.1016/j.aap.2023.107378 PMID: 37976634

Allen, J., Woolford, M., Livingston, P. M., Lobchuk, M., Muldowney, A., & Hutchinson, A. M. (2023). Informal carer support needs, facilitators and barriers in transitional care for older adults from hospital to home: A scoping review. *Journal of Clinical Nursing*, *32*(19-20), 6773–6795. DOI: 10.1111/jocn.16767 PMID: 37272211

Almada, A. L., Casquinha, P., Cotovio, V., Santos, M. H. D., & Caixeiro, A. (2018). The potential role of psychosocial rehabilitation in palliative care. *Journal of the Royal College of Physicians of Edinburgh*, *48*(4), 311–317. DOI: 10.4997/jrcpe.2018.405 PMID: 30488884

Alodhialah, A. M., Almutairi, A. A., & Almutairi, M. (2024). Exploring nurses' emotional resilience and coping strategies in palliative and End-of-Life care settings in Saudi Arabia: A qualitative study. In *Healthcare* (Vol. 12, No. 16, p. 1647). MDPI. DOI: 10.3390/healthcare12161647

Alzheimer's Association. (2021). 2021 Alzheimer's disease facts and figures. *Alzheimer's & Dementia*, *17*(3), 327–406. DOI: 10.1002/alz.12328 PMID: 33756057

American Art Therapy Association. (n.d.). *What is Art Therapy? Fact Sheet.* Retrieved 3 September 2025, from https://arttherapy.org/what-is-art-therapy/

American Music Therapy Association. (2020). *Definition and Scope of Music Therapy Practice 2020*. AMTA.

Aminabee, S. (2024). The future of healthcare and patient-centric care: Digital innovations, trends, and predictions. In *Emerging technologies for health literacy and medical practice* (pp. 240–262). IGI Global Scientific Publishing., DOI: 10.4018/979-8-3693-1214-8.ch012

Anandarajah, G., Mennillo, H. A., Rachu, G., Harder, T., & Ghosh, J. (2020). Lifestyle medicine interventions in patients with advanced disease receiving palliative or hospice care. *American Journal of Lifestyle Medicine*, *14*(3), 243–257. DOI: 10.1177/1559827619830049 PMID: 32477022

Anderson, K. A., Dabelko-Schoeny, H., & Johnson, T. D. (2017). The state of adult day services: Findings and implications from the MetLife National Study of Adult Day Services. *The Gerontologist*, *57*(2), 331–340. DOI: 10.1093/geront/gnv099

Androutsou, T., Kouris, I., Anastasiou, A., Pavlopoulos, S., Mostajeran, F., Bamiou, D.-E., Genna, G. J., Costafreda, S. G., & Koutsouris, D. (2020). A smartphone application designed to engage the elderly in home-based rehabilitation. *Frontiers in Digital Health*, *2*, 15. DOI: 10.3389/fdgth.2020.00015 PMID: 34713028

Angelopoulou, E., Bougea, A., Hatzimanolis, A., Stefanis, L., Scarmeas, N., & Papageorgiou, S. (2024). Mild Behavioral Impairment in Parkinson's Disease: An Updated Review on the Clinical, Genetic, Neuroanatomical, and Pathophysiological Aspects. *Medicina (Kaunas, Lithuania)*, *60*(1), 115. DOI: 10.3390/medicina60010115 PMID: 38256375

Anttonen, A., & Karsio, O. (2016). Eldercare service redesign in Finland: Deinstitutionalization of long-term care. *Journal of Social Service Research*, *42*(2), 151–166. DOI: 10.1080/01488376.2015.1129017

Archbold, P. G., Stewart, B. J., Greenlick, M. R., & Harvath, T. A. (2018). Mutuality and preparedness as predictors of caregiver role strain. *Research in Nursing & Health*, *33*(2), 103–116. DOI: 10.1002/nur.20365 PMID: 2270302

Armat, M. R., Emami Zeydi, A., Mokarami, H., Nakhlband, A., & Hojjat, S. K. (2022). The impact of laughter yoga on depression and anxiety among retired women: A randomized controlled clinical trial. *Journal of Women & Aging*, *34*(1), 31–42. DOI: 10.1080/08952841.2020.1774225 PMID: 32552530

Ashburner, J., Ziviani, J., & Rodger, S. (2013). Sensory processing and classroom emotional, behavioural, and educational outcomes in children with autism spectrum disorder. *The American Journal of Occupational Therapy*, *67*(5), 562–573. DOI: 10.5014/ajot.2013.008821

Aslan, K. S. Ü., & Altın, S. (2022). Aromatherapy and foot massage on happiness, sleep quality, and fatigue levels in patients with stroke: A randomized controlled trial. *European Journal of Integrative Medicine*, *54*, 102164. DOI: 10.1016/j.eujim.2022.102164

Bag, B. (2020). Therapeutic Use of Humor in Psychiatric Care. *Psikiyatride Güncel Yaklasimlar*, *12*(4), 519–533. DOI: 10.18863/pgy.689943

Bandieri, E., Borelli, E., Gilioli, F., Bigi, S., Mucciarini, C., Ferrari, U., Eliardo, S., Pinto, L., Porro, C. A., Efficace, F., Luppi, M., & Potenza, L. (2023). Stigma of palliative care among patients with advanced cancer and their caregivers on early palliative care. *Cancers (Basel)*, *15*(14), 3656. DOI: 10.3390/cancers15143656 PMID: 37509317

Bandila, R. K. (2022). Concerns of Elderly Women's Wellbeing: Some Policy Issues. In *Research Anthology on Supporting Healthy Aging in a Digital Society* (pp. 1621–1630). IGI Global Scientific Publishing., DOI: 10.4018/978-1-6684-5295-0.ch093

Bandura, A. (1997). Self-efficacy: The exercise of control. *The Freeman.*

Banerjee, A., Maji, D., Datta, R., Barman, S., Samanta, D., & Chattopadhyay, S. (2022). SHUBHCHINTAK: An efficient remote health monitoring approach for elderly people. *Multimedia Tools and Applications*, *81*(26), 37137–37163. DOI: 10.1007/s11042-022-13539-y PMID: 35968413

Başdaş, Ö., Özbey, H., Oğul, G., & Güneş, T. (2024). Effects of aromatherapy on pain, stress, and behaviors of newborns: A randomized controlled trial. *Alternative Therapies in Health and Medicine*, *30*(12), 43–47. PMID: 39480678

Bassul, C., Gannon, J., Kelly, Y., Williams, M., Morrissey, D., McKee, J., O'Rourke, N., & Flynn, R. (2025). How to achieve person-centered care for people using home care services: A narrative review. *Home Health Care Management & Practice*, *37*(2), 129–139. DOI: 10.1177/10848223241267874

Basu, A., & Patnaik, S. (2023). Digital health adoption in rural India: Challenges and opportunities for telemedicine. *Indian Journal of Public Health Research & Development*, *14*(2), 115–122.

Bate, P., & Robert, G. (2006). Experience-based design: From redesigning the system around the patient to co-designing services with the patient. *Quality & Safety in Health Care, 15*(5), 307–310. DOI: 10.1136/qshc.2005.016527 PMID: 17074863

Beech, R., Ong, B. N., Jones, S., & Edwards, V. (2017). Delivering person-centred holistic care for older people. *Quality in Ageing : Policy, Practice and Research, 18*(2), 157–167. DOI: 10.1108/QAOA-05-2016-0019

Bergstraesser, E. (2013). Pediatric palliative care—When quality of life becomes the main focus of treatment. *European Journal of Pediatrics, 172*(2), 139–150. DOI: 10.1007/s00431-012-1710-z PMID: 22476440

Beswick, A. D., Rees, K., Dieppe, P., Ayis, S., Gooberman-Hill, R., Horwood, J., & Ebrahim, S. (2008). Complex interventions to improve physical function and maintain independent living in elderly people: A systematic review and meta-analysis. *Lancet, 371*(9614), 725–735. DOI: 10.1016/S0140-6736(08)60342-6 PMID: 18313501

Bhattacharyya, K. K. (2021). *Rethinking the Aging Transition*. Springer., DOI: 10.1007/978-3-030-88870-1

Bhuvaneswari, K., & Deb, S. (2016). Efficacy of Family-Based Care as Compared with Institutional Care: A Careful Review. *Institutionalised Children Exploration and Beyond, 3*(2), 161–181. DOI: 10.1177/2349301120160204

Bialon, L. N., & Coke, S. (2012). A study on caregiver burden: Stressors, challenges, and possible solutions. *The American Journal of Hospice & Palliative Care, 29*(3), 210–218. DOI: 10.1177/1049909111416494 PMID: 21803785

Bieligmeyer, S., Kesselring, A., Kleinschmidt, R., & Bardenheuer, H. (2018). Feeling the sound – Short-term effect of a vibroacoustic music intervention on well-being and subjectively assessed warmth distribution in cancer patients. *Complementary Therapies in Medicine, 40*, 171–178. DOI: 10.1016/j.ctim.2018.03.002 PMID: 30219444

Bífárìn, O., Quinn, C., Breen, L., Wu, C., Ke, M., Yu, L., & Oyebode, J. (2023). Stressors and coping mechanisms of family care-givers of older relatives living with long-term conditions in mainland China: A scoping review of the evidence. *Ageing and Society, 43*(4), 952–989. DOI: 10.1017/S0144686X21000817

Binette, J., & Vasold, K. (2018). *Home and community preferences: A national survey of adults age 18-plus*. AARP Research.

Blard, F., Erraud, J., Bonnet, M., Auzou, N., & Tison, F. (2024). Mindfulness in Parkinson's disease: A French national survey and a pilot intervention feasibility trial using the MBSR program (M-Park). Revue neurologique, S0035-3787(24)00521-6. Advance online publication. https://doi.org/DOI: 10.1016/j.neurol.2024.03.013

Boise, L., Congleton, L., & Shannon, K. (2005). Empowering family caregivers: The powerful tools for caregivers program. *Educational Gerontology*, *31*(7), 573–586. DOI: 10.1080/03601270590962523

Boyde, C., Thaut, M., Roeser, J., Riedl, A., Klein, P., & von Georgi, R. (2024). Interaction-focused music therapy with cancer-affected children and their significant others (INMUT). *Pilot and Feasibility Studies*, *10*(86), 1–15. PMID: 38807165

Brandell, J. R., & George, L. J. (2015). Social Work and Psychodynamic Thought. In *International Encyclopedia of the Social & Behavioral Sciences* (2nd ed., pp. 761–768). Elsevier Inc., DOI: 10.1016/B978-0-08-097086-8.28117-8

Bressington, D., Mui, J., Yu, C., Leung, S. F., Cheung, K., Wu, C. S. T., Bollard, M., & Chien, W. T. (2019). Feasibility of a group-based laughter yoga intervention as an adjunctive treatment for residual symptoms of depression, anxiety and stress in people with depression. *Journal of Affective Disorders*, *248*, 42–51. DOI: 10.1016/j.jad.2019.01.030 PMID: 30711868

Brimblecombe, N., Piccardt, L., King, D., Knapp, M., & Stevens, M. (2018). Perceptions of unmet needs for community social care services in England: A qualitative study of older people, carers and professionals. *Health & Social Care in the Community*, *26*(3), e241–e249. DOI: 10.1111/hsc.12522

Bro, M. L., Johansen, C., Vuust, P., Enggaard, L., Himmelstrup, B., Mourits-Andersen, T., Brown, P., d'Amore, F., Andersen, E., Abildgaard, N., & Gram, J. (2019). Effects of live music during chemotherapy in lymphoma patients: A randomized controlled trial. *Supportive Care in Cancer*, *27*(10), 3887–3896. DOI: 10.1007/s00520-019-04666-8 PMID: 30762141

Brown, R. M., Brown, S. L., & Johnson, A. S. (2015). Helping others as a means of reducing caregiver burden. *Journal of Applied Gerontology*, *34*(3), 221–242. DOI: 10.1177/0733464812465988

Cain, C. L., Surbone, A., Elk, R., & Kagawa-Singer, M. (2018). Culture and palliative care: Preferences, communication, meaning, and mutual decision making. *Journal of Pain and Symptom Management*, *55*(5), 1408–1419. DOI: 10.1016/j.jpainsymman.2018.01.007 PMID: 29366913

Campbell, J., Ikegami, N., & Gibson, M. (2019). Lessons from Japan's long-term care insurance system. *Health Affairs*, *38*(6), 912–919.

Carey, T. A., Schouten, K., Wakerman, J., Humphreys, J. S., Miegel, F., Murphy, S., & Arundell, M. (2016). Improving the quality of life of palliative and chronic disease patients and carers in remote Australia with the establishment of a day respite facility. *BMC Palliative Care*, *15*(1), 62. DOI: 10.1186/s12904-016-0136-1 PMID: 27430257

Carman, K. L., Dardess, P., & Maurer, M.. (2016). Patient and family engaged care: A framework for understanding the elements of engagement. *Health Affairs*, *35*(4), 595–603. PMID: 27044957

Case, C., Dalley, T., & Reddick, D. (2022). The handbook of art therapy. In *The Handbook of Art Therapy* (4th ed.). Taylor and Francis., DOI: 10.4324/9781003197850

Cassie, K. M., Snyder, M., & McClure, R. (2022). Caring in place: A framework for inclusive home environments. *Journal of Housing for the Elderly*, *36*(1), 74–93. DOI: 10.1080/02763893.2021.1944985

Chaisomboon, M., Jomnonkwao, S., & Ratanavaraha, V. (2020). Elderly users' satisfaction with public transport in Thailand using different importance performance analysis approaches. *Sustainability (Basel)*, *12*(21), 9066. DOI: 10.3390/su12219066

Chakrabarti, S. (2016). Family caregivers in India: Issues and perspectives. *Indian Journal of Psychiatry*, *58*(2), 217–223.

Chandra, S., & Banerjee, D. (2020). Caregiver burden and home care challenges in India: A narrative review. *Indian Journal of Social Psychiatry*, *36*(3), 208–214.

Chan, E. A., Wong, F., Cheung, M. Y. C., & Lam, W. (2012). Using narrative inquiry and ethnography to understand the impact of culture on caregiving. *Journal of Advanced Nursing*, *68*(3), 584–593. DOI: 10.1111/j.1365-2648.2011.05801.x

Chan, E. Y., Lim, W. S., & Tan, J. (2021). Carer Matters: A hospital-initiated programme to support caregivers during care transition. *BMC Geriatrics*, *21*(1), 1–12. PMID: 33388045

Chaudhuri, K. R., Azulay, J. P., Odin, P., Lindvall, S., Domingos, J., Alobaidi, A., Kandukuri, P. L., Chaudhari, V. S., Parra, J. C., Yamazaki, T., Oddsdottir, J., Wright, J., & Martinez-Martin, P. (2024). Economic Burden of Parkinson's Disease: A Multinational, Real-World, Cost-of-Illness Study. *Drugs - Real World Outcomes*, *11*(1), 1–11. DOI: 10.1007/s40801-023-00410-1 PMID: 38193999

Chelly, F., Kacem, I., Moussa, A., Ghenim, A., Krifa, I., Methamem, F., Chouachane, A., Aloui, A., Brahem, A., Kalboussi, H., El Maalel, O., Chatti, S., Maoua, M., Bannanou, S., & Mrizak, N. (2022). Healing humor: The use of humor in the nurse-patient relationship. *Occupational Diseases and Environmental Medicine*, *10*(3), 217–231. DOI: 10.4236/odem.2022.103017

Cheng, C., Elamin, M. E., May, H., & Kennedy, M. (2023). Drawing on emotions: The evolving role of art therapy. *Irish Journal of Psychological Medicine*, *40*(3), 500–502. DOI: 10.1017/ipm.2021.20 PMID: 33870885

Chen, J., Lin, Y., Yan, J., Wu, Y., & Hu, R. (2018). The effects of spiritual care on quality of life and spiritual well-being among patients with terminal illness: A systematic review. *Palliative Medicine*, *32*(7), 1167–1179. DOI: 10.1177/0269216318772267 PMID: 29708010

Chen, L. M., Inoue, M., & Buckley, N. (2024). Case studies on community care in Japan: Considerations for mitigating social isolation and loneliness in older adults with dementia. *Frontiers in Public Health*, *12*, 1411217. DOI: 10.3389/fpubh.2024.1411217 PMID: 39651466

Chenoweth, L., & McAuliffe, D. (2012). *Road to Social Work and Human Service Practice*. Cengage Learning Australia.

Chen, Y. C., Lin, Y. C., & Huang, L. (2021). HOLISTIC study: A home-based longitudinal investigation of integrated care. *Journal of Advanced Nursing*, *77*(4), 1982–1993.

Chen, Y., Li, X., Wang, J., Liu, M., Cai, C., & Shi, Y. (2023). Research on the application of fuzzy Bayesian network in risk assessment of catenary construction. *Mathematics*, *11*(7), 1719. DOI: 10.3390/math11071719

Cheung, M., & Leung, C. A. (2020). LYas a social work intervention. *Smith College Studies in Social Work*, *90*(4), 288–301. DOI: 10.1080/00377317.2020.1819938

Chew, E. Y. H., Ong, Z. L., Glass, G. F.Jr, & Chan, E. Y. (2022). '24/7'Caregiving: A Qualitative Analysis of an Emerging Phenomenon of Interest in Caregiving. *International Journal of Environmental Research and Public Health*, *19*(24), 17046. DOI: 10.3390/ijerph192417046 PMID: 36554924

Chiaramonte, D. R., & Adler, S. R. (2020). Integrative palliative care: A new transformative field to alleviate suffering. *Journal of Alternative and Complementary Medicine (New York, N.Y.)*, *26*(9), 761–765. DOI: 10.1089/acm.2020.0366 PMID: 32924551

Chien, L. Y., Chu, H., Guo, J. L., Liao, Y. M., Chang, L. I., Chen, C. H., & Chou, K. R. (2011). Caregiver support groups in patients with dementia: A meta-analysis. *International Journal of Geriatric Psychiatry, 26*(10), 1089–1098. DOI: 10.1002/gps.2660 PMID: 21308785

Chi, N. C., & Demiris, G. (2015). A systematic review of telehealth tools and interventions to support family caregivers. *Journal of Telemedicine and Telecare, 21*(1), 37–44. DOI: 10.1177/1357633X14562734 PMID: 25475220

Chobtham, K., Constantinou, A. C., & Kitson, N. K. (2023). Hybrid Bayesian network discovery with latent variables. *Data Mining and Knowledge Discovery, 37*(1), 476–520. DOI: 10.1007/s10618-022-00882-9

Cho, E., Kim, H., Kim, J., Lee, K., Meghani, S. H., & Chang, S. J. (2017). Older adult residents' perceptions of daily lives in nursing homes. *Journal of Nursing Scholarship, 49*(5), 495–503. DOI: 10.1111/jnu.12314 PMID: 28605167

Chung, M. L., Chen, Y., & Chou, K. R. (2021). Effects of caregiving burden, resilience, and social support on family caregivers' physical and mental health. *Archives of Psychiatric Nursing, 35*, 87–94. DOI: 10.1016/j.apnu.2021.01.004

Church, F. C. (2021). Treatment Options for Motor and Non-Motor Symptoms of Parkinson's Disease. *Biomolecules, 11*(4), 612. DOI: 10.3390/biom11040612 PMID: 33924103

Cıhan, P., & Coskun, H. (2021, June). Performance comparison of machine learning models for diabetes prediction. In *2021 29th Signal Processing and Communications Applications Conference (SIU)* (pp. 1–4). IEEE. https://doi.org/DOI: 10.1109/SIU53274.2021.9477824

Ciurea, A. V., Mohan, A. G., Covache-Busuioc, R. A., Costin, H. P., Glavan, L. A., Corlatescu, A. D., & Saceleanu, V. M. (2023). Unraveling Molecular and Genetic Insights into Neurodegenerative Diseases: Advances in Understanding Alzheimer's, Parkinson's, and Huntington's Diseases and Amyotrophic Lateral Sclerosis. *International Journal of Molecular Sciences, 24*(13), 10809. DOI: 10.3390/ijms241310809 PMID: 37445986

Clair, A. A., & Ebberts, A. G. (1997). The effects of music therapy on interactions between family caregivers and their care receivers with late-stage dementia. *Journal of Music Therapy, 34*(3), 148–164. DOI: 10.1093/jmt/34.3.148

Coady, N., & Lehmann, P. (2008). *Theoretical Perspectives for Direct social Work practice: A generalist-eclectic Approach* (2nd ed.). Springer.

Collins, R. N., Kishita, N., & Rymer, S. (2018). Psychological interventions for dementia caregivers: A systematic review and meta-analysis. *Aging & Mental Health, 22*(12), 1612–1630. DOI: 10.1080/13607863.2017.1370689

Compen, F. R.. (2018). Mindfulness-based cognitive therapy for cancer patients delivered via eHealth: A randomized controlled trial. *Psycho-Oncology, 27*(4), 1172–1179. DOI: 10.1002/pon.4642 PMID: 29266524

Connolly, M., & Harms, L. (2011a). Ecosystems theories. In *Social Work: From Theory to Practice* (pp. 47–72). Cambridge University Press. DOI: 10.1017/CBO9781139192521

Constantinou, A. C., Guo, Z., & Kitson, N. K. (2023). The impact of prior knowledge on causal structure learning. *Knowledge and Information Systems, 65*(8), 3385–3434. DOI: 10.1007/s10115-023-01858-x

Crouch, E., Probst, J. C., & Bennett, K. (2017). Rural-urban differences in caregiver burden: Implications for policy and practice. *The Journal of Rural Health, 33*(1), 32–40. DOI: 10.1111/jrh.12173 PMID: 26449177

Czaja, S. J., Boot, W. R., Charness, N., Rogers, W. A., & Sharit, J. (2018). Improving social support for older adults through technology: Findings from the PRISM randomized controlled trial. *The Gerontologist, 58*(3), 467–477. DOI: 10.1093/geront/gnw249 PMID: 28201730

D'Amelio, M., Terruso, V., Palmeri, B., Di Benedetto, N., Famoso, G., Cottone, P., Aridon, P., Ragonese, P., & Savettieri, G. (2009). Predictors of caregiver burden in partners of patients with Parkinson's disease. Neurological sciences: official journal of the Italian Neurological Society and of the Italian Society of Clinical Neurophysiology, 30(2), 171–174. https://doi.org/DOI: 10.1007/s10072-009-0024-z

Danucalov, M. A. D., Kozasa, E. H., Afonso, R. F., Galduroz, J. C. F., & Leite, J. R. (2013). Yoga and heart rate variability: A comprehensive review of the literature. *International Journal of Yoga, 6*(1), 76–83. DOI: 10.4103/0973-6131.105948 PMID: 23439856

Das, S. (2024). Why restructuring residential care matters: A global perspective. In *Care of Older Persons* (pp. 59–72). Routledge India. DOI: 10.4324/9781003528432-6

DeCaro, D. S., & Constantine Brown, J. L. (2016). Laughter Yoga, Adults Living With Parkinson s Disease, and Caregivers: A Pilot Study. *Explore (New York, N.Y.), 12*(3), 196–199. DOI: 10.1016/j.explore.2016.02.005 PMID: 27033323

Dehghan, N., Forouzi, M. A., Etminan, A., Roy, C., & Dehghan, M. (2022). The effects of lavender, rosemary and orange essential oils on memory problems and medication adherence among patients undergoing hemodialysis: A parallel randomized controlled trial. *Explore (New York, N.Y.)*, *18*(5), 559–566. DOI: 10.1016/j.explore.2021.10.004 PMID: 34736874

Demir, V., Eryürek, S., & Savaş, E. (2024). The effect of mindfulness-based art therapy on psychological symptoms and happiness levels in patients with migraine: A pilot study. *Current Psychology (New Brunswick, N.J.)*, *43*(19), 17664–17672. DOI: 10.1007/s12144-024-05634-0

Denham, A. C., & Kistler, C. E. (2023). Home-and Community-Based Care. In *Chronic Illness Care: Principles and Practice* (pp. 269–283). Springer International Publishing., DOI: 10.1007/978-3-031-29171-5_20

Deshields, T. L., Wells-Di Gregorio, S., Flowers, S. R., Irwin, K. E., Nipp, R., Padgett, L., & Zebrack, B. (2021). Addressing distress management challenges: Recommendations from the consensus panel of the American Psychosocial Oncology Society and the Association of Oncology Social Work. *CA: a Cancer Journal for Clinicians*, *71*(5), 407–436. DOI: 10.3322/caac.21672 PMID: 34028809

Deshmukh, L., Janghel, U., Sonkuwar, A., & Thakur, R. (2024). Exploring the Synergy between Yoga and Mindfulness Sport Practices: Enhancing Mental and Physical Well-Being. *Indian Journal of YOGA Exercise & Sport Science and Physical Education*, 26-32. DOI: 10.58914/ijyesspe.2024-9.1.4

Dev, P. S., Eljo, J. J. G., & Srinivasan, S. (2025). Intergenerational Caregiving on Grandparents Health: A Case Study. In *Perspectives on the Economics of Aging* (pp. 205-236). IGI Global Scientific Publishing. DOI: DOI: 10.4018/979-8-3693-7753-6.ch008

Dev, P. S., Eljo, J. J. G., & Srinivasan, S. (2025). Navigating Mental Health Challenges in the Care of Elderly With Disabilities in Kerala: A Gerontological Social Work Perspective. In *Modern Digital Approaches to Care Technologies for Individuals With Disabilities* (pp. 33-56). IGI Global Scientific Publishing. DOI: 10.4018/979-8-3693-7560-0.ch003

Dilhani, W. N. S., Mitchell, S., Dale, J., Toor, K., Javaid, M., & MacArtney, J. I. (2024). A mixed-methods systematic review investigating the use of digital health interventions to provide palliative and end-of-life care for patients in low-and middle-income countries. *Palliative Care and Social Practice*, *18*, 26323524241236965. DOI: 10.1177/26323524241236965 PMID: 38617095

Dilworth-Anderson, P., Williams, I. C., & Gibson, B. E. (2002). Issues of race, ethnicity, and culture in caregiving research: A 20-year review. *The Gerontologist, 42*(2), 237–272. DOI: 10.1093/geront/42.2.237 PMID: 11914467

Donovan, N. J., & Blazer, D. (2020). Social isolation and loneliness in older adults: Review and commentary of a national academies report. *The American Journal of Geriatric Psychiatry, 28*(12), 1233–1244. DOI: 10.1016/j.jagp.2020.08.005 PMID: 32919873

Dos Santos, F. C., Snigurska, U. A., Keenan, G. M., Lucero, R. J., & Modave, F. (2023). Clinical decision support systems for palliative care management: A scoping review. *Journal of Pain and Symptom Management, 66*(2), e205–e218. DOI: 10.1016/j.jpainsymman.2023.03.006 PMID: 36933748

Doty, P. (2010). The evolving balance of formal and informal, institutional and non-institutional long-term care for older Americans: A thirty-year perspective. *The Public Policy and Aging Report, 20*(1), 3–9. DOI: 10.1093/ppar/20.1.3

Dratsiou, I., Villacañas, O., Cooper, S., Isaris, P., Serras, M., Unzueta, L., & Fernandez-Carbajales, V. (2021, June). *Assistive technologies for supporting well-being of older adults. Proceedings of the 14th PErvasive Technologies Related to Assistive Environments Conference*, 338–341. DOI: 10.1145/3453892.3461352

Duncan, B., & Miller, S. (2001). Using the Client's Theory of Change: Research and practice. *Psychotherapy in Australia, 8*, 16–23.

Dunér, A., Bjälkebring, P., & Johansson, B. (2019). Autonomy, choice and control for older users of home care services: Current developments in Swedish eldercare. *Journal of Social Service Research, 45*(1), 129–141. DOI: 10.1080/01488376.2018.1479677

Du, Z., Guo, S., Sun, Y., Zhou, Q., Jiang, Y., Shen, Y., Zhu, H., Zhou, Z., & Zhou, H. (2023). Causal relationships between dietary habits and five major mental disorders: A two-sample Mendelian randomization study. *Journal of Affective Disorders, 340*, 607–615. DOI: 10.1016/j.jad.2023.08.098 PMID: 37598719

Efendi, A., Ammarullah, M. I., Isa, I. G. T., Sari, M. P., Izza, J. N., Nugroho, Y. S., Nasrullah, H., & Alfian, D. (2025). IoT-based elderly health monitoring system using Firebase cloud computing. *Health Science Reports, 8*(3), e70498. DOI: 10.1002/hsr2.70498 PMID: 40041774

El Arab, R. A., Abu-Mahfouz, M. S., Abuadas, F. H., Alzghoul, H., Almari, M., Ghannam, A., & Seweid, M. M. (2025). Bridging the gap…. *Healthcare (Basel), 13*(7), 701. DOI: 10.3390/healthcare13070701 PMID: 40217999

Ellermann, A. (1998). Can discourse analysis enable reflective social work practice? *Social Work Education, 17*(1), 35–44. DOI: 10.1080/02615479811220041

Elliott, D., McKinley, S., Alison, J., Aitken, L. M., King, M., Leslie, G. D., Kenny, P., Taylor, P., Foley, R., & Burmeister, E. (2011). Health-related quality of life and physical recovery after a critical illness: A multi-centre randomised controlled trial of a home-based physical rehabilitation program. *Critical Care, 15*(3), R142. DOI: 10.1186/cc10265 PMID: 21658221

Elliott, S., Golds, S., Sissons, I., & Wilson, H. (2015). Long-term care: A review of global funding models. *British Actuarial Journal, 20*(1), 167–208. DOI: 10.1017/S1357321714000300

El-Mallakh, P., & Findlay, J. (2015). Strategies to improve medication adherence in patients with schizophrenia: The role of support services. *Neuropsychiatric Disease and Treatment,* •••, 1077–1090. DOI: 10.2147/NDT.S56107 PMID: 25931823

El-Sayed, M. M., Hafez, S. A., Nashwan, A. J., Khedr, M. A., & El-Ashry, A. M. (2024). Feasibility of a group-based laughter yoga therapy on anxiety and happiness among community-dwelling older adults: A quasi-experimental study. *International Journal of Africa Nursing Sciences, 20,* 100675. DOI: 10.1016/j.ijans.2024.100675

Emilia, C. (2021a). Art therapy with children surviving cancer used to relieve symptoms associated with death, loss and pain. *European Psychiatry : the Journal of the Association of European Psychiatrists, 64*(S1), S682–S683. DOI: 10.1192/j.eurpsy.2021.1809

Emilia, C. (2021b). Implementing new digital options in education/ occupational/ play/ art therapy as tools for self- knowledge, self-managements, self-esteem. *European Psychiatry : the Journal of the Association of European Psychiatrists, 64*(S1), S681–S682. DOI: 10.1192/j.eurpsy.2021.1808

Emon, M. U., Keya, M. S., Kaiser, M. S., Islam, M. A., Tanha, T., & Zulfiker, M. S. (2021, March). Primary stage of diabetes prediction using machine learning approaches. In *2021 International Conference on Artificial Intelligence and Smart Systems (ICAIS)* (pp. 364–367). IEEE. https://doi.org/DOI: 10.1109/ICAIS50930.2021.9395968

Ene, J. C., Chukwu, N. E., & Ajibo, H. T. (2022). Exploring care management for older adults with illnesses as family members' responsibility. The need for social workers' support services in Nigeria. *European Journal of Mental Health, 17*(3), 38–51. https://www.ceeol.com/search/article-detail?id=1090051. DOI: 10.5708/EJMH.17.2022.3.3

Engel, G. L. (1977). The need for a new medical model: A challenge for biomedicine. *Science, 196*(4286), 129–136. DOI: 10.1126/science.847460 PMID: 847460

Etemadi, M., Abkenar, S. B., Ahmadzadeh, A., Kashani, M. H., Asghari, P., Akbari, M., & Mahdipour, E. (2023). A systematic review of healthcare recommender systems. *Expert Systems with Applications, 213*, 118823. DOI: 10.1016/j.eswa.2022.118823

Etkind, S. N., Bone, A. E., Lovell, N., Cripps, R. L., Harding, R., Higginson, I. J., & Sleeman, K. E. (2020). The role and response of palliative care and hospice services in epidemics and pandemics: A rapid review to inform practice during the COVID-19 pandemic. *Journal of Pain and Symptom Management, 60*(1), e31–e40. DOI: 10.1016/j.jpainsymman.2020.03.029 PMID: 32278097

Fan, S. Y., Lin, I. M., Hsieh, J. G., & Chang, C. J. (2017). Psychosocial care provided by physicians and nurses in palliative care: A mixed methods study. *Journal of Pain and Symptom Management, 53*(2), 216–223. DOI: 10.1016/j.jpainsymman.2016.08.019 PMID: 27756622

Farias, I. P. S. E., Sousa, S. A. D., Almeida, L. D. F. D. D., Santiago, B. M., Pereira, A. C., & Cavalcanti, Y. W. (2020). Does non-institutionalized elders have a better oral health status compared to institutionalized ones? A systematic review and meta-analysis. *Ciencia & Saude Coletiva, 25*(6), 2177–2192. DOI: 10.1590/1413-81232020256.18252018 PMID: 32520263

Faydalı, S., & Çetinkaya, F. (2018). The effect of aromatherapy on sleep quality. *Alternative Therapies in Health and Medicine, 24*(3), 42–48. PMID: 29210873

Feerick, F., Coughlan, E., Knox, S., Murphy, A., Grady, I. O., & Deasy, C. (2025). Barriers to paramedic professionalisation: A qualitative enquiry across the UK, Canada, Australia, USA and the republic of Ireland. *BMC Health Services Research, 25*(1), 993. DOI: 10.1186/s12913-025-13196-5 PMID: 40734170

Feinberg, L. F. (2019). *Breaking new ground: Supporting family caregivers in the workplace*. AARP Public Policy Institute.

Feldwisch, R. P. (2022). History, profession, and ethics of art therapy. In *Foundations of Art Therapy* (pp. 3–30). Elsevier., DOI: 10.1016/B978-0-12-824308-4.00007-7

Fields, N. L., Anderson, K. A., & Dabelko-Schoeny, H. (2011). Ready or not: Transitioning from institutional care to community care. *Journal of Housing for the Elderly, 25*(1), 3–17. DOI: 10.1080/02763893.2011.545330

Fleszar-Pavlovic, S. E., McConnell, T., Schmid, W., & Pavlicevic, M. (2024). eHealth mindfulness-based music therapy for patients undergoing allogeneic stem cell transplantation: A pilot randomized controlled trial protocol. *Supportive Care in Cancer, 31*(9), 4512–4522. PMID: 38763308

Flieger, S. P., Chui, K., & Koch-Weser, S. (2020). Lack of awareness and common misconceptions about palliative care among adults: Insights from a national survey. *Journal of General Internal Medicine, 35*(7), 2059–2064. DOI: 10.1007/s11606-020-05730-4 PMID: 32157652

Gallagher-Thompson, D., Solano, N., McGee, J. S., & Kurylo, M. (2003). Coping with caregiving: Reducing stress and improving your quality of life (2nd ed.). *Aging and Mental Health, 7*(3), 235–245. DOI: 10.1080/1360786031000101175

Gao, F., Chui, P. L., Che, C. C., Xiao, L., & Zhang, Q. (2024). Advance care planning readiness among community-dwelling older adults and the influencing factors: A scoping review. *BMC Palliative Care, 23*(1), 255. DOI: 10.1186/s12904-024-01583-4 PMID: 39491026

Gasse, M., Aussem, A., & Elghazel, H. (2014). A hybrid algorithm for Bayesian network structure learning with application to multi-label learning. *Expert Systems with Applications, 41*(15), 6755–6772. DOI: 10.1016/j.eswa.2014.04.032

Geerlings, A. D., Kapelle, W. M., Sederel, C. J., Tenison, E., Wijngaards-Berenbroek, H., Meinders, M. J., Munneke, M., Ben-Shlomo, Y., Bloem, B. R., & Darweesh, S. K. L. (2023). Caregiver burden in Parkinson's disease: A mixed-methods study. *BMC Medicine, 21*(1), 247. DOI: 10.1186/s12916-023-02933-4 PMID: 37424022

Gérain, P., & Zech, E. (2019). Informal caregiver burnout? Development of a theoretical framework to understand the impact of caregiving. *Frontiers in Psychology, 10*, 466359. DOI: 10.3389/fpsyg.2019.01748 PMID: 31428015

Gerdner, L. A. (2012). Music therapy in dementia care.[56]. *Perspectives in Psychiatric Care, 48*(2), 77–78. DOI: 10.1111/j.1744-6163.2012.00332.x

Ghoshal, A., & Damani, A. (2025). Home-Based Care Services. In *The Palgrave Encyclopedia of Disability* (pp. 1–11). Springer Nature Switzerland., DOI: 10.1007/978-3-031-40858-8_535-1

Gibson, C. A., Lichtenthal, W., Berg, A., & Breitbart, W. (2006). Psychologic issues in palliative care. *Anesthesiology Clinics of North America, 24*(1), 61–80. DOI: 10.1016/j.atc.2005.12.001 PMID: 16487896

Gilmartin, M. J. (2023). Nurses improving care for health systems elders (NICHE). *Geriatric Nursing, 53*, 310–312. DOI: 10.1016/j.gerinurse.2023.08.002 PMID: 37689486

Gitlin, L. N., Reever, K., Dennis, M. P., Mathieu, E., & Hauck, W. W. (2006). Enhancing quality of life of families who use adult day services: Short- and long-term effects of the Adult Day Services Plus Program. *The Gerontologist, 46*(5), 630–639. DOI: 10.1093/geront/46.5.630 PMID: 17050754

Gladstone, J., Dumbrill, G., Leslie, B., Koster, A., Young, M., & Ismaila, A. (2014). Understanding worker-parent engagement in child protection casework. *Children and Youth Services Review, 44*, 56–64. DOI: 10.1016/j.childyouth.2014.06.002

Glajchen, M. (2012). Physical well-being of oncology caregivers: an important quality-of-life domain. In *Seminars in oncology nursing* (Vol. 28, No. 4, pp. 226-235). WB Saunders. DOI: 10.1016/j.soncn.2012.09.005

Glueckauf, R. L.. (2012). Online cognitive-behavioral therapy for dementia caregivers: A pilot study. *The Gerontologist, 52*(4), 472–478. DOI: 10.1093/geront/gnr119 PMID: 22241808

Gomes, B., Calanzani, N., Curiale, V., McCrone, P., Higginson, I. J., & de Brito, M. (2013). Effectiveness and cost-effectiveness of home palliative care services for adults with advanced illness and their caregivers. *Cochrane Database of Systematic Reviews, 2022*(6). Advance online publication. DOI: 10.1002/14651858.CD007760.pub2 PMID: 23744578

Gomes, B., Calanzani, N., & Higginson, I. (2021). Effectiveness of home palliative care services: A systematic review. *Cochrane Database of Systematic Reviews, 2*, 1–62.

Gonot-Schoupinsky, F. N., & Garip, G. (2018). Laughter and humour interventions for well-being in older adults: A systematic review and intervention classification. *Complementary Therapies in Medicine, 38*, 85–91. DOI: 10.1016/j.ctim.2018.04.009 PMID: 29857886

Gonzales, E., Lee, K., & Harootyan, B. (2020). Voices from the field: Ecological factors that promote employment and health among low-income older adults with implications for direct social work practice. *Clinical Social Work Journal, 48*(2), 211–222. DOI: 10.1007/s10615-019-00719-x

Gordon, A. (2018). Institutional and non-institutional long-term care. In *Learning geriatric medicine: a study guide for medical students* (pp. 329–335). Springer International Publishing., DOI: 10.1007/978-3-319-61997-2_32

Gorfinkiel, M. D., San Miguel, B. E., & Peterson, E. (2025). Home-based care services for elderly dependent adults. A comparative analysis of Madrid and Stockholm. *Investigaciones Regionales= Journal of Regional Research*, (61), 17-30. https://dialnet.unirioja.es/servlet/articulo?codigo=10051205

Gorman, M. (2017). Development and the rights of older people. In *The ageing and development report* (pp. 3–21). Routledge. DOI: 10.4324/9781315071541-2

Graham, C. L., Scharlach, A. E., & Price Wolf, J. (2014). The impact of the "village" model on health, well-being, service access, and social engagement of older adults. *Health Education & Behavior*, *41*(1, suppl), 91S–97S. DOI: 10.1177/1090198114532290 PMID: 24799128

Grech, S. (2019). Disabled families: The impacts of disability and care on family labour and poverty in rural Guatemala. *Societies (Basel, Switzerland)*, *9*(4), 76. DOI: 10.3390/soc9040076

Greer, J. A., Applebaum, A. J., Jacobsen, J. C., Temel, J. S., & Jackson, V. A. (2020). Understanding and addressing the role of coping in palliative care for patients with advanced cancer. *Journal of Clinical Oncology*, *38*(9), 915–925. DOI: 10.1200/JCO.19.00013 PMID: 32023161

Grinde, B., & Patil, G. G. (2009). Biophilia: Does visual contact with nature impact on health and well-being? *International Journal of Environmental Research and Public Health*, *6*(9), 2332–2343. DOI: 10.3390/ijerph6092332 PMID: 19826546

Gronda, H. (2008). Case Management for People Experiencing Homelessness: What Makes It Work? Evidence for Practice. *Parity*, *21*(10). http://www.yp4.org.au/

Gupta, S. (2020). Institutional Care for Elderly. In *Ageing Issues and Responses in India* (pp. 143–155). Springer Singapore., DOI: 10.1007/978-981-15-5187-1_9

Gutiérrez, R., & Ramos, J. (2024). The Well-Teach framework: Integrating evidence-based education into caregiving. *Journal of Holistic Nursing*, *42*(1), 45–59.

Hailu, G. N., Gebru, H. B., Hagos, G. G., Weldemariam, A. H., Tadesse, D. B., & Mebrahtom, G. (2025). The role of family caregivers in supporting older adults in Africa: Systematic review. *BMC Geriatrics*, *25*(1), 1–15. DOI: 10.1186/s12877-025-06154-7 PMID: 40610950

Haleem, A., Javaid, M., Singh, R. P., & Suman, R. (2023). Exploring the revolution in healthcare systems through the applications of digital twin technology. *Biomedical Technology*, *4*, 28–38. DOI: 10.1016/j.bmt.2023.02.001

Hammar, T., Rissanen, P., & Perälä, M. L. (2008). Home-care clients' need for help, and use and costs of services. *European Journal of Ageing*, *5*(2), 147–160. DOI: 10.1007/s10433-008-0078-4 PMID: 28798569

Han, S., Zhang, L., Li, Q., Wang, X., & Lian, S. (2023). The Effects of Laughter Yoga on Perceived Stress, Positive Psychological Capital, and Exercise Capacity in Lung Cancer Chemotherapy Patients: A Pilot Randomized Trial. *Integrative Cancer Therapies*, *22*, 15347354231218271. DOI: 10.1177/15347354231218271 PMID: 38102816

Haramshahi, M., Babaie, S., Shahnazi, M., Kafil, B., Farshbaf-Khalili, A., & Naghdi, M. (2024). The efficacy of oral Lavandula angustifolia Mill. essential oil on menopausal symptoms, serum lipid profile, and cortisol concentration in postmenopausal women: A triple-blind, randomized, controlled trial. *Complementary Therapies in Medicine*, *82*, 103050. DOI: 10.1016/j.ctim.2024.103050 PMID: 38754638

Harms, L. (2010). A multidimensional approach. In Harms, L. (Ed.), *Understanding human development* (2nd ed., pp. 3–35). Oxford University Press.

Harris, D. M., O'Bryan, S. J., & Latella, C. (2024). Non-invasive brain stimulation as treatment for motor impairment in people with Parkinson's disease: Protocol for an umbrella review. *PLoS One*, *19*(6), e0304717. DOI: 10.1371/journal.pone.0304717 PMID: 38870241

Harris-Kojetin, L., Sengupta, M., Park-Lee, E., Valverde, R., Caffrey, C., Rome, V., & Lendon, J. (2016). Long-term care providers and services users in the United States: Data from the National Study of Long-Term Care Providers, 2013–2014.

Harris, R., Sims, S., & Parr, J. (2020). Evidence-based home healthcare: Global trends and outcomes. *Journal of Community Health Nursing*, *37*(1), 22–33.

Hasan, N., & Ahmed, M. (2024). *Wearable technology for elderly care: Integrating health monitoring and emergency alerts*. Journal of Computer Networks and Communications. *Article, 5593708*. Advance online publication. DOI: 10.1155/2024/5593708

Hassan, A. Y. I. (2020). Challenges and recommendations for the deployment of information and communication technology solutions for informal caregivers: Scoping review. *JMIR Aging*, *3*(2), e20310. DOI: 10.2196/20310 PMID: 32723720

Hatzipapas, I., Visser, M. J., & Janse van Rensburg, E. (2017). Laughter therapy as an intervention to promote psychological well-being of volunteer community care workers working with HIV-affected families. *SAHARA J : Journal of Social Aspects of HIV/AIDS Research Alliance*, *14*(1), 202–212. DOI: 10.1080/17290376.2017.1402696 PMID: 29169302

Hayslip, B.Jr, & Kaminski, P. L. (2005). Grandparents raising their grandchildren: A review of the literature and suggestions for practice. *The Gerontologist*, *45*(2), 262–269. DOI: 10.1093/geront/45.2.262 PMID: 15799992

He, W., & Kinsella, K. (2020). Global aging in the new millennium. *The cultural context of aging: Worldwide perspectives, 27.*

Head, B. A., Schapmire, T. J., Earnshaw, L., Chenault, J., Pfeifer, M., Sawning, S., & Shaw, M. A. (2016). Improving medical graduates' training in palliative care: Advancing education and practice. *Advances in Medical Education and Practice*, •••, 99–113. DOI: 10.2147/AMEP.S94550 PMID: 26955298

Hebert, R. S., Dang, Q., & Schulz, R. (2007). Religious beliefs and practices are associated with better mental health in family caregivers. *The Gerontologist*, *47*(6), 703–710. DOI: 10.1093/geront/47.6.703 PMID: 17158632

Heidari, M., Ghodusi Borujeni, M., Rezaei, P., Kabirian Abyaneh, S., & Heidari, K. (2020). Effect of Laughter Therapy on Depression and Quality of Life of the Elderly Living in Nursing Homes. *The Malaysian Journal of Medical Sciences : MJMS*, *27*(4), 119–129. DOI: 10.21315/mjms2020.27.4.11 PMID: 32863751

Heidelburg, K., Parker, J., & Casella, J. (2024). Strategies for using technology to develop novice school psychology consultants' multicultural consultation skills. *Journal of Educational & Psychological Consultation*, *34*(4), 350–372. DOI: 10.1080/10474412.2024.2315092

Heo, E. H., Kim, S., Park, H. J., & Kil, S. Y. (2016). The effects of a simulated laughter programme on mood, cortisol levels, and health-related quality of life among haemodialysis patients. *Complementary Therapies in Clinical Practice*, *25*, 1–7. DOI: 10.1016/j.ctcp.2016.07.001 PMID: 27863598

Hepworth, D. H., Rooney, R. H., Rooney, G. D., Strom-Gottfried, K., & Larsen, J. (2010). *Direct Social Work Practice: Theory and Skills* (8th ed.). Cengage Learning.

Herz, R. S. (2009). Aromatherapy facts and fictions: A scientific analysis of olfactory effects on mood, physiology and behavior. *The International Journal of Neuroscience*, *119*(2), 263–290. DOI: 10.1080/00207450802333953 PMID: 19125379

Hillcoat-Nallétamby, S. (2014). The meaning of "independence" for older people in different residential settings. *The Journals of Gerontology. Series B, Psychological Sciences and Social Sciences*, *69*(3), 419–430. DOI: 10.1093/geronb/gbu008 PMID: 24578371

Hilton, C. (2017). Psychiatric Hospitals and Older People: Status Quo or Making Changes? In *Improving Psychiatric Care for Older People: Barbara Robb's Campaign 1965-1975* (pp. 19–55). Springer International Publishing., DOI: 10.1007/978-3-319-54813-5_2

Hirsch, C., Davoli, L., Grosu, R., & Ferrari, G. (2023). DynGATT: A dynamic GATT-based data synchronization protocol for BLE networks. *Computer Networks, 222*, 109560. DOI: 10.1016/j.comnet.2023.109560

Hodgetts, S., Nicholas, D., Zwaigenbaum, L., & McConnell, D. (2013). Parents' and professionals' perceptions of family-centered care for children with autism spectrum disorder across service sectors. *Social Science & Medicine, 96*, 138–146. DOI: 10.1016/j.socscimed.2013.07.012 PMID: 24034961

Höglinger, G., Bähr, M., Becktepe, J., Berg, D., Brockmann, K., Buhmann, C., Ceballos-Baumann, A., Claßen, J., Deuschl, C., Deuschl, G., Dodel, R., Ebersbach, G., Eggers, C., van Eimeren, T., Fanciulli, A., Fimm, B., Folkerts, A.-K., Gausepohl, M., Hasan, A., & Trenkwalder, C.German Parkinson's Guidelines Committee. (2024). Diagnosis and treatment of Parkinson's disease (guideline of the German Society for Neurology). *Neurological Research and Practice, 6*(1), 30. DOI: 10.1186/s42466-024-00325-4 PMID: 38845028

Hohman, M. (2012). *Motivational interviewing in Social work Practice*. The Guilford Press.

Ho, K.. (2020). Artificial intelligence in caregiving: Opportunities, challenges, and policy implications. *Journal of Medical Internet Research, 22*(8), e15666. DOI: 10.2196/15666

Holroyd-Leduc, J., Resin, J., Ashley, L., Barwich, D., Elliott, J., Huras, P., France, L., Mahoney, M., Maybee, A., McNeil, H., Pullman, D., Sawatzky, R., Stolee, P., & Muscedere, J. (2016). Giving voice to older adults living with frailty and their family caregivers: Engagement of older adults living with frailty in research, health care decision making, and in health policy. *Research Involvement and Engagement, 2*(1), 23. DOI: 10.1186/s40900-016-0038-7 PMID: 29062523

Hosu, L.-M. (2022). Art therapy focused on stimulating the emotional and expressive skills of the atypical children. *European Psychiatry : the Journal of the Association of European Psychiatrists, 65*(S1), S236–S237. DOI: 10.1192/j.eurpsy.2022.612

Hosu, L.-M. (2023). Environmental manipulation and stimulation of atypical children through art therapy. *European Psychiatry : the Journal of the Association of European Psychiatrists, 66*(S1), S820–S821. DOI: 10.1192/j.eurpsy.2023.1738

Hua, A. (2025). Integrating Community-Based and Smart Care Models: Strategies for Advancing China's Elderly Care Industry Amid Demographic Challenges. *International Journal of Asian Social Science Research, 2*(1), 77–84. DOI: 10.70267/6f3z9930

Huang, Y., Aronson, J. P., Pilitsis, J. G., Gee, L., Durphy, J., Molho, E. S., & Ramirez-Zamora, A. (2018). Anatomical Correlates of Uncontrollable Laughter With Unilateral Subthalamic Deep Brain Stimulation in Parkinson's Disease. *Frontiers in Neurology, 9*, 341. DOI: 10.3389/fneur.2018.00341 PMID: 29887826

Huang, Y., Li, Y., Pan, H., & Han, L. (2023). Global, regional, and national burden of neurological disorders in 204 countries and territories worldwide. *Journal of Global Health, 13*, 04160. DOI: 10.7189/jogh.13.04160 PMID: 38018250

Hui, D., Heung, Y., & Bruera, E. (2022). Timely palliative care: Personalizing the process of referral. *Cancers (Basel), 14*(4), 1047. DOI: 10.3390/cancers14041047 PMID: 35205793

Hung, J. (2022). Smart elderly care services in China: Challenges, progress, and policy development. *Sustainability (Basel), 15*(1), 178. DOI: 10.3390/su15010178

Hu, Z., Abd Rahman, N. H., & Hanafi, H. (2025). Non-governmental Organizations' Role in Promoting Life Satisfaction Among the Elderly Within the Active Aging Strategy. *Voluntas, 36*(3), 337–351. DOI: 10.1007/s11266-025-00728-0

Ibáñez, V., Silva, J., & Cauli, O. (2018). A survey on sleep assessment methods. *PeerJ, 6*, e4849. DOI: 10.7717/peerj.4849 PMID: 29844990

Imrie, R., & Luck, R. (2014). Designing inclusive environments: Rehabilitating the body and the relevance of universal design. *Disability and Rehabilitation, 36*(16), 1315–1319. DOI: 10.3109/09638288.2014.936191 PMID: 24989068

International Labour Organization (ILO). (2021). *Unpaid caregiving and economic contribution in India*. ILO India Report.

Izullah, F. R., Koivisto, M., & Nieminen, V. .a. (2022). Aging and sleep deprivation affect different neurocognitive stages of spatial information processing during a virtual driving task – An ERP study, *Transportation Research Part F: Traffic Psychology and Behaviour*, Vol 89.

Jafari, M., Raoofi, S., Zarnaq, R. K., Mobasseri, K., & Ghasemyani, S. (2024). Infrastructure analysis of long-term care for elderly adults in Iran: A qualitative study. *Int J Agin, 2*, e22. DOI: 10.34172/ija.2024.e22

Jaiswal, R., Alici, Y., & Breitbart, W. (2014). A comprehensive review of palliative care in patients with cancer. *International Review of Psychiatry (Abingdon, England)*, *26*(1), 87–101. DOI: 10.3109/09540261.2013.868788 PMID: 24716503

Jethva, D. D., Patel, B. C., Sundar, S., Patel, J. B., Vora, H. H., & Sanghavi, P. R. (2025). Harmonising hope: Impact of music therapy on cancer pain and palliative care. *Indian Journal of Palliative Care*, *31*(1), 21–28. DOI: 10.25259/IJPC_235_2024 PMID: 40027977

Kabat-Zinn, J. (1990). *Full catastrophe living: Using the wisdom of your body and mind to face stress, pain, and illness*. Delacorte.

Kalia, L. V., & Lang, A. E. (2015). Parkinson's disease. *Lancet*, *386*(9996), 896–912. DOI: 10.1016/S0140-6736(14)61393-3 PMID: 25904081

Kang, H. Y., Ahn, H. Y., Kang, M. J., & Hur, M. H. (2023). Effects of aromatherapy on sore throat, nasal symptoms and sleep quality in adults infected with COVID-19: A randomized controlled trial. *Integrative Medicine Research*, *12*(4), 101001. DOI: 10.1016/j.imr.2023.101001 PMID: 38024288

Kapp, S. K. (Ed.). (2020). *Autistic community and the neurodiversity movement: Stories from the frontline*. Springer., DOI: 10.1007/978-981-13-8437-0

Kasmaei, M. S., Freeman, S., Banner, D., Klassen-Ross, T., & Martin-Khan, M. (2025). The Impact of the COVID-19 Pandemic on Care Aides' Job Satisfaction in Long-Term Care Facilities in Northern British Columbia: A Qualitative Study. *COVID*, *5*(9), 157. DOI: 10.3390/covid5090157

Kataria, M. (2018). *Laughter yoga: Daily laughter practices for health and happiness*. Penguin Random House India Private Limited.

Kaye, H. S., & Harrington, C. (2015). Long-term services and supports in the community: Toward a research agenda. *Disability and Health Journal*, *8*(1), 3–8. DOI: 10.1016/j.dhjo.2014.09.003 PMID: 25445015

Keykhahoseinpoor, A., Rahnama, N., & Chitsaz, A. (2013). Effects of eight weeks LYtraining on motor function, balance, and flexibility in subjects with PD's disease. Journal of research in rehabilitation sciences, 9(1), 39-47. https://doi.org/DOI: 10.22122/jrrs.v9i1.856

Khaleel, F. A., & Al-Bakry, A. M. (2021). Diagnosis of diabetes using machine learning algorithms. *Materials Today: Proceedings*, *47*(14), 4851–4854. DOI: 10.1016/j.matpr.2021.07.196

Khanam, J. J., & Foo, S. Y. (2021). A comparison of machine learning algorithms for diabetes prediction. *ICT Express*, *7*(4), 432–439. DOI: 10.1016/j.icte.2021.02.004

Kiecolt-Glaser, J. K., McGuire, L., Robles, T. F., & Glaser, R. (2002). Psychoneuroimmunology and psychosomatic medicine: Back to the future. *Psychosomatic Medicine*, *64*(1), 15–28. DOI: 10.1097/00006842-200201000-00004 PMID: 11818582

Kim, S. H., Kim, Y. H., & Kim, H. J. (2015). Laughter and stress relief in cancer patients: A pilot study. *Evidence-Based Complementary and Alternative Medicine : eCAM*, *2015*, 1–6. DOI: 10.1155/2015/864739 PMID: 26064177

Kissane, D., & Yates, P. (2018). Psychological and existential distress. *Palliative care nursing*, 229-243.

Kitson, N. K., Constantinou, A. C., Guo, Z., Liu, Y., & Chobtham, K. (2023). A survey of Bayesian network structure learning. *Artificial Intelligence Review*, *56*(8), 8721–8814. DOI: 10.1007/s10462-022-10351-w

Kitwood, T. (1997). *Dementia reconsidered: The person comes first.* Open University Press.

Klingbeil, J., Wawrzyniak, M., Stockert, A., Brandt, M. L., Schneider, H. R., Metelmann, M., & Saur, D. (2021). Pathological laughter and crying: Insights from lesion network-symptom-mapping. *Brain*, *144*(10), 3264–3276. DOI: 10.1093/brain/awab224 PMID: 34142117

Knaul, F. M., Arreola-Ornelas, H., Kwete, X. J., Bhadelia, A., Rosa, W. E., Touchton, M., Méndez-Carniado, O., Enciso, V. V., Pastrana, T., Friedman, J. R., Connor, S. R., Downing, J., Jamison, D. T., Krakauer, E. L., Watkins, D., Anyosa, R. C., Garcia-Santisteban, R., Nargund, R. S., Cleary, J., & Radbruch, L. (2025). The evolution of serious health-related suffering from 1990 to 2021: An update to The Lancet Commission on global access to palliative care and pain relief. *The Lancet. Global Health*, *13*(3), e422–e436. https://www.thelancet.com/journals/langlo/article/PIIS2214-109X(24)00476-5/fulltext. DOI: 10.1016/S2214-109X(24)00476-5 PMID: 40021301

Koehler, F., Martin, Z.-S., Hertrampf, R.-S., Gäbel, C., Kessler, J., Ditzen, B., & Warth, M. (2021). Music therapy in the psychosocial treatment of adult cancer patients: A systematic review and meta-analysis. *Frontiers in Psychology*, *11*, 651. DOI: 10.3389/fpsyg.2020.00651 PMID: 32373019

Korostiy, V., & Hmain, S. (2013). Art Therapy In The Treatment Of Patients With Depressive Disorder. *European Psychiatry : the Journal of the Association of European Psychiatrists*, *28*(S1), 1. DOI: 10.1016/S0924-9338(13)77177-3

Koshmaganbetova, G., Zhylkybekova, A., Abenova, N. A., & Glushkova, N. (2024). Gender Disparities in Care Allocation among Informal Elderly Caregivers: A literature Review. *The Journal of Health Design*, *1*(55), 40–49. DOI: 10.32921/2225-9929-2024-1-55-40-49

Kouli, A., Torsney, K. M., & Kuan, W. L. (2018). Parkinson's Disease: Etiology, Neuropathology, and Pathogenesis. In T. B. Stoker (Eds.) et al., Parkinson's Disease: Pathogenesis and Clinical Aspects. Codon Publications. DOI: 10.15586/codonpublications.parkinsonsdisease.2018.ch1

Kozhyna, H., Korostiy, V., Hmain, S., & Mykhaylov, V. (2017). The use of art therapy in complex treatment on the quality of remission in patients with melancholy in major depressive disorder. *European Psychiatry : the Journal of the Association of European Psychiatrists*, *41*(S1), s777–s777. DOI: 10.1016/j.eurpsy.2017.01.1473

Kraun, L., De Vliegher, K., Vandamme, M., Holtzheimer, E., Ellen, M., & van Achterberg, T. (2022). Older peoples' and informal caregivers' experiences, views, and needs in transitional care decision-making: A systematic review. *International Journal of Nursing Studies*, *134*, 104303. DOI: 10.1016/j.ijnurstu.2022.104303 PMID: 35797843

Kroemeke, A., & Gruszczynska, E. (2016). Well-being and institutional care in older adults: Cross-sectional and time effects of provided and received support. *PLoS One*, *11*(8), e0161328. DOI: 10.1371/journal.pone.0161328 PMID: 27548721

Kruse, C., Betancourt, J., Ortiz, S., Luna, S. M. V., Bamrah, I. K., & Segovia, N. (2019). Barriers to the use of mobile health in improving health outcomes in developing countries: Systematic review. *Journal of Medical Internet Research*, *21*(10), e13263. DOI: 10.2196/13263 PMID: 31593543

Kuhlthau, K. A., O'Connor, K., & Perrin, J. M. (2022). Caring for children with autism spectrum disorder: The experience of caregivers. *Journal of Autism and Developmental Disorders*, *52*(3), 1408–1420. DOI: 10.1007/s10803-021-05052-8 PMID: 33909211

Kumar, R., Singh, R., & Sharma, V. (2024). Protective potential of LYand clapping exercises on stress level and motor functions in PD patients with type 2 diabetes. *PDism & Related Disorders*, *122*. Advance online publication. DOI: 10.1016/j.parkreldis.2024.106915

Kumar, S. (2018). Community-led home palliative care: The Kerala model. *Indian Journal of Palliative Care*, *24*(3), 237–244.

Kurasz, A. M., Smith, G. E., Curiel, R. E., Barker, W. W., Behar, R. C., Ramirez, A., & Armstrong, M. J. (2022). Patient values in healthcare decision making among diverse older adults. *Patient Education and Counseling*, *105*(5), 1115–1122. DOI: 10.1016/j.pec.2021.08.031 PMID: 34509339

Kuru Alici, N., & Arikan Dönmez, A. (2020). A systematic review of the effect of laughter yoga on physical function and psychosocial outcomes in older adults. *Complementary Therapies in Clinical Practice*, *41*, 101252. DOI: 10.1016/j.ctcp.2020.101252 PMID: 33217706

Kutner, J. S., Smith, M. C., Corbin, L., Hemphill, L., Benton, K., Mellis, B. K., Beaty, B., Felton, S., Yamashita, T. E., Bryant, L. L., & Fairclough, D. L. (2008). Massage therapy versus simple touch to improve pain and mood in patients with advanced cancer: A randomized trial. *Annals of Internal Medicine*, *149*(6), 369–379. DOI: 10.7326/0003-4819-149-6-200809160-00003 PMID: 18794556

Kwon, S., Kim, H., & Yeo, W.-H. (2021). Recent advances in wearable sensors and portable electronics for sleep monitoring. *iScience*, *24*(5), 102461. DOI: 10.1016/j.isci.2021.102461 PMID: 34013173

LaGoy, A. D., Mayeli, A., Smagula, S. F., & Ferrarelli, F. (2022). Relationships between rest-activity rhythms, sleep, and clinical symptoms in individuals at clinical high risk for psychosis and healthy comparison subjects. *Journal of Psychiatric Research*, *155*, 465–470. DOI: 10.1016/j.jpsychires.2022.09.009 PMID: 36183600

Lalani, N., Duggleby, W., & Olson, J. (2018). Spirituality among family caregivers in palliative care: An integrative literature review. *International Journal of Palliative Nursing*, *24*(2), 80–91. DOI: 10.12968/ijpn.2018.24.2.80 PMID: 29469645

Lalani, N., Osei, E. A., Yang, S., Katare, B., & Wagle, S. (2025). Financial health and well-being of rural female caregivers of older adults with chronic illnesses. *BMC Geriatrics*, *25*(1), 239. DOI: 10.1186/s12877-025-05853-5 PMID: 40211160

LaManna, J. B., Unruh, L., Chisholm, L., Pericles, P., & Fotovvat, H. (2020). Perceptions of health and well-being among older adult caregivers: Comparisons of current caregivers with former and never caregivers. *Geriatric Nursing*, *41*(4), 429–435. DOI: 10.1016/j.gerinurse.2020.01.015 PMID: 32044146

Lane, B., Cannella, K., Bowen, C., Copelan, D., Nteff, G., Barnes, K., Poudevigne, M., & Lawson, J. (2012). Examination of the effectiveness of peppermint aromatherapy on nausea in women post C-section.[57]. *Journal of Holistic Nursing*, *30*(2), 90–104. DOI: 10.1177/0898010111423419 PMID: 22034523

Lazar, M., & Davenport, L. (2018). Barriers to health care access for low income families: A review of literature. *Journal of Community Health Nursing*, *35*(1), 28–37. DOI: 10.1080/07370016.2018.1404832 PMID: 29323941

Lee-Cheong, S., Amanullah, S., & Jardine, M. (2022). New assistive technologies in dementia and mild cognitive impairment care: A PubMed review. *Asian Journal of Psychiatry*, *73*, 103135. DOI: 10.1016/j.ajp.2022.103135 PMID: 35569363

Lee, J., & Son, J. (2025). Development of a Sustainable Elderly Care System Leveraging ICT Technologies and Big Data. In *Big Data and Data Science Engineering* (Vol. 8, pp. 81–92). Springer Nature Switzerland., DOI: 10.1007/978-3-031-87061-3_7

Lee, Y., Pokharel, S., Muslim, A. A., Kc, D. B., Lee, K. H., & Yeo, W. H. (2023). Deep learning-based fall monitoring among older adults with skin-wearable electronics. *Sensors (Basel)*, *23*(8), 3983. DOI: 10.3390/s23083983 PMID: 37112326

Legault, Z., Znaty, A., Smith, S., & Boudrias, M. H. (2021). Yoga Interventions Used for the Rehabilitation of Stroke, Parkinson's Disease, and Multiple Sclerosis: A Scoping Review of Clinical Research. *Journal of Alternative and Complementary Medicine (New York, N.Y.)*, *27*(12), 1023–1057. DOI: 10.1089/acm.2021.0003 PMID: 34185577

Leon, N., & Xu, H. (2023). Implementation considerations for non-communicable disease-related integration in primary health care: A rapid review of qualitative evidence. *BMC Health Services Research*, *23*(1), 169. DOI: 10.1186/s12913-023-09151-x PMID: 36803143

Lewis, B., Purser, K., & Mackie, K. (2020). *The human rights of older persons*. Springer Singapore., DOI: 10.1007/978-981-15-6735-3

Liang, J. H., Lu, L., Li, J. Y., Qu, X. Y., Li, J., Qian, S., Wang, Y., Jia, R., Wang, C., & Xu, Y. (2020). Contributions of modifiable risk factors to dementia incidence: A Bayesian network analysis. *Journal of the American Medical Directors Association*, *21*(11), 1592–1599. DOI: 10.1016/j.jamda.2020.04.006 PMID: 32563753

Li, F., Harmer, P., Fitzgerald, K., Eckstrom, E., Stock, R., Galver, J., Maddalozzo, G. F., & Batya, S. S. (2014). Tai chi and postural stability in patients with Parkinson's disease. *The New England Journal of Medicine*, *366*(6), 511–519. DOI: 10.1056/NEJMoa1107911 PMID: 22316445

Li, J., Liao, Y., Zhang, S. Y., Jin, L., Congdon, N., Fan, Z., Zeng, Y., Zheng, Y., Liu, Z., Liu, Y., & Liang, L. (2024). Effect of laughter exercise versus 0.1% sodium hyaluronic acid on ocular surface discomfort in dry eye disease: Non-inferiority randomised controlled trial. *BMJ (Clinical Research Ed.), 386*, e080474. DOI: 10.1136/bmj-2024-080474 PMID: 39260878

Li, J., Zhang, J., Kong, B., Chen, L., Yuan, J., He, M., Wang, Y., Wei, S., Chen, W., Tang, Y., Zhu, X., & Yao, P. (2023). Abdominal obesity mediates the causal relationship between depression and the risk of gallstone disease.... *Journal of Psychosomatic Research, 174*, 111474. DOI: 10.1016/j.jpsychores.2023.111474 PMID: 37689051

Lillehei, A. S., Halcon, L. L., Savik, K., & Reis, R. (2015). Effect of inhaled lavender and sleep hygiene on self-reported sleep issues. *Journal of Alternative and Complementary Medicine (New York, N.Y.), 21*(7), 430–438. DOI: 10.1089/acm.2014.0327 PMID: 26133206

Lindeman, D. A.. (2020). Telehealth and remote caregiving: Expanding the role of digital health in supporting families. *Frontiers in Public Health, 8*, 201–218. DOI: 10.3389/fpubh.2020.00189

Lin, Y. C., & Huang, C. J. (2022). Impact of caregiver inclusion in home health systems: Evidence from the HOLISTIC study. *Geriatric Nursing, 43*, 56–64.

Lin, Y., Lange, D., & Seligmann, B. J. (2023). Causal network topology analysis (CaNeTA) as a tool for risk assessment in fire safety engineering. *Fire Safety Journal, 140*, 103880. DOI: 10.1016/j.firesaf.2023.103880

Lin, Y., & Yang, F. (2023). Intervention of emotional interaction in college art and design courses for autism patients' emotions. *CNS Spectrums, 28*(S2), S124. DOI: 10.1017/S1092852923005667

Li, T., Soh, K. L., Zakaria, N. F., Pang, Y., Wang, P., & Hu, N. (2024). Effects of LYon Patients Receiving Hemodialysis: A Systematic Review. *Holistic Nursing Practice, 38*(4), 202–212. DOI: 10.1097/HNP.0000000000000650 PMID: 38900006

Liu, T., Hao, X., & Zhang, Z. (2016). Identifying community healthcare supports for the elderly and the factors affecting their aging care model preference: Evidence from three districts of Beijing. *BMC Health Services Research, 16*(S7, Suppl 7), 626. DOI: 10.1186/s12913-016-1863-y PMID: 28185601

Li, W. W., Chhabra, J., & Singh, S. (2021). Palliative care education and its effectiveness: A systematic review. *Public Health, 194*, 9. DOI: 10.1016/j.puhe.2021.02.033 PMID: 33873061

Li, Y., Zhang, L., Chen, X., Wang, J., & Zhou, H. (2025). The effect of music therapy on anxiety, depression, pain and sleep quality of lung cancer patients: A systematic review and meta-analysis. *Supportive Care in Cancer, 33*(3), 169. DOI: 10.1007/s00520-025-09213-2 PMID: 39928168

Llop-Medina, L., Fu, Y., Garcés-Ferrer, J., & Doñate-Martínez, A. (2022). Palliative care in older people with multimorbidities: A scoping review on the palliative care needs of patients, carers, and health professionals. *International Journal of Environmental Research and Public Health, 19*(6), 3195. DOI: 10.3390/ijerph19063195 PMID: 35328881

Lloyd-Jukes, H., Gibson, O. J., Wrench, T., Odunlade, A., & Tarassenko, L. (2021). Vision-based patient monitoring and management in mental health settings. *Journal of Clinical Engineering, 46*(1), 36–43. DOI: 10.1097/JCE.0000000000000447

Losada, A., Márquez-González, M., & Romero-Moreno, R. (2011). Cognitive-behavioral therapy (CBT) for dementia caregivers: A systematic review. *International Psychogeriatrics, 23*(7), 1002–1018. DOI: 10.1017/S1041610210002231

Lu, P.-Y., Wu, H.-Y., Chen, L.-H., Liu, C.-Y., & Chiou, A.-F. (2023). The effects of self-aromatherapy massage on pain and sleep quality in patients with rheumatoid arthritis: A randomized controlled trial. *Pain Management Nursing, 24*(2), e52–e60. DOI: 10.1016/j.pmn.2023.02.009 PMID: 36990808

Lu, W., Silvera-Tawil, D., Yoon, H. J., Higgins, L., Zhang, Q., Karunanithi, M., Bomke, J., Byrnes, J., Hewitt, J., Smallbon, V., Freyne, J., Prabhu, D., & Varnfield, M. (2025). Impact of the Smarter Safer Homes solution.... *Journal of Medical Internet Research, 27*, e59921. DOI: 10.2196/59921 PMID: 39608020

Maguraushe, K., & Ndlovu, B. M. (2024). The use of smart technologies for enhancing palliative care: A systematic review. *Digital Health, 10*, 20552076241271835. DOI: 10.1177/20552076241271835 PMID: 39493628

Mahdood, B., Imani, B., & Khazaei, S. (2022). Effects of inhalation aromatherapy with Rosa damascena (Damask rose) on the state anxiety and sleep quality of operating room personnel during the COVID-19 pandemic: A randomized controlled trial. *Journal of Perianesthesia Nursing, 37*(4), 493–500. DOI: 10.1016/j.jopan.2021.09.011 PMID: 35256247

Mahmood, A. (2024). Integrating Palliative Care into Non-Communicable Disease Management: A Holistic Approach. *Non-Communicable Diseases and Care, 1*(2), 53-65. https://researchcorridor.org/index.php/ncdc/article/view/381

Malakar, Y., Peeters, L. J., Walton, A., & O'Sullivan, D. (2023). A causal network approach using a community well-being framework.... *Environmental Impact Assessment Review*, *102*, 107188. DOI: 10.1016/j.eiar.2023.107188

Mallon, A., Hasson, F., Casson, K., Slater, P., & McIlfatrick, S. (2021). Young adults understanding and readiness to engage with palliative care: extending the reach of palliative care through a public health approach: a qualitative study. *BMC Palliative Care*, *20*(1), 120. DOI: 10.1186/s12904-021-00808-0 PMID: 34320961

Mamdiwar, S. D., R, A., Shakruwala, Z., Chadha, U., Srinivasan, K., & Chang, C.-Y. (2021). Recent advances on IoT-assisted wearable sensor systems for healthcare monitoring. *Biosensors (Basel)*, *11*(10), 372. DOI: 10.3390/bios11100372 PMID: 34677328

Mani, R. K., Bhatnagar, S., Butola, S., Gursahani, R., Mehta, D., Simha, S., Divatia, J. V., Kumar, A., Iyer, S. K., Deodhar, J., Bhat, R. S., Salins, N., Thota, R. S., Mathur, R., Iyer, R. K., Gupta, S., Kulkarni, P., Murugan, S., Nasa, P., & Myatra, S. N. (2024). Indian society of critical care medicine and Indian association of palliative care expert consensus and position statements for end-of-life and palliative care in the intensive care unit. *Indian Journal of Critical Care Medicine : Peer-Reviewed, Official Publication of Indian Society of Critical Care Medicine*, *28*(3), 200–250. DOI: 10.5005/jp-journals-10071-24661 PMID: 38477011

Manninen, S., Tuominen, L., Dunbar, R. I., Karjalainen, T., Hirvonen, J., Arponen, E., Hari, R., Jääskeläinen, I. P., Sams, M., & Nummenmaa, L. (2017). Social Laughter Triggers Endogenous Opioid Release in Humans. *The Journal of Neuroscience : The Official Journal of the Society for Neuroscience*, *37*(25), 6125–6131. DOI: 10.1523/JNEUROSCI.0688-16.2017 PMID: 28536272

Marella, D., & Vicard, P. (2022). Bayesian network structural learning from complex survey data. *Statistical Methods & Applications*, *31*(4), 981–1013. DOI: 10.1007/s10260-021-00618-x

Marquine, M. J., Maldonado, Y., Zlatar, Z., Moore, R. C., Martin, A. S., Palmer, B. W., & Jeste, D. V. (2015). Differences in life satisfaction among older community-dwelling Hispanics and non-Hispanic Whites. *Aging & Mental Health*, *19*(11), 978–988. DOI: 10.1080/13607863.2014.971706 PMID: 25402813

Marshall, C., Virdun, C., & Phillips, J. L. (2024). Patient and family perspectives on rural palliative care models: A systematic review and meta-synthesis. *Palliative Medicine*, *38*(9), 935–950. DOI: 10.1177/02692163241269796 PMID: 39254116

Martins, M. D. L. D. C., & Pinto, S. (2023). Analysis of a telephone hotline for palliative care patients at home and their families. *International Journal of Palliative Nursing, 29*(12), 571–577. DOI: 10.12968/ijpn.2023.29.12.571 PMID: 38085617

Massari, E. L. H., Mhammedi, S., Sabouri, Z., & Gherabi, N. (2022). Ontology based machine learning to predict diabetes patients. In *Advances in information, communication and cybersecurity* (pp. 437–445). Springer, Cham. https://doi.org/ DOI: 10.1007/978-3-030-91738-8_40

McCauley, R., McQuillan, R., Ryan, K., & Foley, G. (2021). Mutual support between patients and family caregivers in palliative care: A systematic review and narrative synthesis. *Palliative Medicine, 35*(5), 875–885. DOI: 10.1177/0269216321999962 PMID: 33794713

McDonald, C. (2006). Challenging social work, the politics of change. In *Challenging social work: The context of practice* (1st ed., pp. 61–75). DOI: 10.1007/978-0-230-50549-0_4

McLaughlan, R., & Richards, K. (2023). Realizing homeliness in palliative care: Inpatient and family perspectives on designing the built environment. *Design for Health (Abingdon, England), 7*(2), 138–157. DOI: 10.1080/24735132.2023.2228599

Meier, M., Wirz, L., Dickinson, P., & Pruessner, J. C. (2021). Laughter yoga reduces the cortisol response to acute stress in healthy individuals. *Stress (Amsterdam, Netherlands), 24*(1), 44–52. DOI: 10.1080/10253890.2020.1766018 PMID: 32393092

Memarian, A., Sanatkaran, A., & Bahari, S. M. (2017). The effect of LYexercises on anxiety and sleep quality in patients suffering from PD's disease. *Biomedical Research and Therapy, 4*(07), 1463–1479. DOI: 10.15419/bmrat.v4i07.200

Menekli, T., & Doğan, R. (2021). The relationship between humor style and death anxiety of palliative care patients. *International Journal of Health Services Research and Policy, 6*(3), 369–379. DOI: 10.33457/ijhsrp.996104

Mennella, C., Maniscalco, U., De Pietro, G., & Esposito, M. (2024). Ethical and regulatory challenges of AI technologies in healthcare: A narrative review. *Heliyon, 10*(4), e26297. DOI: 10.1016/j.heliyon.2024.e26297 PMID: 38384518

Mennella, C., Maniscalco, U., Masala, G. L., & Esposito, M. (2024). Editorial: Artificial intelligence and robotic applications for smart monitoring and assistance in healthcare services. *Frontiers in Robotics and AI, 11*, 1527773. DOI: 10.3389/frobt.2024.1527773 PMID: 39687348

Micco, A., Carpentieri, E., Di Sorbo, A., Chetta, A., & Del Donno, M. (2023). Palliative care and end of life management in patients with idiopathic pulmonary fibrosis. *Multidisciplinary Respiratory Medicine, 18*, 896. DOI: 10.4081/mrm.2023.896 PMID: 36909932

Mills, J., Fox, J., Damarell, R., Tieman, J., & Yates, P. (2021). Palliative care providers' use of digital health and perspectives on technological innovation: A national study. *BMC Palliative Care, 20*(1), 124. DOI: 10.1186/s12904-021-00822-2 PMID: 34364379

Minhaj, U., & Rauf, K. (2023). The psychology of art therapy: An effective approach for mental disorders. *Pakistan Journal of Psychology, 54*(1), 47–63.

Mini, P. (2024). Comparative analysis of financial flows in healthcare systems of Germany, Austria, and Czechia. *ACTA VŠFS, 18*(2), 180–197. DOI: 10.37355/acta-2024/2-05

Ministry of Health and Family Welfare (MoHFW). (2022). *National Programme for Palliative Care: Implementation Report*. Government of India.

Mishra, R., & Sondhi, V. (2019). Fostering resilience among orphaned adolescents through institutional care in India. *Residential Treatment for Children & Youth, 36*(4), 314–337. DOI: 10.1080/0886571X.2018.1535286

Mitrani, V. B., Feaster, D. J., Weiss-Laxer, N., & Szapocznik, J. (2006). Longitudinal effects of a family therapy intervention for caregivers of individuals with dementia. *Family Process, 45*(3), 451–465. DOI: 10.1111/j.1545-5300.2006.00179.x

Mittelman, M. S., Papayannopoulou, P., Vernooij-Dassen, M., Moniz-Cook, E., & Jeon, Y.-H. (2018). The unforgettables: A chorus for people with dementia and their family caregivers. *International Psychogeriatrics, 30*(6), 779–789. DOI: 10.1017/S1041610217001867 PMID: 29375037

Mohajer, S., Mazlum, S. R., Rajabzadeh, M., & Namazinia, M. (2022). The effect of laughter yoga on depression in cancer patients undergoing chemotherapy: A randomized clinical trial. *Hayat (Tihran), 28*(3), 284–295. DOI: 10.30699/hayat.28.3.284

MoHFW. (2023). *eSanjeevani Telemedicine: Annual Report 2023*. New Delhi: Government of India.

Moilanen, T., Kangasniemi, M., Papinaho, O., Mynttinen, M., Siipi, H., Suominen, S., & Suhonen, R. (2021). Older people's perceived autonomy in residential care: An integrative review. *Nursing Ethics, 28*(3), 414–434. DOI: 10.1177/0969733020948115 PMID: 33000683

Mo, J., Vickerstaff, V., Minton, O., Tavabie, S., Taubert, M., Stone, P., & White, N. (2022). How effective is virtual reality technology in palliative care? A systematic review and meta-analysis. *Palliative Medicine*, *36*(7), 1047–1058. DOI: 10.1177/02692163221099584 PMID: 35635018

Mondanaro, J. F., Sara, G. A., Thoma, M. V., & Loewy, J. V. (2021). The effects of clinical music therapy on resiliency in adults undergoing infusion. *Journal of Pain and Symptom Management*, *61*(6), 1099–1108. DOI: 10.1016/j.jpainsymman.2020.10.032 PMID: 33152443

Montesi, L., & Calestani, M. (2021). *Managing chronicity in unequal states: ethnographic perspectives on caring*. UCL Press., DOI: 10.14324/111.9781800080287

Moore, E. (2009). *Case Management for Community Practice*. Oxford University Press., www.touchingthecorners.com/index.htm

Moore, S. (1992). Case Management and the Integration of Services: How Service Delivery Systems Shape Case Management. *Social Work*, *37*(5), 418. DOI: 10.1093/sw/37.5.418

Moraes, A., Jermana, L., (2018). Advances in Photopletysmography Signal Analysis for Biomedical Applications, *Sensors*, Basel, Switzerland.

Morita, P., Sahu, K., & Oetomo, A. (2023). Health monitoring using smart home technologies: Scoping review. *JMIR mHealth and uHealth*, *11*, e37347. DOI: 10.2196/37347 PMID: 37052984

Moro, T. T., Savage, T. A., & Gehlert, S. (2017). Agency, social and healthcare supports for adults with intellectual disability at the end of life in out-of-home, non-institutional community residences in Western nations: A literature review. *Journal of Applied Research in Intellectual Disabilities*, *30*(6), 1045–1056. DOI: 10.1111/jar.12374 PMID: 28585240

Mosca, I., van der Wees, P. J., Mot, E. S., Wammes, J. J., & Jeurissen, P. P. (2016). Sustainability of long-term care: Puzzling tasks ahead for policy-makers. *International Journal of Health Policy and Management*, *6*(4), 195–205. DOI: 10.15171/ijhpm.2016.109 PMID: 28812803

Mostafa, M. (2014). Architecture for autism: Autism ASPECTSS™ in school design. *Archnet-IJAR*, *8*(1), 143–158. DOI: 10.26687/archnet-ijar.v8i1.314

Moxley, D. (1997). Sorting out the purpose of case management. In *Case management by design: Reflections on principles and Practices*. Nelson-Hall.

Mujumdar, A., & Vaidehi, V. (2019). Diabetes prediction using machine learning algorithms. *Procedia Computer Science, 165*, 292–299. DOI: 10.1016/j.procs.2020.01.047

Muleiro Alvarez, M., Cano-Herrera, G., Osorio Martínez, M. F., Vega Gonzales-Portillo, J., Monroy, G. R., Murguiondo Pérez, R., Torres-Ríos, J. A., van Tienhoven, X. A., Garibaldi Bernot, E. M., Esparza Salazar, F., & Ibarra, A. (2024). A Comprehensive Approach to Parkinson's Disease: Addressing Its Molecular, Clinical, and Therapeutic Aspects. *International Journal of Molecular Sciences, 25*(13), 7183. DOI: 10.3390/ijms25137183 PMID: 39000288

Muller, E. (2023). 7 Common Remote Patient Monitoring Devices https://www.healthrecoverysolutions.com/blog/7-common-remote-patient-monitoring-devices

Mulukuntla, S. (2025). Monitoring and Remote Patient Management with Immersive Technologies. In *Augmented Wellness: Exploring the Power of VR and AR in Healthcare* (pp. 197-218). Singapore: Springer Nature Singapore. DOI: 10.1007/978-981-96-2952-7_9

Murthy, G. V. S., Gupta, S., Ellwein, L. B., Munoz, S. R., Bachani, D., & Dada, V. K. (2001). A population-based eye survey of older adults in a rural district of Rajasthan: I. Central vision impairment, blindness, and cataract surgery. *Ophthalmology, 108*(4), 679–685. DOI: 10.1016/S0161-6420(00)00579-0 PMID: 11297483

Nair, H., & Prasad, R. (2021). Integration of evidence and Ayurveda in chronic illness management. *AYU Journal, 42*(2), 91–98.

Nair, P. R., & Prasad, R. (2021). Cultural perceptions and delays in evidence-based caregiving in rural India. *Indian Journal of Community Medicine : Official Publication of Indian Association of Preventive & Social Medicine, 46*(3), 352–358.

Namisango, E., Onyeka, T., Esther, N., Luyirika, E. B., Ali, Z., & Powell, R. A. (2024). Creating the evidence base for palliative care in cancer–models and strategies to build research capacity. *ecancermedicalscience, 18*, 1819. DOI: 10.3332/ecancer.2024.1819

Narayanan, R. (2021). Gender and informal caregiving in Indian households. *Indian Journal of Gender Studies, 28*(4), 507–524.

National Alliance for Caregiving. (2020). *Caregiving in the U.S. 2020*. National Alliance for Caregiving and AARP.

National Association for Holistic Aromatherapy. (n.d.). *What is aromatherapy?* https://naha.org/explore-aromatherapy/about-aromatherapy/what-is-aromatherapy/

National Center for Complementary and Integrative Health (NCCIH). (2018). *Complementary, alternative, or integrative health: What's in a name?* Retrieved from https://www.nccih.nih.gov/health/complementary-alternative-or-integrative-health-whats-in-a-name

National Institute for Health and Care Excellence (NICE). (2019). *Home care for adults with complex health needs.* NICE Guidelines.

National Institution for Transforming India (NITI Aayog). (2021). *India's National Strategy for Home-based Healthcare.*

Nearney, H. (2006). Art therapy: A senior house officer's perspective. *Psychiatric Bulletin, 30*(3), 109–110. DOI: 10.1192/pb.30.3.109

Neves, B. B., Sanders, A., & Kokanović, R. (2019). "It's the worst bloody feeling in the world": Experiences of loneliness and social isolation among older people living in care homes. *Journal of Aging Studies, 49*, 74–84. DOI: 10.1016/j.jaging.2019.100785 PMID: 31229221

Nicholson, C. J., Combes, S., Mold, F., King, H., & Green, R. (2023). Addressing inequity in palliative care provision for older people living with multimorbidity. Perspectives of community-dwelling older people on their palliative care needs: A scoping review. *Palliative Medicine, 37*(4), 475–497. DOI: 10.1177/02692163221118230 PMID: 36002975

Nogueira, A. R., Pugnana, A., Ruggieri, S., Pedreschi, D., & Gama, J. (2022). Methods and tools for causal discovery and causal inference. *Wiley Interdisciplinary Reviews. Data Mining and Knowledge Discovery, 12*(2), e1449. DOI: 10.1002/widm.1449

Northouse, L. L., Katapodi, M. C., Schafenacker, A. M., & Weiss, D. (2012). The impact of caregiving on the psychological well-being of family caregivers and cancer patients. In *Seminars in oncology nursing* (Vol. 28, No. 4, pp. 236-245). WB Saunders. DOI: 10.1016/j.soncn.2012.09.006

Nouira, M., Souayeh, N., Kanzari, S. A., Rouis, H., Lika, A., Mbarki, C., Rahali, F. Z., & Bettaieb, H. (2024). Aromatherapy using lavender oil effectiveness on pain and anxiety after C-section: A randomized controlled trial. *Journal of Epidemiology and Global Health, 14*(4), 1536–1544. DOI: 10.1007/s44197-024-00305-6 PMID: 39400653

Noureldein, M. H., & Eid, A. A. (2018). Homeostatic effect of laughter on diabetic cardiovascular complications: The myth turned to fact. *Diabetes Research and Clinical Practice, 135*, 111–119. DOI: 10.1016/j.diabres.2017.11.014 PMID: 29162513

Nwameme, A. U., Tabong, P. T. N., & Adongo, P. B. (2018). Implementing community-based health planning and services in impoverished urban communities: Health workers' perspective. *BMC Health Services Research, 18*(1), 186. DOI: 10.1186/s12913-018-3005-1 PMID: 29554964

O'Brien, K., Bracht, M., & Robson, K. (2018). Family Integrated Care (FICare): Engaging parents in NICU-based evidence-driven care. *The Lancet. Child & Adolescent Health*, *2*(4), 245–254. DOI: 10.1016/S2352-4642(18)30039-7 PMID: 30169298

Oechsle, K. (2019). Current advances in palliative & hospice care: Problems and needs of relatives and family caregivers during palliative and hospice care—An overview of current literature. *Medical Science*, *7*(3), 43. DOI: 10.3390/medsci7030043 PMID: 30871105

Oken, B. S., Fonareva, I., Haas, M., Wahbeh, H., Lane, J. B., Zajdel, D., & Amen, A. (2010). Pilot controlled trial of mindfulness meditation and education for dementia caregivers. *Journal of Alternative and Complementary Medicine (New York, N.Y.)*, *16*(10), 1031–1038. DOI: 10.1089/acm.2009.0733 PMID: 20929380

Oladehinde-Omodona, B., & Okusi, O. (2025). Stress mangement on professional health care givers. https://www.theseus.fi/handle/10024/886095

Oliver, M., & Barnes, C. (2012). *The new politics of disablement*. Palgrave Macmillan. DOI: 10.1007/978-0-230-39244-1

Orkibi, H., & Keisari, S. (2023). Creative Arts Therapies - Processes and Outcomes for Emotional Well-Being. In Ivcevic, Z., Hoffmann, J. D., & Kaufman, J. C. (Eds.), *The Cambridge Handbook of Creativity and Emotions* (pp. 411–433). Cambridge University Press., DOI: 10.1017/9781009031240.027

Oswald, F., & Rowles, G. D. (2017). Beyond the relocation trauma in old age: New trends in elders' residential decisions. In *New dynamics in old age* (pp. 127–152). Routledge.

Otis-Green, S., & Juarez, G. (2012). Enhancing the social well-being of family caregivers. In *Seminars in oncology nursing* (Vol. 28, No. 4, pp. 246-255). WB Saunders. DOI: 10.1016/j.soncn.2012.09.007

Ott, T., Heckel, M., Öhl, N., Steigleder, T., Albrecht, N. C., Ostgathe, C., & Dabrock, P. (2023). Palliative care and new technologies. The use of smart sensor technologies and its impact on the Total Care principle. *BMC Palliative Care*, *22*(1), 50. DOI: 10.1186/s12904-023-01174-9 PMID: 37101258

Özer, Z., & Ateş, S. (2021). Effects of laughter yoga on hemodialysis patients' plasma-beta endorphin levels, pain levels and sleep quality: A randomized controlled trial. *Complementary Therapies in Clinical Practice*, *43*, 101382. DOI: 10.1016/j.ctcp.2021.101382 PMID: 33831803

Ozturk, F. O., & Tezel, A. (2021). Effect of laughter yoga on mental symptoms and salivary cortisol levels in first-year nursing students: A randomized controlled trial. *International Journal of Nursing Practice*, *27*(2), e12924. DOI: 10.1111/ijn.12924 PMID: 33580606

Palmer, J. B., Lane, D., Mayo, D., Schluchter, M., & Leeming, R. (2015). Effects of music therapy on anesthesia requirements and anxiety in women undergoing ambulatory breast surgery for cancer diagnosis and treatment: A randomized controlled trial. *Journal of Clinical Oncology*, *33*(28), 3162–3168. DOI: 10.1200/JCO.2014.59.6049 PMID: 26282640

Pan, Q., Brulin, D., & Campo, E. (2023). Evaluation of a Wireless Home Sleep Monitoring System Compared to Polysomnography. *Ingénierie et Recherche Biomédicale : IRBM = Biomedical Engineering and Research*, *44*(2), 100735. DOI: 10.1016/j.irbm.2022.09.002

Papa, A., Mital, M., Pisano, P., & Del Giudice, M. (2020). E-health and wellbeing monitoring using smart healthcare devices: An empirical investigation. *Technological Forecasting and Social Change*, *153*, 119226. DOI: 10.1016/j.techfore.2018.02.018

Papanikolaou, E., Stratouli, E., Lianou, M., & Georgiadi, E. (2023). Guided imagery and music in the treatment for breast and gynecologic cancer: A randomized controlled trial. *Journal of Music Therapy*, *60*(4), 410–434. DOI: 10.1093/jmt/thad011 PMID: 37503863

Parchmann, N., Hansen, D., Orzechowski, M., & Steger, F. (2024). An ethical assessment of professional opinions on concerns, chances, and limitations.... *GeroScience*, *46*(6), 6269–6282. DOI: 10.1007/s11357-024-01229-6 PMID: 38834930

Parker, M. W., Davis, C., White, K., Johnson, D., Golden, M., & Zola, S. (2022). Reduced care burden and improved quality of life in African American family caregivers: Positive impact of personalized assistive technology. *Technology and Health Care*, *30*(2), 379–387. DOI: 10.3233/THC-213049 PMID: 34334439

Paul, R., & Sinha, R. (2022). Evidence-based nursing in home care: Role of Indian nurses. *Nursing Journal of India*, *113*(6), 284–290.

Pearl, J. (2024). Advances in causal inference in AI. *Journal of Medical Internet Research, 2024–2025*. Advance online publication. 10.2196

Peeler, A., Afolabi, O., Adcock, M., Evans, C., Nkhoma, K., van Breevoort, D., Farrant, L., & Harding, R. (2024). Primary palliative care in low-and middle-income countries: A systematic review and thematic synthesis of the evidence for models and outcomes. *Palliative Medicine*, *38*(8), 776–789. DOI: 10.1177/02692163241248324 PMID: 38693716

Pereira, A. V., Vaz, A., Paúl, C., Santiago, L., & Rosendo, I. (2025). Comprehensive geriatric assessment in primary healthcare: A scoping review protocol. *BMJ Open*, *15*(6), e091095. DOI: 10.1136/bmjopen-2024-091095 PMID: 40467309

Perpiñá-Galvañ, J., Orts-Beneito, N., Fernández-Alcántara, M., García-Sanjuán, S., García-Caro, M. P., & Cabañero-Martínez, M. J. (2019). Level of burden and health-related quality of life in caregivers of palliative care patients. *International Journal of Environmental Research and Public Health*, *16*(23), 4806. DOI: 10.3390/ijerph16234806 PMID: 31795461

Peshkova, M., Yumasheva, V., Rudenko, E., Kretova, N., Timashev, P., & Demura, T. (2023). Digital twin concept: Healthcare, education, research. *Journal of Pathology Informatics*, *14*, 100313. DOI: 10.1016/j.jpi.2023.100313 PMID: 37168801

Petrovic, M., & Gaggioli, A. (2020). Digital mental health tools for caregivers of older adults—a scoping review. *Frontiers in Public Health, 8*, 128. Petrovic, M., & Gaggioli, A. (2020). Digital mental health tools for caregivers of older adults—a scoping review. *Frontiers in Public Health*, *8*, 128. DOI: 10.3389/fpubh.2020.00128 PMID: 32411643

Pharr, J. R., Francis, C. D., Terry, C., Clark, M. C., & Lee, D. J. (2014). Culture, caregiving, and health: Exploring the influence of culture on family caregiver experiences. *ISRN Public Health*, *2014*, 1–8. DOI: 10.1155/2014/689826

Philips, N. J., Joshi, S., Nimbalkar, K., & Suryawanshi, A. (2025). Vision-based monitoring system for elderly care using CNN + BiLSTM. *Journal of Information Systems Engineering & Management*, *10*(55), 11425.

Pinto, S., Fumincelli, L., Mazzo, A., Caldeira, S., & Martins, J. C. (2017). Comfort, well-being and quality of life: Discussion of the differences and similarities among the concepts. *Porto Biomedical Journal*, *2*(1), 6–12. DOI: 10.1016/j.pbj.2016.11.003 PMID: 32258577

Pourshaikhian, M., Moghadamnia, M. T., Kazemnezhad Leyli, E., & Shafiei Kisomi, Z. (2024). Effects of aromatherapy with Matricaria chamomile essential oil on anxiety and hemodynamic indices in patients with acute coronary syndrome, 2021: A randomized controlled trial. *BMC Complementary Medicine and Therapies*, *24*(1), 17. DOI: 10.1186/s12906-023-04326-9 PMID: 38172912

Putri, N. R. I. A. T., Cahyaningrum, E. D., Wurdaningsih, T. K., Syangadah, Z., & Mesayu, S. F. (2025). Evaluation of coloring therapy as an anxiety reduction strategy in the older adults in the community area. *BIO Web of Conferences, 152*. DOI: 10.1051/bioconf/202515201032

Qu, L., Cao, Y., Wang, M., Song, D., & Huang, G. (2025). Effects of laughter therapy on improving physical and psychological symptoms among cancer patients: a systematic review and meta-analysis. Supportive care in cancer: official journal of the Multinational Association of Supportive Care in Cancer, 33(3), 230. https://doi.org/1DOI: 10.1007/s00520-025-09276-

Rabinowitch, T.-C., Aberg, L., & Meltzer, L. J. (2023). Outcomes and experiences of an online Balance-Space music therapy intervention for cancer patients. *The Arts in Psychotherapy*, *82*, 101998. DOI: 10.1016/j.aip.2023.101998 PMID: 36713463

Rabow, M. W., Hauser, J. M., & Adams, J. (2004). Supporting family caregivers at the end of life: They don't know what they don't know. *Journal of the American Medical Association*, *291*(4), 483–491. DOI: 10.1001/jama.291.4.483 PMID: 14747506

Rady, M., Moussa, K., Mostafa, M., Elbasry, A., Ezzat, Z., & Medhat, W. (2021, October). Diabetes prediction using machine learning: A comparative study. In *2021 3rd Novel Intelligent and Leading Emerging Sciences Conference (NILES)* (pp. 279–282). IEEE. https://doi.org/DOI: 10.1109/NILES53778.2021.9600091

Rajagopal, M., & Joad, A. (2020). Informal caregiving and palliative care gaps in India. *Journal of Pain and Symptom Management*, *59*(1), 102–109.

Rajagopal, M., & Palat, G. (2020). Overcoming policy barriers to palliative care in India. *Health Policy and Planning*, *35*(2), 184–192.

Rantz, M. J., Skubic, M., Abbott, C., Galambos, C., Alexander, G., Popescu, M., & Keller, J. (2015). Automated technology to promote aging in place using sensor networks. *Journal of Gerontological Nursing*, *41*(7), 10–17. DOI: 10.3928/00989134-20150615-03

Rao, S. R., Salins, N., Joshi, U., Patel, J., Remawi, B. N., Simha, S., Preston, N., & Walshe, C. (2022). Palliative and end-of-life care in intensive care units in low-and middle-income countries: A systematically constructed scoping review. *Journal of Critical Care*, *71*, 154115. DOI: 10.1016/j.jcrc.2022.154115 PMID: 35907272

Rastogi, M., Paige Feldwisch, R., Pate, M., & Scarce, J. (2022). Foundations of Art Therapy: Theory and Applications. In *Foundations of Art Therapy: Theory and Applications*. Academic Press.

Rath, K. C., Khang, A., Rath, S. K., Satapathy, N., Satapathy, S. K., & Kar, S. (2024). Artificial intelligence (AI)-enabled technology in medicine-advancing holistic healthcare monitoring and control systems. In *Computer vision and AI-integrated IoT technologies in the medical ecosystem* (pp. 87–108). CRC Press. DOI: 10.1201/9781003429609-6

Reinhard, S. C., Levine, C., & Samis, S. (2019). Home alone revisited: Family caregivers providing complex care. AARP Public Policy Institute. https://www.aarp.org/content/dam/aarp/ppi/2019/04/home-alone-revisited-family-caregivers-providing-complex-care.pdf

Reinhard, S. C., Feinberg, L. F., Choula, R., & Houser, A. (2019). *Valuing the invaluable: 2019 update—Charting a path forward.* AARP Public Policy Institute.

Reis, A., Pedrosa, A., Dourado, M., & Reis, C. (2013). Information and communication technologies in long-term and palliative care. *Procedia Technology*, *9*, 1303–1312. DOI: 10.1016/j.protcy.2013.12.146

Ricker, M. A., & Haas, W. C. (2017). Anti-inflammatory diet in clinical practice: A review. *Nutrition in Clinical Practice*, *32*(3), 318–325. DOI: 10.1177/0884533617700353 PMID: 28350517

Riedler, K., Hecker, A., Bauer, B., Tax, C., Gmainer, D. G., Pignet, A.-L., Kamolz, L.-P., & Lumenta, D. B. (2023). The efficacy of regeneration oil and almond oil on split-thickness skin graft donor sites: A single-blinded randomized controlled trial. *Clinics and Practice*, *13*(3), 648–655. DOI: 10.3390/clinpract13030059 PMID: 37366928

Riegel, M., Randall, S., Ranse, K., & Buckley, T. (2021). Healthcare professionals' values about and experience with facilitating end-of-life care in the adult intensive care unit. *Intensive & Critical Care Nursing*, *65*, 103057. DOI: 10.1016/j.iccn.2021.103057 PMID: 33888382

Robertson, R., Robertson, A., Jepson, R., & Maxwell, M. (2012). Walking for depression or depressive symptoms: A systematic review and meta-analysis. *Mental Health and Physical Activity*, *5*(1), 66–75. DOI: 10.1016/j.mhpa.2012.03.002

Robison, J., Shugrue, N., Porter, M., Fortinsky, R. H., & Curry, L. A. (2012). Transition from home care to nursing home: Unmet needs in a home-and community-based program for older adults. *Journal of Aging & Social Policy*, *24*(3), 251–270. DOI: 10.1080/08959420.2012.676315 PMID: 22720886

Rodin, G., An, E., Shnall, J., & Malfitano, C. (2020). Psychological interventions for patients with advanced disease: Implications for oncology and palliative care. *Journal of Clinical Oncology*, *38*(9), 885–904. DOI: 10.1200/JCO.19.00058 PMID: 32023159

Rong, C., Wu, Q. H., Xu, H. Y., Chang, M., Zhang, L., & Xie, R. R. (2024). The evaluation and enhancement strategies of core competencies for older adult caregivers in integrated medical and older adult care institutions. *Frontiers in Public Health*, *12*, 1407496. DOI: 10.3389/fpubh.2024.1407496 PMID: 38957206

Rothman, J. (1991). A Model of Case Management: Toward Empirically Based Practice. *Social Work*, *36*(6), 520–528. DOI: 10.1093/sw/36.6.520 PMID: 1754929

Rouhi, S., Etemadi, S., & Pooraghajan, M. (2020). Laughter in combination with yoga exercises: Changes in psychological distress and quality of life in patients with coronary heart disease (CHD). *The Open Psychology Journal*, *13*(1), 144–150. Advance online publication. DOI: 10.2174/1874350102013010144

Ruch, W., & Raskin, V. (2008). Psychology of humor (No. 8, pp. 17-100). Mouton de Gruyter.

Rumbold, B., & Aoun, S. M. (2021). Palliative and end-of-life care service models: To what extent are consumer perspectives considered? In *Healthcare* (Vol. 9, No. 10, p. 1286). MDPI. DOI: 10.3390/healthcare9101286

Russell, R. (2007). Men doing "women's work": Elderly men caregivers and the gendered construction of care work. *Journal of Men's Studies*, *15*(1), 1–18. DOI: 10.3149/jms.1501.1

Sabouri, Z., Maleh, Y., & Gherabi, N. (2022). Benchmarking classification algorithms for measuring the performance on maintainable applications. In *Advances in information, communication and cybersecurity* (pp. 173–179). Springer., DOI: 10.1007/978-3-030-91738-8_17

Saleebey, D. (2006). Power in the People. In *The strengths perspective in social work practice* (4th ed., pp. 1–24). Pearson/Allyn & Bacon.

Salins, N., Deodhar, J., & Goel, S. (2022). Home-based cancer palliative care in India: Outcomes and challenges. *Indian Journal of Cancer*, *59*(2), 234–241.

Same, A., McBride, H., Liddelow, C., Mullan, B., & Harris, C. (2020). Motivations for volunteering time with older adults: A qualitative study. *PLoS One*, *15*(5), e0232718. DOI: 10.1371/journal.pone.0232718 PMID: 32365081

Sánchez, J. C., Echeverri, L. F., Londoño, M. J., Ochoa, S. A., Quiroz, A. F., Romero, C. R., & Ruiz, J. O. (2017). Effects of a Humor Therapy Program on Stress Levels in Pediatric Inpatients. *Hospital Pediatrics*, *7*(1), 46–53. DOI: 10.1542/hpeds.2016-0128 PMID: 27908974

Şancı, Y., Yıldız, S., Ayçiçek, A., & Möhür, N. (2023). Effect of peppermint-lemon aromatherapy on nausea-vomiting and quality of life in pediatric patients with leukemia: A randomized controlled trial. *Journal of Pediatric Nursing*, *72*, e217–e227. DOI: 10.1016/j.pedn.2023.07.001 PMID: 37453895

Sangeeth, S., & Solomon, M. D. (2015). Quality of Life Among Elderly in Non-Institusional Care. *International Journal of Science and Research, Chennai*, 1462-1467.

Sarmento, V. P., Higginson, I. J., Ferreira, P. L., & Gomes, B. (2016). Past trends and projections of hospital deaths to inform the integration of palliative care in one of the most ageing countries in the world. *Palliative Medicine*, *30*(4), 363–373. DOI: 10.1177/0269216315594974 PMID: 26163531

Sarwar, M. A., Kamal, N., Hamid, W., & Shah, M. A. (2018, September). Prediction of diabetes using machine learning algorithms in healthcare. In *2018 24th International Conference on Automation and Computing (ICAC)* (pp. 1–6). IEEE. https://doi.org/DOI: 10.23919/IConAC.2018.8748992

Satsangi, A. K., & Brugnoli, M. P. (2018). Anxiety and psychosomatic symptoms in palliative care: From neuro-psychobiological response to stress, to symptoms' management with clinical hypnosis and meditative states. *Annals of Palliative Medicine*, *7*(1), 7511–7111. DOI: 10.21037/apm.2017.07.01 PMID: 28866901

Savage, B. M., Lujan, H. L., Thipparthi, R. R., & DiCarlo, S. E. (2017). Humor, laughter, learning, and health! A brief review. *Advances in Physiology Education*, *41*(3), 341–347. DOI: 10.1152/advan.00030.2017 PMID: 28679569

Schrag, A., Hovris, A., Morley, D., Quinn, N., & Jahanshahi, M. (2006). Caregiver-burden in parkinson's disease is closely associated with psychiatric symptoms, falls, and disability. *Parkinsonism & Related Disorders*, *12*(1), 35–41. DOI: 10.1016/j.parkreldis.2005.06.011 PMID: 16271496

Schulz, R., & Eden, J. (2016). Committee on family caregiving for older adults board on health care services health and medicine division. *Families caring for an aging. America*, •••, 1–366. https://www.ncbi.nlm.nih.gov/books/NBK396401/pdf/Bookshelf_NBK396401.pdf

Schulz, R., & Eden, J. (Eds.). (2016). *Families caring for an aging America*. National Academies Press., DOI: 10.17226/23606

Schulz, R., & Sherwood, P. R. (2008). Physical and mental health effects of family caregiving.[58]. *The American Journal of Nursing*, *108*(9, Suppl), 23–27. DOI: 10.1097/01.NAJ.0000336406.45248.4c PMID: 18797217

Schweighoffer, R., Reeves, E., & Liebig, B. (2020). Collaborative networks in primary and specialized palliative care in Switzerland-Perspectives of doctors and nurses. *The Open Public Health Journal*, *13*(1), 36–43. Advance online publication. DOI: 10.2174/1874944502013010036

Sebastian, S. (2020). *Abuse and Neglect, Perceived Burden and Quality of Life of Elders Seeking Treatment for Mental Disorders and Elders Residing in Institutional Care: A Comparative Study* (Master's thesis, Central Institute of Psychiatry (India)).

Seibel, K., Rios, C. L. O., Sparna, T., Becker, C., Gaertner, J., Becker, G., & Boehlke, C. (2024). Implementation of a digital distress detection system in palliative care: Qualitative data on perspectives of a multiprofessional palliative care team. *BMC Palliative Care*, *23*(1), 203. DOI: 10.1186/s12904-024-01530-3 PMID: 39113031

Sengupta, J., & Chatterjee, S. C. (2017). Dying in intensive care units of India: Commentaries on policies and position papers on palliative and end-of-life care. *Journal of Critical Care*, *39*, 11–17. DOI: 10.1016/j.jcrc.2016.12.017 PMID: 28104546

Shaheen, R., & Salim, H. (2025). Role of artificial intelligence in healthcare. In *Intersection of Human Rights and AI in Healthcare* (pp. 173–200). IGI Global Scientific Publishing., DOI: 10.4018/979-8-3693-7051-3.ch007

Shahidi, M., Mojtahed, A., Modabbernia, A., Mojtahed, M., Shafiabady, A., Delavar, A., & Honari, H. (2011). Laughter yoga versus group exercise program in elderly depressed women: A randomized controlled trial. *International Journal of Geriatric Psychiatry*, *26*(3), 322–327. DOI: 10.1002/gps.2545 PMID: 20848578

Shakhovska, N., Fedushko, S., Shvorob, I., & Syerov, Y. (2019). Development of mobile system for medical recommendations. *Procedia Computer Science*, *155*, 43–50. DOI: 10.1016/j.procs.2019.08.010

Sharma, M., & Gupta, A. (2021). Impact of yoga-based pulmonary rehabilitation in COPD: A clinical trial. *AIIMS Journal of Medical Sciences*, *75*(3), 112–120.

Sharma, S. (2025). Enhancing patient satisfaction and care. In *Exploration of Transformative Technologies in Healthcare 6.0* (pp. 421–442). IGI Global Scientific Publishing., DOI: 10.4018/979-8-3693-7210-4.ch015

Shrestha, S., Arora, S., Hunter, A., & Debesay, J. (2025). The morality of care: Female family caregivers' motivations for providing care to older migrants. *Qualitative Health Research, 35*(9), 992–1006. DOI: 10.1177/10497323241280239 PMID: 39499504

Singh, M. P., & Keche, Y. N. (2025). Ethical integration of artificial intelligence in healthcare…. *Cureus, 17*(5), e84804. DOI: 10.7759/cureus.84804 PMID: 40568260

Smith, M. C.. (2019). Complementary therapies for caregiver stress management: A systematic review. *Complementary Therapies in Medicine, 45*, 147–155. DOI: 10.1016/j.ctim.2019.02.001

Spasova, S., Baeten, R., Coster, S., Ghailani, D., Peña-Casas, R., & Vanhercke, B. (2018). Challenges in long-term care in Europe. *Eurohealth (London), 24*(4), 7–12. DOI: 10.2767/84573

Srinivasan, S. (2025). Patient-Centric Care in Tuberculosis Management: Addressing Challenges and Improving Health Outcomes. In *Convergence of Population Health Management, Pharmacogenomics, and Patient-Centered Care* (pp. 265-282). IGI Global. DOI: 10.4018/979-8-3693-3260-3.ch012

Srinivasan, S., & Praba Lama (2025). Patient-Centered Care for TB Patients: An Effective Approach to Corporate Social Responsibility. In Corporate Social Responsibility in Health and Social Care (pp. 183-218).IGI Global. DOI: 10.4018/979-8-3693-5991-4.ch008

Srinivasan, S., Vallipriya, R., & Singh, A. K. (2025). An Analysis Health and Psychological General Well-Being Among Convicts Central Prison of Tamil Nadu. In *Sustainable Development Goals (SDG) and Its Intersection With Health and Well-Being* (pp. 1-38). IGI Global Scientific Publishing. DOI: 10.4018/979-8-3693-9755-8.ch001

Srinivasan, S., Vallipriya, R., & Singh, A. K. (2025). Spiritual Well-Being Index for Incarcerated Populations: An Exploratory Study. In *Sustainable Development Goals (SDG) and Its Intersection With Health and Well-Being* (pp. 425-460). IGI Global Scientific Publishing. DOI: 10.4018/979-8-3693-9755-8.ch015

Srinivasan, S., & Rajavel, N. (2025). Artificial Intelligence Approach to Psychological Wellbeing Among the Ageing Population. In *AI Technologies and Advancements for Psychological Well-Being and Healthcare* (pp. 187–218). IGI Global., DOI: 10.4018/979-8-3693-9158-7.ch008

Srinivasan, S., & Rajavel, N. (2025). Technology Improves the Quality of Life for Elderly People. In *Perspectives on the Economics of Aging* (pp. 109–150). IGI Global Scientific Publishing., DOI: 10.4018/979-8-3693-7753-6.ch005

Srinivasan, S., Rajavel, N., & Mahmoudi-Dehaki, M. (2025). Elderly Inmates Living With Dementia in Central Prisons. In *Assistive Technology Solutions for Aging Adults and Individuals With Disabilities* (pp. 343–404). IGI Global Scientific Publishing., DOI: 10.4018/979-8-3693-6308-9.ch015

Srivastava, M., & Ghosh, A. (2024). Societal impact of death anxiety and mental health among nurses in India. *Societal Impacts*, *4*, 100095. DOI: 10.1016/j.socimp.2024.100095

Steinhardt, T. L., Mortvedt, S., & Trondalen, G. (2021). Music therapy in the hospital-at-home: A practice for children in palliative care. *British Journal of Music Therapy*, *35*(2), 53–62. DOI: 10.1177/13594575211029109

Stevenson, H., & Alzyood, M. (2025). Healing through art: A thematic synthesis within a quasi-systematic review of art's impact on adult mental well-being during the COVID-19 pandemic. *BMC Public Health*, *25*(1), 1641. Advance online publication. DOI: 10.1186/s12889-025-22741-0 PMID: 40319249

Stolberg, M., Kennedy, L., & Unglaub, L. (2017). *History of palliative care, 1500-1970* (Vol. 123). Springer., DOI: 10.1007/978-3-319-54178-5

Stummer, F. O., Mayrhofer, M., Szabo, N., & Hoffmann, K. (2025). Barriers to and potential of remote consultations in general practice: Insights from the SARS-CoV-2 pandemic in Austria. *BMC Digital Health*, *3*(1), 33. DOI: 10.1186/s44247-025-00176-2

Suarez-Iglesias, D., Santos, L., Sanchez-Lastra, M. A., & Ayan, C. (2022). Systematic review and meta-analysis of randomised controlled trials on the effects of yoga in people with PD's disease. *Disability and Rehabilitation*, *44*(21), 6210–6229. DOI: 10.1080/09638288.2021.1966522 PMID: 34533097

Substance Abuse and Mental Health Services Administration. (2014). SAMHSA's concept of trauma and guidance for a trauma-informed approach. https://ncsacw.samhsa.gov/userfiles/files/SAMHSA_Trauma.pdf

Sultana, A., Tasnim, S., Sharma, R., Pawar, P., Bhattcharya, S., & Hossain, M. M. (2021). Psychosocial challenges in palliative care: Bridging the gaps using digital health. *Indian Journal of Palliative Care*, *27*(3), 442–447. DOI: 10.25259/IJPC_381_20 PMID: 34898939

Sumneangsanor, T., Thitipattanapong, S., & Thongruang, S. (2022). The effects of a biofeedback and music training programme in reducing stress in Thai patients living with cancer receiving palliative care. *International Journal of Palliative Nursing*, *28*(10), 453–463. DOI: 10.12968/ijpn.2022.28.10.453 PMID: 36269291

Sun, J., Xiu, K., Wang, Z., Hu, N., Zhao, L., Zhu, H., Kong, F., Xiao, J., Cheng, L., & Bi, X. (2023). Multifunctional wearable humidity and pressure sensors based on biocompatible graphene/bacterial cellulose bio aerogel for wireless monitoring and early warning of sleep apnea syndrome. *Nano Energy*, *108*, 108215. DOI: 10.1016/j.nanoen.2023.108215

Sun, X., Zhang, G., Yu, Z., Li, K., & Fan, L. (2024). The meaning of respect and dignity for intensive care unit patients: A meta-synthesis of qualitative research. *Nursing Ethics*, *31*(4), 652–669. DOI: 10.1177/09697330231222598 PMID: 38147009

Swartz, K., & Collins, L. G. (2019). Caregiver care. *American Family Physician*, *99*(11), 699–706. https://www.aafp.org/pubs/afp/issues/2019/0601/p699.html PMID: 31150177

Syse, A., Artamonova, A., Thomas, M., & Veenstra, M. (2022). Do characteristics of family members influence older persons' transition to long-term healthcare services? *BMC Health Services Research*, *22*(1), 362. DOI: 10.1186/s12913-022-07745-5 PMID: 35303891

Tajudeen, F. P., Bahar, N., Tan, M. P., Peer Mustafa, M. B., Saedon, N. I., & Jesudass, J. (2022). Understanding user requirements for a senior-friendly mobile health application. *Geriatrics (Basel, Switzerland)*, *7*(5), 110. DOI: 10.3390/geriatrics7050110 PMID: 36286212

Tanaka, A., Tokuda, N., & Ichihara, K. (2018). Psychological and physiological effects of LYsessions in Japan: A pilot study. *Nursing & Health Sciences*, *20*(3), 304–312. DOI: 10.1111/nhs.12562 PMID: 30156373

Tandon, N., & Sharma, S. (2020). Ayurveda and home-based care practices: Evidence and gaps. *Journal of Ayurveda and Integrative Medicine*, *11*(4), 518–526.

Tan, E. W., Chai, S. C., Sankai, Y., Shingu, M., Razaob, N. A., & Hussain, H. (2025). Single joint hybrid assistive limb…. *PLoS One*, *20*(4), e0322191. DOI: 10.1371/journal.pone.0322191 PMID: 40273196

Tan, Y., Liang, X., Ming, W., Xing, H., Wang, Y., & Gao, Y. (2024). A scoping review of digital technology applications in palliative care. *BMC Palliative Care*, *23*(1), 290. DOI: 10.1186/s12904-024-01626-w PMID: 39707313

Tariq, J., Zakar, R., Ali, M. V., Zakar, M. Z., Sajjad, A., & Fischer, F. (2023). Determinants of physical, psychological, and social well-being in older adults: A cross-sectional study in senior care facilities of Pakistan (2019/20). *BMC Geriatrics*, *23*(1), 349. DOI: 10.1186/s12877-023-04014-w PMID: 37277717

Tavakoli, T., Davoodi, N., Jafar Tabatabaee, T. S., Rostami, Z., Mollaei, H., Salmani, F., Ayati, S., & Tabrizi, S. (2019). Comparison of Laughter Yoga and Anti-Anxiety Medication on Anxiety and Gastrointestinal Symptoms of Patients with Irritable Bowel Syndrome. *Middle East Journal of Digestive Diseases, 11*(4), 211–217. DOI: 10.15171/mejdd.2019.151 PMID: 31824624

Terzoni, S., De Vita, A., Ferrara, P., Sacchini, F., Cangelosi, G., Mancin, S., Petrelli, F., Lopane, D., Milani, A., Parozzi, M., & Lusignani, M. (2025). Biological effects of music therapy in end-of-life care: A narrative review. *Medicina, 61*(9), 1690. DOI: 10.3390/medicina61091690 PMID: 41011081

Thomas, A., Denis, A., Robert, W., Kabiito, S. P., Morish, Z., Samuel, A., Sallam, M., & Adamopoulos, I. (2025). Artificial Intelligence-Powered Robotic Technology for Transforming Palliative Care. *Mesopotamian Journal of Artificial Intelligence in Healthcare, 2025*, 58–84. DOI: 10.58496/MJAIH/2025/007

Thomas, J. (2007). Optimizing opioid management in palliative care. *Journal of Palliative Medicine, 10*(Supplement_1), S-1–S-18. DOI: 10.1089/jpm.2007.9828 PMID: 18052750

Thomas, S., Edwards, E., & Kobylecki, C. (2024, August 13). (2024). Parkinson's Nurses Are Crucial for the Management of Parkinson's Disease: 2007-2024. *Journal of Parkinson's Disease, 14*(s1), S209–S217. Advance online publication. DOI: 10.3233/JPD-230224 PMID: 38578901

Tian, Y. J., Felber, N. A., Pageau, F., Schwab, D. R., & Wangmo, T. (2024). Benefits and barriers associated with the use of smart home health technologies in the care of older persons: A systematic review. *BMC Geriatrics, 24*(1), 152. DOI: 10.1186/s12877-024-04702-1 PMID: 38355464

Tičinović, M., & Tomasović Mrčela, N. (2023). Self-assessed needs of the elderly for the non-institutional care services of gerontological centers in relation to their functional ability. *Hrvatski časopis zdravstvenih znanosti, 3*(1), 33-40. DOI: 10.48188/hczz.3.1.5

Tilbury, D. E. F. (1977). *Casework in Context*. Elsevier., DOI: 10.1016/C2013-0-05717-9

Tohidi, S., Kordvarkaneh, Z., Shayan, A., Oshvandi, K., Abbasi, M., Moradkhani, S., & Ahmadinia, H. (2022). Comparison of aromatherapy with lavender and damask rose essential oils on nausea rate in patients undergoing chemotherapy: A randomised control trial. *Australian Journal of Herbal and Naturopathic Medicine, 34*(2), 60–66. DOI: 10.33235/ajhnm.34.2.60-66

Tolosa, E., Garrido, A., Scholz, S. W., & Poewe, W. (2021). Challenges in the diagnosis of Parkinson's disease. *Lancet Neurology*, *20*(5), 385–397. DOI: 10.1016/S1474-4422(21)00030-2 PMID: 33894193

Toroghi, L. M. (2015). The Effectiveness of Art Therapy On Housewives General Health, Anxiety and Self-efficacy in Tehran. *European Psychiatry : the Journal of the Association of European Psychiatrists*, *30*, 852. Advance online publication. DOI: 10.1016/S0924-9338(15)30665-9

Tosin, M. H., Goetz, C. G., & Stebbins, G. T. (2024). Patient With Parkinson Disease and Care Partner Perceptions of Key Domains Affecting Health-Related Quality of Life: Systematic Review. *Neurology*, *102*(3), e208028. DOI: 10.1212/WNL.0000000000208028 PMID: 38215353

Travers, J. L., Hirschman, K. B., & Naylor, M. D. (2020). Adapting Andersen's expanded behavioral model of health services use to include older adults receiving long-term services and supports. *BMC Geriatrics*, *20*(1), 58. DOI: 10.1186/s12877-019-1405-7 PMID: 32059643

Trevithick, P. (2003). Effective relationship-based practice: A theoretical exploration. *Journal of Social Work Practice*, *17*(2), 163–176. DOI: 10.1080/026505302000145699

Triscott, J. A. C., Dobbs, B., Charles, L., Huang, J., Moores, D., & Tian, P. G. J. (2021). The care-of-the-elderly health guide. *Journal of Primary Care & Community Health*, *12*, 21501327211044058. DOI: 10.1177/21501327211044058 PMID: 34486428

Turcotte, P. L., Larivière, N., Desrosiers, J., Voyer, P., Champoux, N., Carbonneau, H., Carrier, A., & Levasseur, M. (2015). Participation needs of older adults having disabilities and receiving home care: Met needs mainly concern daily activities, while unmet needs mostly involve social activities. *BMC Geriatrics*, *15*(1), 95. DOI: 10.1186/s12877-015-0077-1 PMID: 26231354

Tziraki, C., Grimes, C., Ventura, F., O'Caoimh, R., Santana, S., Zavagli, V., Varani, S., Tramontano, D., Apóstolo, J., Geurden, B., Luca, V. D., Tramontano, G., Romano, M. R., Anastasaki, M., Lionis, C., Rodríguez-Acuña, R., Capelas, M. L., & Afonso, T. (2020). Rethinking palliative care in a public health context: Addressing the needs of persons with non-communicable chronic diseases. *Primary Health Care Research and Development*, *21*, e32. DOI: 10.1017/S1463423620000328 PMID: 32928334

U.S. Department of Health and Human Services (2011). *Your Guide to Healthy Sleep,* NIH Publication, Nr. 11-5271.

Ullrich, A., Ascherfeld, L., Marx, G., Bokemeyer, C., Bergelt, C., & Oechsle, K. (2017). Quality of life, psychological burden, needs, and satisfaction during specialized inpatient palliative care in family caregivers of advanced cancer patients. *BMC Palliative Care, 16*(1), 31. DOI: 10.1186/s12904-017-0206-z PMID: 28486962

Ulrich, R. S. (1984). View through a window may influence recovery from surgery.[59]. *Science, 224*(4647), 420–421. DOI: 10.1126/science.6143402 PMID: 6143402

van der Linden, M. (1996). Effects of music therapy on anxiety in elderly patients. *Age and Ageing, 25*(2), 127–131. DOI: 10.1093/ageing/25.2.127

Van der Wal, C. N., & Kok, R. N. (2019). Laughter-inducing therapies: Systematic review and meta-analysis. *Social Science & Medicine, 232*, 473–488. DOI: 10.1016/j.socscimed.2019.02.018 PMID: 31029483

Vejmelka, L., & Sabolić, T. (2015). The potential of institutions for children without parental care: The perspective of the institutional caregivers. *Kriminologija & socijalna integracija: časopis za kriminologiju, penologiju i poremećaje u ponašanju, 23*(1), 99-128. https://hrcak.srce.hr/clanak/218862

Vélez-López, A., Carmona-Torres, J. M., López-González, Á., Laredo-Aguilera, J. A., Callado-Pérez, D., & Rabanales-Sotos, J. (2024). Community-based interventions in people with palliative care needs: an integrative review of studies from 2017 to 2022. In *Healthcare* (Vol. 12, No. 15, p. 1477). MDPI. DOI: 10.3390/healthcare12151477

Verdonschot, M. M. L., de Witte, L. P., Reichrath, E., Buntinx, W. H. E., & Curfs, L. M. G. (2009). Impact of environmental factors on community participation of persons with an intellectual disability: A systematic review. *Journal of Intellectual Disability Research, 53*(1), 54–64. DOI: 10.1111/j.1365-2788.2008.01128.x PMID: 19093982

Verma, R., & Yadav, P. (2021). AIIMS home-based dementia and stroke rehabilitation: Outcomes and caregiver role. *Neurology India, 69*(5), 1253–1260.

Viganò, C., Wenk, M., Ferrara, L., Magnotti, R., & Borsani, S. (2019). The "State of The Art" of Art Therapy in Psychiatry: Reflections on International Evidences and Italian Experiences. *Journal of Complementary Medicine & Alternative Healthcare, 10*(5). Advance online publication. DOI: 10.19080/JCMAH.2019.10.555796

Vijay, D., & Monin, P. (2018). Poisedness for social innovation: The genesis and propagation of community-based palliative care in Kerala (India). *M@ n@ gement, 21*(4), 1329-1356. DOI: 10.3917/mana.214.1329

Vinayak, S., Dehkhoda, F., & Vinayak, R. (2017). The effect of music therapy on sleep quality of cancer patients undergoing chemotherapy or radiotherapy: A randomized control trial. *Journal of Social Sciences (COES&RJ-JSS), 6*(4), 734-743.

Vuksan, M., Williams, A. M., & Crooks, V. A. (2012). The workplace perspective on supporting family caregivers at end of life: Evaluating a new Canadian social program. *Community Work & Family, 15*(3), 317–333. DOI: 10.1080/13668803.2012.664891

Wang, J., Wang, J., Cao, Y., Jia, S., & Wu, B. (2016). Older residents' perspectives of long-term care facilities in China. *Journal of Gerontological Nursing, 42*(8), 34–43. DOI: 10.3928/00989134-20160615-05 PMID: 27319405

Wang, J., Zhang, B., Yahaya, R., & Abdullah, A. (2025). Colors of the mind: A meta-analysis of creative arts therapy as an approach for post-traumatic stress disorder intervention. *BMC Psychology, 13*(32), 32. Advance online publication. DOI: 10.1186/s40359-025-02361-4 PMID: 39799380

Wang, K., Ghafurian, M., Chumachenko, D., Cao, S., Butt, Z. A., Salim, S., Abhari, S., & Morita, P. P. (2024). Application of artificial intelligence.... *Computers in Biology and Medicine, 173*, 108340. DOI: 10.1016/j.compbiomed.2024.108340 PMID: 38555702

Wang, M., & Ding, X. (2025). Integrated palliative care improves the quality of life of advanced cancer patients. *BMC Palliative Care, 24*(1), 162. DOI: 10.1186/s12904-025-01800-8 PMID: 40483417

Wang, Y., Liang, J., Fang, Y., Yao, D., Zhang, L., Zhou, Y., Wang, Y., Hu, L., Lu, Z., Wang, Y., & Xiao, Z. (2023). Burden of common neurologic diseases in Asian countries, 1990–2019: An analysis for the Global Burden of Disease Study 2019. *Neurology, 100*(21), e2141–e2154. DOI: 10.1212/WNL.0000000000207218 PMID: 37015823

Warth, M., Keßler, J., Hillecke, T. K., & Bardenheuer, H. (2015). Music therapy in palliative care – A randomized controlled trial to evaluate effects on relaxation. *Deutsches Ärzteblatt International, 112*, 788–794. PMID: 26806566

Waymouth, M., Siconolfi, D., Friedman, E. M., Saliba, D., Ahluwalia, S. C., & Shih, R. A. (2023). Barriers and facilitators to home-and community-based services access for persons with dementia and their caregivers. *The Journals of Gerontology. Series B, Psychological Sciences and Social Sciences, 78*(6), 1085–1097. DOI: 10.1093/geronb/gbad039 PMID: 36896936

Weaver, D. (2000). Organizational Technology as Institutionalized Ideology: Case Management Practices in Welfare-to-Work Programs. *Administration in Social Work, 24*(1), 1–19. DOI: 10.1300/J147v24n01_01

Weiss, M. E., Sawin, K. J., & Gralton, K. (2020). RAND caregiver integration framework: Implications for home-based care. *Journal of Family Nursing, 26*(3), 215–232.

Wentlandt, K., Seccareccia, D., Kevork, N., Workentin, K., Blacker, S., Grossman, D., & Zimmermann, C. (2016). Quality of care and satisfaction with care on palliative care units. *Journal of Pain and Symptom Management, 51*(2), 184–192. DOI: 10.1016/j.jpainsymman.2015.10.006 PMID: 26598036

Westra, H. A., & Aviram, A. (2013). Core skills in motivational interviewing. *Psychotherapy (Chicago, Ill.), 50*(3), 273–278. DOI: 10.1037/a0032409 PMID: 24000834

Whitebird, R. R., Kreitzer, M. J., & O'Connor, P. J. (2013). Mindfulness-based stress reduction for family caregivers: A randomized controlled trial. *The American Journal of Hospice & Palliative Care, 30*(2), 187–195. DOI: 10.1177/1049909112452622 PMID: 23070934

Wirtz, J., Bateson, J. E., Čaić, M., Frank, D. A., & Veflen, N. (2025). The healthy aging and service firms: The promise of smart technologies. *Journal of Service Management*. Advance online publication. DOI: 10.1108/JOSM-10-2024-0426

Wirtz, J., & Stock-Homburg, R. (2025). Generative AI meets service robots. *Journal of Service Research, 10946705251340487*(4), 527–543. Advance online publication. DOI: 10.1177/10946705251340487

Woods, B., O'Philbin, L., Farrell, E. M., Spector, A. E., & Orrell, M. (2018). Reminiscence therapy for dementia. *Cochrane Database of Systematic Reviews, 3*(3), CD001120. Advance online publication. DOI: 10.1002/14651858.CD001120.pub3 PMID: 29493789

World Health Organization. (2016). *WHO Framework on Integrated People-Centred Health Services*. WHO.

World Health Organization. (2017). *Integrated care for older people: Guidelines on community-level interventions to manage declines in intrinsic capacity*. https://www.ncbi.nlm.nih.gov/books/NBK488250/

World Health Organization. (2020). *Integrative health services: The role of music therapy in palliative and supportive care*. World Health Organization.

World Health Organization. (2022). *Global report on health equity for persons with disabilities*. https://www.who.int/publications/i/item/9789240063600

World Health Organization. (2022). *World Health Statistics 2022: Health Workforce and Ageing*. WHO.

World Health Organization. (2024). *WHO guidance on artificial intelligence in healthcare*. https://www.who.int/publications/i/item/9789240084759

Wright, M., Wood, J., Lynch, T., & Clark, D. (2008). Mapping levels of palliative care development: A global view. *Journal of Pain and Symptom Management, 35*(5), 469–485. DOI: 10.1016/j.jpainsymman.2007.06.006 PMID: 18243637

Yang, G., Wan, L., Dong, H., Liang, X., & He, Y. (2022). Utilisation willingness for institutional care by the disabled elderly and its influencing factors based on Andersen's model: A cross-sectional survey of Henan, China. *BMJ Open, 12*(12), e064949. DOI: 10.1136/bmjopen-2022-064949 PMID: 36600340

Yang, Y., Liang, X., Liu, Q., & Liu, J. (2025). Navigating limited resources: Experiences of caregivers for elderly terminal cancer patients in a region with limited palliative care services. *Supportive Care in Cancer, 33*(3), 207. DOI: 10.1007/s00520-025-09270-7 PMID: 39971822

Yang, Y., Wang, G., Zhang, S., Wang, H., Zhou, W., Ren, F., Liang, H., Wu, D., Ji, X., Hashimoto, M., & Wei, J. (2022). Efficacy and evaluation of therapeutic exercises on adults with Parkinson's disease: A systematic review and network meta-analysis. *BMC Geriatrics, 22*(1), 813. DOI: 10.1186/s12877-022-03510-9 PMID: 36271367

Yao, H., Jingyue, W., Rui, Z., Hou, Y., & Hui, Y. (2025). E-CARE as core competencies for palliative social workers: A systematic review. *BMC Palliative Care, 24*(1), 163. DOI: 10.1186/s12904-025-01735-0 PMID: 40490802

Yildirim, D., Ozdogan, M. H., Erdal, S., Selcuk, S., Guneri, A., Simsek, E. B., Can, T. B., Gunduz, H., & Kuni, A. (2025). The efficacy of lavender oil on fatigue and sleep quality in patients with hematological malignancy receiving chemotherapy: A single-blind randomized controlled trial. *Supportive Care in Cancer, 33*(2), 1–10. DOI: 10.1007/s00520-024-09143-5 PMID: 39775962

Yim, J. (2016). Therapeutic Benefits of Laughter in Mental Health: A Theoretical Review. *The Tohoku Journal of Experimental Medicine, 239*(3), 243–249. DOI: 10.1620/tjem.239.243 PMID: 27439375

Zarit, S. H., Kim, K., Femia, E. E., Almeida, D. M., & Klein, L. C. (2014). The effects of adult day services on family caregivers' daily stress, affect, and health: Outcomes from the Daily Stress and Health (DaSH) study. *The Gerontologist, 54*(4), 570–579. DOI: 10.1093/geront/gnt045 PMID: 23690056

Zeng, Z., Jiang, X., & Neapolitan, R. (2016). Discovering causal interactions using Bayesian network scoring and information gain. *BMC Bioinformatics, 17*(1), 1–14. DOI: 10.1186/s12859-016-1084-8 PMID: 27230078

Zhang, K., Yuan, H., & Fang, Y. (2022). Evaluation of smart agitation prediction and management for dementia care and novel universal village oriented solution for integration, resilience, inclusiveness and sustainability. In *2022 6th International Conference on Universal Village (UV)* (pp. 1-34). IEEE. DOI: 10.1109/UV56588.2022.10185497

Zhang, L., Cui, Z., Huffman, L. G., & Oshri, A. (2023). Sleep mediates the effect of stressful environments on youth development of impulsivity: The moderating role of within default mode network resting-state functional connectivity. *Sleep Health, 9*(4), 503–511. DOI: 10.1016/j.sleh.2023.03.005 PMID: 37270396

Zhang, M., & Cheng, Q. (2024). Becoming a self-reliant elder: Fading intergenerational reciprocity and pursuing active aging among middle-class seniors in urban China. *SAGE Open, 14*(2), 21582440241259161. DOI: 10.1177/21582440241259161

Zhang, Q., Varnfield, M., Higgins, L., Smallbon, V., Bomke, J., O'Dwyer, J., Byrnes, J. M., Sum, M., Hewitt, J., Lu, W., & Karunanithi, M. (2022). Protocol for a stratified randomized controlled trial…. *JMIR Research Protocols, 11*(1), e31970. DOI: 10.2196/31970 PMID: 35072640

Zhang, Y., Liu, S., Xu, K., Zhou, Y., Shen, Y., Liu, Z., Bai, Y., & Wang, S. (2024). Non-pharmacological therapies for treating non-motor symptoms in patients with Parkinson's disease: A systematic review and meta-analysis. *Frontiers in Aging Neuroscience, 16*, 1363115. DOI: 10.3389/fnagi.2024.1363115 PMID: 38737585

Zhao, L., Chang, B., Hu, Q., Chen, X., Du, J., & Shao, S. (2025). The health care needs of multidimensional frail elderly patients with multimorbidity in primary health-care settings: A qualitative study. *BMC Primary Care, 26*(1), 128. DOI: 10.1186/s12875-025-02836-8 PMID: 40281402

Zimbroff, R. M., Ornstein, K. A., & Sheehan, O. C. (2021). Home-based primary care: A systematic review of the literature, 2010–2020. *Journal of the American Geriatrics Society, 69*(10), 2963–2972. DOI: 10.1111/jgs.17365 PMID: 34247383

Zovko, K., Šerić, L., & Perković, T. a. (2023). IoT and health monitoring wearable devices as enabling technologies for sustainable enhancement of life quality in smart environments, *Journal of Cleaner Production*, ISSN 0959-6526.

About the Contributors

Tuong-Minh Ly-Le holds a Ph.D. in Communication from Bond University, Australia, and a Master of Health Science in Integrative Care from Northwestern Health Sciences University, U.S. With a unique academic and professional background that bridges communication, health sciences, and public advocacy, Dr. Ly-Le is deeply committed to advancing the field of integrative health through more effective and evidence-based communication strategies. Dr. Ly-Le has published extensively on topics related to public relations, health communication, and the sociocultural dimensions of media influence. A consistent advocate for science-backed communication, Dr. Ly-Le's current work focuses on a cross-disciplinary approach, combining insights from communication theory, behavioral health, and clinical care to inform how integrative practices are understood and adopted by the public. She aims to bridge the gap between scientific evidence and daily health practices through culturally sensitive and practically grounded communication. This book is the culmination of her ongoing mission to democratize knowledge of integrative care for a global audience of caregivers, healthcare professionals, and patient advocates.

***

Burcu Akpınar Söylemez, PhD, RN, Professor Department of Internal Medicine Nursing, Dokuz Eylul University Faculty of Nursing, Inciralti, Izmir, Türkiye ORCID: 0000-0002-9643-0325

Aishwarya Arya is pursuing Ph.D. in Management, Accomplished her Bachelor's and Master's from Institute of Hotel Management and Catering Technology, Lucknow in Hospitality Administration thereafter another Master's in Travel & Tourism Management. She started her academic career in the year 2019 from IHM Lucknow, previously worked with Babu Banarsi Das University,

Lucknow as Assistant Professor. She presented and attended many National and International Conferences, seminars and webinars. Her area of specialization includes Room Division, Hospitality Management & Sales and Marketing. She has patents published in Under the office of the controller General of Patents, Designs and Trademarks Department of Industrial Policy and Promotions, Ministry of Commerce and Industry, Government of India.

Shravani Bhalerao is a Student at Ajeenkya D Y Patil School of Engineering, studying in T.E in Bachelor's in Engineering in Artificial Intelligence & Data Science Department.

Omkar Bholankar is a Student at Ajeenkya D Y Patil School of Engineering, studying in T.E in Bachelor's in Engineering in Artificial Intelligence & Data Science Department.

Subhashini Durai is a research enthusiast, and she serves LEAD College of Management, Kerala.

Jipson Joseph has a PhD in Ethics from DVK Bangalore. Currently, he is a Research Scholar in the School of Law at Christ University, Bangalore. His research interests encompass the fields of ethics, gender studies, constitutional law, human rights, human security, environmental justice, BRICS countries, development policies, and global poverty. He has published six books, co-edited one book, and contributed scholarly articles to numerous international and national journals and edited volumes, including those published by IGI Global Scientific Publishing.

Ankit Kumar is currently pursuing PhD in Management from C.S.J.M. University, Kanpur. I have experience in academic as well in Hospitality Industries. My Industry and Teaching experience has been very satisfying and I have continuously upgraded my skills in my respective field. I have a patent published in Under the office of the controller General of Patents, Designs and Trademarks Department of Industrial Policy and Promotions, Ministry of Commerce and Industry, Government of India. I have many papers published in Peer reviewed Journal and UGC listed Journal.

Krishna M is a passionate and curious learner with a solid academic foundation in computer applications and data science. I hold a Bachelor’s degree in Computer Applications (BCA), which provided me with a strong grounding in programming, database management, and software development. Driven by a desire to explore deeper into the world of data, I am currently pursuing a Master of Science (MSc) in Data Science, where I am gaining hands-on experience in machine learning, data analytics, big data technologies, and statistical modeling. Throughout my academic journey, I have developed a keen interest in research, particularly in using data-driven approaches to solve real-world problems. I am fascinated by the potential of data science in diverse fields such as healthcare, social sciences, finance, and artificial intelligence. My goal is to contribute to the advancement of knowledge through meaningful research that blends theory with practical impact. I am constantly seeking opportunities to engage in academic and industry research projects, collaborate with fellow learners and professionals, and stay updated with the latest trends and tools in data science. With a commitment to continuous learning and innovation, I aspire to pursue a research-oriented career that allows me to contribute to data-driven solutions and societal development.

Geetha Manoharan is currently working in Telangana as an assistant professor at SR University. She is the university-level PhD program coordinator and has also been given the additional responsibility of In Charge Director of Publications and Patents under the Research Division at SR University.

Ahmed J. Obaid, is a Asst. Professor at the Department of Computer Science, Faculty of Computer Science and Mathematics, University of Kufa, Iraq. Dr. Ahmed holds a Bachelor in Computer Science, degree in – Information Systems from College of Computers, University of Anbar, Iraq (2001-2005), and a Master Degree (M. TECH) of Computer Science Engineering (CSE) from School of Information Technology, Jawaharlal Nehru Technological University, Hyderabad, India (2010-2013), and a Doctor of Philosophy (PhD) in Web Mining from College of Information Technology, University of University of Babylon, Iraq (2013-2017). He is a Certified Web Mining Consultant with over 14 years of experience in working as Faculty Member in University of Kufa, Iraq. He has taught courses in Web Designing, Web Scripting, JavaScript, VB.Net, MATLAB Toolbox's, and other courses on PHP, CMC, and DHTML from more than 10 international organizations and institutes from USA, and India. Dr. Ahmed is a member of Statistical and Information Consultation Center (SICC), University of Kufa, Iraq.

Ecem Özgül, PhD, RN, Research Assistant Izmir University of Economics, Faculty of Health Sciences, Department of Nursing, İzmir, Türkiye ORCID: 0000-0002-1294-9446

Sabyasachi Pramanik is a professional IEEE member. He obtained a PhD in Computer Science and Engineering from Sri Satya Sai University of Technology and Medical Sciences, Bhopal, India. Presently, he is an Associate Professor, Department of Computer Science and Engineering, Haldia Institute of Technology, India. He has many publications in various reputed international conferences, journals, and book chapters (Indexed by SCIE, Scopus, ESCI, etc). He is doing research in the fields of Artificial Intelligence, Data Privacy, Cybersecurity, Network Security, and Machine Learning. He also serves on the editorial boards of several international journals. He is a reviewer of journal articles from IEEE, Springer, Elsevier, Inderscience, IET and IGI Global. He has reviewed many conference papers, has been a keynote speaker, session chair, and technical program committee member at many international conferences. He has authored a book on Wireless Sensor Network. He has edited 8 books from IGI Global, CRC Press, Springer and Wiley Publications.

Hariharan S is a highly committed and enthusiastic graduate with a strong ambition to contribute significantly to the field of wearable healthcare technologies. His core areas of interest include IoMT system design, biosignal processing, medical image analysis, and Artificial Intelligence-driven healthcare solutions. Throughout his academic and research journey, he has gained substantial experience working with prestigious institutions, including the Dr. Shyama Prasad Mukherjee International Institute of Information Technology. He has published his research findings in reputed international and national journals, conference proceedings, and has also contributed to a book chapter, reflecting his strong academic and technical impact. He has filed a patent for his innovative work titled "Intelligent EDGE-Enabled Fall Tracking System for Geriatrics."

Shivansu Sachan is pursuing Ph.D. in Management, a Master's holder from Integral University, Lucknow, Bachelor's from IHM, Lucknow. Academic and professional accomplishments of 6 years with renowned organizations and institutes. His Teaching Career has been very satisfying and have continuously upgraded the skills and knowledge by attending many courses and training programs, seminars, conferences organized by different organizations and also delivered many lectures as a Hospitality sector. He is working as an Assistant Professor at Chhatrapati Shahu ji Maharaj University Kanpur .

Mohammad Badruddoza Talukder is an Associate Professor and Chairman at the College of Tourism and Hospitality Management at the International University of Business Agriculture and Technology (IUBAT) in Dhaka, Bangladesh. Holding a PhD from Lovely Professional University, India, he is renowned for his innovative integration of cutting-edge technologies such as Artificial Intelligence (AI), the Internet of Things (IoT), and Blockchain into tourism and hospitality management. His research explores the transformative impact of these technologies on smart tourism, cloud kitchens, and the broader industry landscape. As a prolific author, Dr. Talukder has published numerous scholarly articles and books, with forthcoming titles that address AI innovations in hospitality, the evolution of cloud kitchens, and the enhancement of digital literacy within hospitality education. His work shapes contemporary tourism and hospitality practices, skillfully marrying technological advancements with practical industry applications. Since 2008, Dr. Talukder has imparted his knowledge through a diverse array of courses in tourism and hospitality across various universities in Bangladesh.

Srinivasan Vasan is an Assistant Professor in the Department of Humanities and Social Sciences at Graphic Era (Deemed to be University), with 14 years of teaching and field expertise. He has served in the Ministry of Health and Family Welfare, as a Guest Faculty, and as a Mobilization Training Specialist with the State Government. Recently, he contributed to a tuberculosis project funded by GFATM and USAID. He has published 60 papers, with 20 more under peer review in UGC-CARE and SCOPUS journals.

Sweta Wankhade is an Assistant Professor, Department of Artificial Intelligence & Data Science Engineering, Ajeenkya DY Patil School of Engineering, Lohegaon, Pune, Maharashtra

Index

A

B

C

D

E

F

H

I

K

L

M

N

O

P

Q

R

S

T

U